AF594977

The Identification of Drug Abuse

The Identification of Drug Abuse

Editor

Maria Pieri

MDPI • Basel • Beijing • Wuhan • Barcelona • Belgrade • Manchester • Tokyo • Cluj • Tianjin

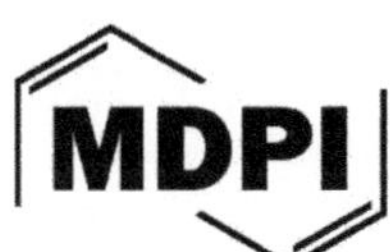

Editor
Maria Pieri
Department of Advanced
Biomedical Science-Legal
Medicine Section,
University of Naples
"Federico II",
Naples, Italy

Editorial Office
MDPI
St. Alban-Anlage 66
4052 Basel, Switzerland

This is a reprint of articles from the Special Issue published online in the open access journal *Toxics* (ISSN 2305-6304) (available at: https://www.mdpi.com/journal/toxics/special_issues/Drug_Abuse_Identification).

For citation purposes, cite each article independently as indicated on the article page online and as indicated below:

LastName, A.A.; LastName, B.B.; LastName, C.C. Article Title. *Journal Name* **Year**, *Volume Number*, Page Range.

ISBN 978-3-0365-7966-5 (Hbk)
ISBN 978-3-0365-7967-2 (PDF)

Contents

About the Editor

Maria Pieri

Prof. Maria Pieri graduated in Industrial Chemistry in 2000 at the University of Naples "Federico II" (Italy). In 2004, Prof. Maria Pieri completed the Ph.D. course in Occupational Medicine, Environmental Hygiene, and Ergonomics at the University of Bari (Italy), with a final thesis on "Urinary mercapturic acids as exposure biomarkers for assessing occupational exposure to genotoxic agents".

Since 2021, Prof. Pieri has been Associate Professor and directs the Forensic Toxicology Laboratory of the Department of Advanced Biomedical Science, Legal Medicine Section of the University of Naples "Federico II". Since 2018, Prof. Pieri has been the executive of the forensic laboratory of the "Federico II" Hospital of Naples. Since 2011, Prof Pieri has been a member of the Italian Forensic Toxicologist Association, now part of the Board of the same Association, as National Secretary. Since 2019, Prof. Pieri has been a member of the International Academy of Legal Medicine (IALM).

The research activity is documented by several articles published in both international peer-reviewed journals, Italian journals, and conference proceedings. The research activity has been focused on the characterization/quantitative determination of biological molecules and macromolecules by means of Liquid and Gas Chromatography coupled with Mass Spectrometry or other detectors such as UV-VIS, Fluorescence, Flame Ionization, and Electron Capture. In particular, the area of expertise comprises:

- Application of proteomics in Forensic Toxicology for the definition of circumstances of death and the correct identification of biological traces;
- Study of post-mortem degenerative and decomposing processes of the peripheral nervous system for the definition of the post-mortem interval;
- Study and application of immunochemical techniques for the determination of drugs of abuse in biological matrices (urine, blood, cheratinic matrices, and organ and tissue fragments);
- Forensic toxicological analysis of drugs of abuse and psychotic substances in both samples from street seizures and biological ones (both from autopsy and living);
- Ethics and privacy within workplace drug testing;
- Medical legal aspects of cosmetics.

Preface to "The Identification of Drug Abuse"

Over the last decades, interest in forensic toxicology has continually increased. Consequently, the discipline assumed a leading role, becoming one of the reference sciences for elucidating events of judicial importance. The need to reconcile analytical problems (e.g., relating to the qualitative/quantitative analysis of substances of abuse in complex biological matrices) with judicial requirements (i.e., providing data that can be used as documentary evidence in proceedings) makes the discipline unique among all "analytical" sciences. Thus, the availability of validated procedures, the constant monitoring of analytical performance through quality assurance protocols, the availability of certified "in matrix" standards, and the analytical problems underlying the analysis of new psychoactive substances in the blood and other biological fluids represent the challenges of modern forensic toxicology. The correct interpretation of analytical data, especially to elucidate the extent of impairment induced by a certain substance, and "old" issues related to the correct interpretation of post-mortem data (given the impossibility of translating the therapeutic ranges defined in vivo) represent further areas of research and debate among scientists. Finally, the possibility of interacting with other disciplines (such as proteomics and social sciences) allows for extending the concept of analytical data acquisition/interpretation beyond the classical limits of forensic toxicology (for example, considering the influence of gender when interpreting the effect of a substance).

I am pleased to present you this Special Issue of *Toxics* on forensic toxicology, focused on problems related to data acquisition/interpretation, with particular emphasis on post-mortem data, new psychoactive substances, and strategies for an appropriate impairment judgment.

Maria Pieri
Editor

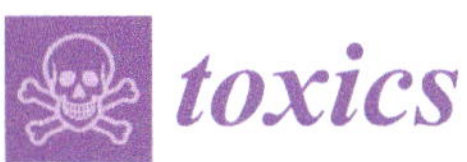 MDPI

Editorial

The Identification of Drug Abuse

Maria Pieri

Department of Advanced Biomedical Science-Legal Medicine Section, University of Naples "Federico II", Via S. Pansini, 5, 80131 Naples, Italy; maria.pieri@unina.it; Tel.: +39-0817463474; Fax: +39-0817464726

Forensic toxicology has played a central role since its development in defining mechanisms of acute intoxication, often with a lethal outcome. In its modern declination, the discipline has seen a constant evolution not only in the object of study—today extended to almost all psychoactive/psychotropic substances or any case capable of inducing morbid and/or toxic manifestations once absorbed by the organism—but also in its possible fields of application.

Analytical difficulties related to the need to highlight the presence of trace-level substances (i.e., a few nanograms or micrograms per mL) in complex biological samples are, in fact, only the first challenge in modern forensic toxicology. The constant improvement in analytical performance, linked to the optimization of purification procedures, the development of systems based on liquid or gaseous chromatography coupled to mass spectrometry, the availability of instruments that are capable of performing multiple scans of ionic signals of multiple substances within the same analytical run and the availability of constantly updated database libraries assist with the acquisition process of analytical data. The analytical aspect is, however, only the first part of the work required of a forensic toxicologist. Analytical purposes make it essential to correctly contextualize the analytical data in order to respond fully and exhaustively to the question posed by the Judicial Authority. The correct interpretation of analytical data is the most complex and debated aspect of forensic chemical-toxicological analysis. Difficulties derive from the need to integrate analytical results with evidence from all the other evaluations that the case under study requires.

Furthermore, the difficulties deriving from post-mortal modifications make the acquisition and correct interpretation of forensic toxicological analysis in the thanatological field profoundly different and significantly more complex than any analyses performed "on a living person".

The availability of data in the literature obtained through validated analytical methods and results integrated with circumstantial, anamnestic and anatomopathological data represent a direction on which to develop a forensic chemical-toxicological analysis in line with the principles underlying the discipline, as well as legal requirements. Only a datum that has been characterized by analytical precision and correctly contextualized in the light of the main characteristics of the case under study is able to make a useful contribution to the resolution of the forensic problem that leads to an analytical request itself.

This Special Issue aims to present the analytical-interpretative difficulties that underlie the determination of different types of substances. The authors contribute with "real cases" and also address strategies through which it may be possible to resolve or at least contribute to the definition of possible causes of intoxication. Thirteen contributions (articles, case reports and reviews) are published.

Iqbali and Coll. present a UPLC-MS/MS method for the identification and quantification of lemborexant, a novel dual orexin receptor antagonist, that was recently approved for the treatment of insomnia [1]. Due to its potential for abuse, lemborexant is scheduled in the IV class by the United States Drug Enforcement Administration. The method presented here was previously validated according to the "Scientific Working Group for Toxicology" guidelines and subsequently cross-validated in rat plasma samples to be applied in pharmacokinetic studies.

Citation: Pieri, M. The Identification of Drug Abuse. *Toxics* **2023**, *11*, 444. https://doi.org/10.3390/toxics11050444

Received: 20 April 2023
Revised: 26 April 2023
Accepted: 4 May 2023
Published: 8 May 2023

Manetti and Coll. present a fatality involving an atypical transdermal patch consumption [2], starting from the results of a case report revealing the presence of fentanyl in a man with a history of illicit drug consumption. The authors review the literature on fatalities involving such synthetic opioids.

Carfora and Coll. present the case of a suicide involving helium, whose detection made it necessary for the development of adequate analytical procedures [3]. For an adequate sampling, the authors optimized the use of a special gas-inlet system provided with a vacuum, through which the sampled gas could be transferred to the mass spectrometer.

Fernández-López and Coll. present a post-mortem study on the overdose caused by carbamazepine in a patient with psychiatric illness [4]. The analytical procedure to determine carbamazepine on human bone is presented and discussed.

Two articles focus on fatal pesticide outcomes, an occurrence still frequent in developing countries and also present in Western ones among agricultural workers. Simonelli and Coll. present a study on phorate ingestion that resulted in fatal outcomes [5]. Post-mortem data obtained from a 24-year-old Bengali male are described and commented on with respect to the literature. Basilicata and Coll. present the case of suicidal diquat ingestion in a 50-year-old man [6]. The subject was promptly rescued and transferred to the emergency department before they died the following day. The authors also focus also on the misconduct of sanitary staff during hospitalization, resulting in a decrease in the patient's chances of survival and consequent professional liabilities.

In the studies of Hernandez and Coll. [7] and Albano and Coll. [8] the issue of prenatal drug exposure is presented. In the first study, the authors validate an analytical procedure to determine the main substance of abuse and metabolites in meconium [7]. Opioid absorption during intrauterine and prenatal life is then reviewed by Albano and Coll., presenting toxicological, clinical, and forensic issues [8].

Koželj and Prosen present data on the temperature-related degradation of tropanes atropine and scopolamine, highlighting the possible underestimation of GC/MS analysis in such tropane alkaloids as cases of the unintentional or intentional ingestion of plant material [9].

The review by Henríquez-Hernández and coll. discusses health-hazardous doses of psychedelic substances, with particular attention paid to ergolamines, simple tryptamines, and phenylethylamines [10].

Mannocchi and Coll. present their results on fatal intoxication related to acetaminophen, citalopram and trazodone [11]. Data from post-mortem analyses performed on the deceased found that an advanced state of decomposition was presented, which is commented on with respect to the available literature.

Scendoni and Coll. first report results for morphine determination in an unusual post-mortem matrix: in fingernails [12]. Data were first acquired by immunohistochemistry and subsequently confirmed by ultra-high-performance liquid chromatography coupled with high-resolution mass spectrometry.

In the paper from Basilicata and Coll., a case of incongruous midazolam administration in a terminal cancer patient is presented [13]. Toxicological data on different biological specimens are presented, and professional liabilities derived from non-adherence to guidelines on palliative care are discussed.

The items discussed in the present Special Issue highlight critical aspects of forensic toxicological activity with respect to both analytical and interpretative problems. Each contribution aimed to discuss a Special Issue related to drug misuse with respect to the most recent literature, thus representing a reference for those who are involved in the field.

Conflicts of Interest: The author declares no conflict of interest.

References

1. Iqbal, M.; Alshememry, A.; Imam, F.; Kalam, M.A.; Akhtar, A.; Ali, E.A. UPLC-MS/MS Based Identification and Quantification of a Novel Dual Orexin Receptor Antagonist in Plasma Samples by Validated SWGTOX Guidelines. *Toxics* **2023**, *11*, 109. [CrossRef] [PubMed]
2. Manetti, F.; David, M.C.; Gariglio, S.; Consalvo, F.; Padovano, M.; Scopetti, M.; Grande, A.; Santurro, A. Atypical Fentanyl Transdermal Patch Consumption and Fatalities: Case Report and Literature Review. *Toxics* **2023**, *11*, 46. [CrossRef] [PubMed]
3. Carfora, A.; Petrella, R.; Ambrosio, G.; Mascolo, P.; Liguori, B.; Juhnke, C.; Campobasso, C.P.; Keller, T. Helium Suicide, a Rapid and Painless Asphyxia: Toxicological Findings. *Toxics* **2022**, *10*, 424. [CrossRef] [PubMed]
4. Fernández-López, L.; Mancini, R.; Rotolo, M.-C.; Navarro-Zaragoza, J.; Hernández del Rincón, P.; Falcón, M. Carbamazepine Overdose after Psychiatric Conditions: A Case Study for Postmortem Analysis in Human Bone. *Toxics* **2022**, *10*, 322. [CrossRef] [PubMed]
5. Simonelli, A.; Carfora, A.; Basilicata, P.; Liguori, B.; Mascolo, P.; Policino, F.; Niola, M.; Campobasso, C.P. Suicide by Pesticide (Phorate) Ingestion: Case Report and Review of Literature. *Toxics* **2022**, *10*, 205. [CrossRef] [PubMed]
6. Basilicata, P.; Pieri, M.; Simonelli, A.; Capasso, E.; Casella, C.; Noto, T.; Policino, F.; Di Lorenzo, P. Diquat Poisoning: Care Management and Medico-Legal Implications. *Toxics* **2022**, *10*, 166. [CrossRef] [PubMed]
7. Hernandez, A.; Lacroze, V.; Doudka, N.; Becam, J.; Pourriere-Fabiani, C.; Lacarelle, B.; Solas, C.; Fabresse, N. Determination of Prenatal Substance Exposure Using Meconium and Orbitrap Mass Spectrometry. *Toxics* **2022**, *10*, 55. [CrossRef] [PubMed]
8. Koželj, G.; Prosen, H. Thermal (In)stability of Atropine and Scopolamine in the GC-MS Inlet. *Toxics* **2021**, *9*, 156. [CrossRef] [PubMed]
9. Albano, G.D.; La Spina, C.; Pitingaro, W.; Milazzo, V.; Triolo, V.; Argo, A.; Malta, G.; Zerbo, S. Intrauterine and Neonatal Exposure to Opioids: Toxicological, Clinical, and Medico-Legal Issues. *Toxics* **2023**, *11*, 62. [CrossRef] [PubMed]
10. Henríquez-Hernández, L.A.; Rojas-Hernández, J.; Quintana-Hernández, D.J.; Borkel, L.F. Hofmann vs. Paracelsus: Do Psychedelics Defy the Basics of Toxicology?—A Systematic Review of the Main Ergolamines, Simple Tryptamines, and Phenylethylamines. *Toxics* **2023**, *11*, 148. [CrossRef] [PubMed]
11. Mannocchi, G.; Tittarelli, R.; Pantano, F.; Vernich, F.; Pallocci, M.; Passalacqua, P.; Treglia, M.; Marsella, L.T. Forensic Aspects of a Fatal Intoxication Involving Acetaminophen, Citalopram and Trazodone: A Case Report. *Toxics* **2022**, *10*, 486. [CrossRef] [PubMed]
12. Scendoni, R.; Bury, R.; Buratti, E.; Froldi, R.; Cippitelli, M.; Mietti, G.; Cingolani, M. Detection of Morphine and Opioids in Fingernails: Immunohistochemical Analysis and Confirmation with Ultra-High-Performance Liquid Chromatography Coupled with High-Resolution Mass Spectrometry. *Toxics* **2022**, *10*, 420. [CrossRef] [PubMed]
13. Basilicata, P.; Giugliano, P.; Vacchiano, G.; Simonelli, A.; Guadagni, R.; Silvestre, A.; Pieri, M. Forensic Toxicological and Medico-Legal Evaluation in a Case of Incongruous Drug Administration in Terminal Cancer Patients. *Toxics* **2021**, *9*, 356. [CrossRef] [PubMed]

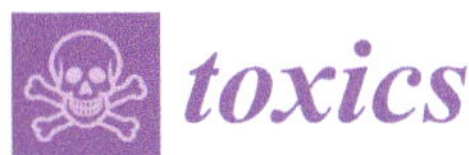

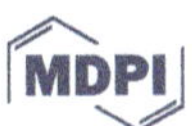

Case Report

Forensic Toxicological and Medico-Legal Evaluation in a Case of Incongruous Drug Administration in Terminal Cancer Patients

Pascale Basilicata [1], Pasquale Giugliano [2], Giuseppe Vacchiano [3], Angela Simonelli [1], Rossella Guadagni [1], Angela Silvestre [1] and Maria Pieri [1,*]

[1] Legal Medicine Section, Department of Advanced Biomedical Science, University of Naples "Federico II", 80131 Naples, Italy; pbasilic@unina.it (P.B.); angela.simonelli@unina.it (A.S.); r.guadagni@unina.it (R.G.); angela.silvestre@unina.it (A.S.)

[2] Legal Medicine Section, AORN "Sant'Anna e San Sebastiano" Caserta, 81100 Caserta, Italy; dottgiugliano@tiscali.it

[3] Department of Law, Economics and Mathematical Methods, University of Sannio, 82100 Benevento, Italy; vacchiano952@gmail.com

* Correspondence: maria.pieri@unina.it; Tel.: +39-0817463474; Fax: +39-0817464726

Citation: Basilicata, P.; Giugliano, P.; Vacchiano, G.; Simonelli, A.; Guadagni, R.; Silvestre, A.; Pieri, M. Forensic Toxicological and Medico-Legal Evaluation in a Case of Incongruous Drug Administration in Terminal Cancer Patients. *Toxics* **2021**, *9*, 356. https://doi.org/10.3390/toxics9120356

Academic Editor: Dirk W. Lachenmeier

Received: 8 November 2021
Accepted: 15 December 2021
Published: 16 December 2021

Abstract: Background: In most cases, palliative care is prescribed to adults diagnosed with cancer. The definition of the most suitable therapy for an effective sedation in terminal cancer patients still represents one of the most challenging goals in medical practice. Due to their poor health, the correct dosing of drugs used for deep palliative sedation in terminal cancer patients, often already on polypharmacological therapy, can be extremely complicated, also considering possible drug-to-drug interactions that could lead to an increased risk of overdose and/or incongruous administration with fatal outcomes. The case of a terminal cancer patient is presented, focusing on the "adequacy" of administered therapy. Materials and Methods: A young male, affected by Ewing sarcoma, attending a palliative care at his own home, died soon after midazolam administration. Toxicological and histological analyses were performed on body fluids and organ fragments. Results and Discussion: Morphological reliefs evidenced a neoplastic mass, composed of lobulated tissue with a lardy, pinkish-gray consistency, extending from the pleural surface to the lung parenchyma, also present at the sacrum region (S1–S5), at the anterior mediastinum level, occupying the entire left pleural cavity, and infiltrating the ipsilateral lung. Metastatic lesions diffused to rachis and lumbar structures. The brain presented edema and congestion. Toxicological analyses evidenced blood midazolam concentrations in the range of 0.931–1.690 μg/mL, while morphine was between 0.266 and 0.909 μg/mL. Death was attributed to cardiorespiratory depression because of a synergic action between morphine and midazolam. The pharmacological interaction between midazolam and morphine is discussed considering the clinical situation of the patient. The opportunity to proceed with midazolam administration is discussed starting from guidelines recommendation. Finally, professional liability outlines are highlighted.

Keywords: deep sedation; drug interaction; midazolam; morphine; palliative care; terminal patient management

1. Introduction

Pain has always been a source of concern for mankind and the subject of a ubiquitous commitment to understand and control it. Remedying suffering and offering relief to the patient mean improving their quality of life and, in general, the quality of the health care provided. When the patient's health conditions worsen and curation is no longer possible, palliative care becomes the only feasible approach, the purpose of which changes as the patient's health conditions change [?]. If the goal is to ensure or improve quality of life, understanding the relationship between comfort and function maintenance is crucial to correctly use sedation: if the patient's condition allows it, sedation is an unintentional consequence of therapy, while during the last moments, it represents the only therapeutic possibility [?]. Since 2002, palliative care has been included in the European Charter of Patients' Rights [?], as point 11 "Right to Avoid Unnecessary Suffering and Pain." De Graeff and Dean recommended the use of palliative sedation therapy for "specific sedative medications to relieve suffering from refractory symptoms by a reduction in patients' consciousness," while refractory symptoms are the ones "for which all possible treatment has failed, or it is estimated that no methods are available for palliation within the time frame and the risk-benefit ratio that the patient can tolerate" [?].

In March 2010, a legislative decree was issued in Italy focusing on palliative care and pain therapy, also introducing the at-home sedation [?]. The Italian Society of Palliative Care underlines the opportunity for the physician to establish an efficient communication with both the patients and the relatives [?]. With respect to the deep sedation, the Italian Commission on Bioethics [?] suggested the following eligibility criteria for access to deep sedation: a patient with an incurable disease in an advanced stage, imminent death, the patient's consent, the presence of acute terminal events or symptoms refractory to treatment causing intolerable suffering to the patient. In a recent review on clinical aspects related to palliative sedation, Arantzamendi and colleagues [?] evidenced that "refractory symptoms most frequently reported were the delirium (41–83%), the pain (25–65%) and dyspnea (16–59%)"; moreover, psychological, and existential distress occurred in 16–59% of patients, with midazolam as the most administered drug.

Terminal cancer patients are among the most fragile and critical and the definition of the most suitable palliative care is still an open challenge: the precarious health conditions that these patients generally present in the terminal stages of their lives, together with therapies (often polytherapy) already prescribed, contribute to complicate the choice of the best approach to ensure adequate quality of life. If sedation must be ensured for a short time period, blood pressure, oxygen saturation, and respiratory rate have to be monitored, as well as the degree of sedation established according to the RAMSEY scale; therapy needs the presence of sanitary personnel during the first 10–15 min.

Finally, palliative care therapy itself can involve the use of several active principles, for which the clinician must carefully evaluate the possible drug-to-drug interactions considering the specific patient's health conditions.

Opiates, mostly morphine, in combination with midazolam and haloperidol, are widely used for symptom control [?]. Drug-to drug interactions occurring in polytherapy involving the simultaneous administration of morphine and benzodiazepines are well documented [?], but additional considerations must be pointed out to approach the correct management of terminal cancer patients requiring the simultaneous administration of such drugs to ensure adequate pain control and/or sedation. All pharmacokinetic (Pk) phases may be subject to nonnegligible variations in terminal cancer patients, resulting in drug bioavailability sensibly divergent from levels that are predictable on the basis of administered doses and "normal" Pk parameters, as determined from studies on healthy volunteers [?]. A modification in metabolism deriving from the advanced illness can modify drugs' pharmacokinetics as well [?]. Franken and colleagues [?] reviewed this item, evidencing that deep modifications in drug absorption rate, bioavailability, metabolism itself can occur in terminal cancer patients, due to changes in hepatic functions or liver blood flow, gastrointestinal problems or symptoms such as nausea and vomiting commonly registered, tissue blood perfusion, and subcutaneous fat content. This last aspect may determine an increased absorption rate, resulting in higher peak concentrations with respect to results of studies performed on healthy volunteers. A continuous and accurate monitoring of the real patient's metabolism is mandatory for a correct and safe pharmacological therapy in terminal cancer subjects approaching the last days of life, and modifications in administered therapy involving the introduction of new drugs or a higher dosage can be decided only in light of a documented worsening of the patient's conditions. It should also not be forgotten that the administered palliative therapy must be discussed and agreed with the patient, until their conditions allow it, or alternatively with relatives and/or legal representatives.

Within this item, the present paper presents the case of a terminal cancer patient who died at their own home in strict temporal relation with a midazolam administration. Toxicological data are discussed in view of guidelines and recommendations for a safe management of terminal cancer patients and possible professional liability.

2. Case Report

A young Italian male was diagnosed with Ewing's sarcoma in the sacral region when he was 24 years old. Despite second- and third-line chemotherapy treatments, as well as radiotherapy, a chest recurrence of sarcoma presented after four years, with costal, pleural, pulmonary, and cardiac involvement. Due to his worsening health conditions and the severity of the painful symptoms, the young man began a treatment of palliative care in an Onco-Hematology Department, including morphine (0.8 mL/min) for analgesia. As the disease worsened, he decided to continue with palliative care at his home and was entrusted to the Territorial Service for Integrated Home Care. The following therapy was prescribed: oxygen, 3 L/min; paracetamol, 1 g iv, at occurrence; morphine, 100 mg at 1.5 mL/h, with continuous infusion; morphine, 3 mg/3 mL infusion in physiological solution, at occurrence; no other drugs were prescribed for patient sedation. The young man died after three days from the arrival at home. Although the clinical diary did not report any worsening of the condition of the young man that justified the implementation of analgesia, empty bottles of midazolam were found in the bedroom. A total of eight empty ampoules (six of 5 mg and two of 15 mg) were found in the bedroom, thus suggesting a possible 60 mg midazolam administration. The parents reported that the physician proceeded with the administration of midazolam (not authorized in Italy for home treatment), moving away immediately after. The parents called the emergency medical services, who reported the death to the Prosecutor Office (P.O.). Both autopsy and toxicological analyses were performed, in an attempt to elucidate the exact cause of death (natural or induced by incongruous drug administration), as well as to verify eventual professional liabilities.

3. Material and Methods

Certified standard solutions of drugs of abuse used for confirmation analysis in gas chromatography/mass spectrometry (GC/MS) were from Cerilliant-Merck (Milan, Italy), *N,O*-bis (trimethylsilyl) trifluoroacetamide (BSTFA) derivatizing agent from Acros (Morris Plains, Morris Count, NJ, USA), and HPLC-grade solvents from Carlo Erba (Milan, Italy).

Enzyme-Linked ImmunoSorbent Assay (ELISA) screening tests were performed on a Dynex-DSX system from Technogenetics (Chantilly, VA, USA), using forensic blood kits from Abbott for AMP/MAMP/MDMA, barbiturates, benzodiazepines, buprenorphine, cannabinoids, cocaine, fentanyl, ketamine, methadone, opiates, oxycodone, tricyclic antidepressants, and zolpidem.

GC/MS analyses were performed using an ISQ single-quadrupole mass spectrometer directly linked to a Trace1300 gas chromatograph equipped with a split-splitless autosampler AI1310, all from ThermoFisher (San José, CA, USA). Gas chromatographic separations were performed with a Rxi®-5MS (30 m × 0.25 mm × 0.25 µm) capillary column (Restek, Bellefonte, PA, USA). Data were processed using the Xcalibur software (version 4.0.27.13) from ThermoFisher.

Headspace gas chromatographic/mass spectrometric (HS-GC/MS) analyses were performed on an HP6890 series gas chromatographer provided with a HP7694E autosampler and a 5973 single-quadrupole mass spectrometer (Hewlett-Packard, Palo Alto, CA, USA); chromatographic separation was accomplished by a CP PorabondQ capillary column (Varian, Agilent, Santa Clara, CA, USA), and data were analyzed using the MSD Chemstation software (D.02.0.275 version) from Agilent Technologies (Santa Clara, CA, USA).

Toxicological Analysis

Biological fluids (left jugular vein, cardiac, portal vein and aorta vein blood, urine, and bile) and organ homogenates (from brain and liver) were used for toxicological analyses; femoral blood, usually used for post-mortem toxicological analyses [?], was not collected, due to body conditions. ELISA screening tests were initially performed on portal vein blood, after dilution (1:10, v:v) of a proper sample aliquot with bidistilled water, according to the manufacturer's specifications. All "nonnegative" results were verified with specific conformation analyses performed on all biological matrices by GC/MS, after appropriate deuterated internal standard addiction and proper purification through solid-phase extraction and eventual derivatization, according to analytical procedures previously validated [? ?]. For GC–MS analyses, all samples were acquired in both *full scan* and selected-ion monitoring mode (GC/MS-SIM). The eventual presence of ethyl alcohol or any other volatile chemicals was also verified, by analyzing portal vein blood by HS-GC/MS.

Toxicological analyses were also performed on liquid residues recovered from the central venous catheter present in the under-right clavicular region of the deceased; solutions of three infusion lines (see Figure **??**, part B) and of the final tract (see Figure **??**, part A) were analyzed in GC/MS.

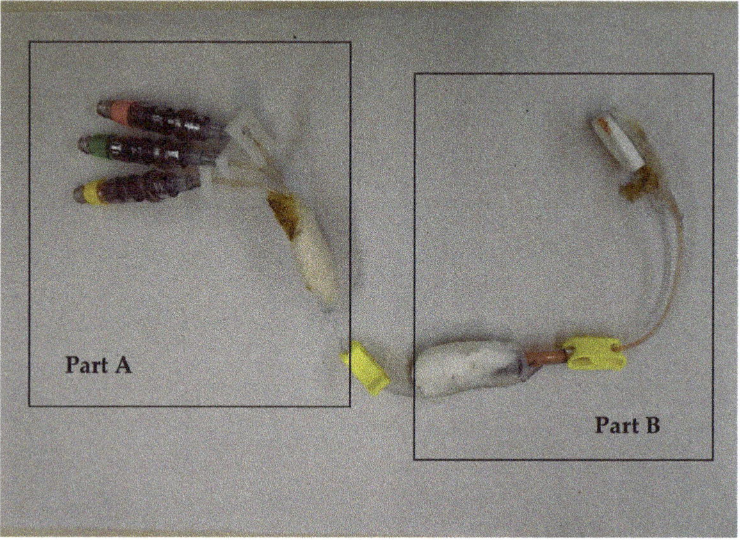

Figure 1. Central venous catheter recovered in deceased' under-right clavicular region.

4. Results

4.1. Autopsy

The autopsy highlighted the presence of a central venous catheter placed in the right clavicular vein, connected distally with three different infusion lines (red, green, and yellow, see Figure **??**). In the left hemithorax, a serious and extensive neoplasm was present. The neoplasm occupied much of the pleural cavity and the left lung had collapsed so that the parenchymal area was highly limited. The neoplastic tissue originated from the ribs of the left hemithorax, showing a thin and pasty tissue from the second and up to the twelfth arc, to testify that the sarcomatous localization affected extensively the costal bony plane. Finally, the pelvis skeleton showed macroscopic morphological findings of the original sarcomatous lesion, which also affected the last lumbar vertebrae (4th on 5th).

4.2. Histological Examinations

Histological investigations confirmed at the left hemithorax the presence of multiple locations of Ewing's sarcoma with large areas of necrosis and hemorrhage and bilateral bronchopneumonitis outbreaks.

A neoplastic localization of Ewing's sarcoma was also highlighted at the level of the trachea. Areas of fibrosis were evidenced on the myocardial tissue, reasonably framed as outcomes of chemotherapy and radiotherapy treatments suffered by the patient.

4.3. Toxicological Analysis

Toxicological screening tests performed on an aliquot of the portal vein blood resulted as "nonnegative" toward benzodiazepines and opiates, and the datum was confirmed by GC/MS. All sampled biological matrices resulted as positive toward morphine; midazolam was detected in all samples but liver homogenate; GC/MS *full scan* analyses resulted as negative toward hydroxymidazolam. Quantification was performed in GC/MS-SIM; the results are presented in Table **??**; morphine quantitative data refer to total morphine, as samples underwent acidic hydrolysis before purification.

Table 1. Morphine and midazolam concentrations detected in analyzed biological matrices.

Matrix	[Midazolam] (μg/mL)	[Morphine] (μg/mL)
left jugular vein blood	1.1	0.6
portal vein blood	0.9	>0.8
cardiac blood	1.3	0.7
aorta vein blood	1.7	0.3
urine	N.D.	>0.8
bile	N.D.	>0.8
brain	1.3 μg/g	0.9 ng/g
liver	N.D.	>0.8 μg/g

The results of toxicological analyses performed on fluids and organ homogenates evidenced positivity toward midazolam and morphine. Midazolam concentrations varied within the range from 0.9 μg/mL (portal vein blood) to 1.7 μg/mL (aorta vein blood); the benzodiazepine was also detected in brain homogenate (1.3 μg/g), while bile, urine, and liver resulted as negative. All analyzed biological matrices resulted as positive to morphine, with concentrations from 0.3 μg/mL (aorta vein blood) up to >0.8 μg/mL (portal vein blood, urine, and bile); the brain and liver presented morphine concentrations of 0.9 ng/g and >0.8 μg/g, respectively.

Results on morphine are in line with pharmacological therapy prescribed to the patient. He presented intense painful symptoms, as the neoplasm infiltrated a large part of the pelvis skeleton, the last lumbar vertebral metamers, numerous costal elements of the left hemithorax in one on the entire pleural surface, and almost all the ipsilateral lung. The prescribed analgesic therapy provided for continuous morphine infusion (and paracetamol at occurrence), justified by a picture of certainly very intense pain, well documented in the medical record.

Different considerations can be made with respect to midazolam concentrations. Regarding the quantitative levels of the drug determined in the different biological matrices, it must be underlined as post-mortem data cannot be simply interpreted by comparison with in vivo therapeutic concentrations. Modifications occurring immediately after death (incomplete drug distribution at the time of death, release from the binding site, passive diffusion) account for significative variations between ante- and post-mortem drug levels [? ?]. Comments on thanatological data must be done with respect to post-mortem studies. Midazolam concentrations highlighted in the case presented here are from 4.2 to 7.7 times higher than the literature datum. Data on midazolam overdoses refer mostly to erroneous administrations by sanitary personnel [?] or to ampoule labeling errors [?] as a major source of iatrogenic injury in hospitalized patients, although they are rarely associated with patients' death [?]. In one case of a "rare midazolam overdose" administered to the victim through an adulterated drink, Wang et al. reported a benzodiazepine concentration, measured in the cardiovascular system, of 0.22 μg/mL [?].

Toxicological analyses performed on solution residues recovered from the central venous catheter evidenced the presence of midazolam in Part A-yellow line and Part B solutions.

5. Discussion

Despite being provided in palliative sedation protocols, simultaneous administration of a sedative-hypnotic benzodiazepine in a terminal cancer patient already under continuous morphine infusion must be carefully evaluated. When administered to healthy patients, sedative-hypnotics induce effects on respiration comparable to those recorded during natural sleep even at hypnotic doses [?]. Conversely, the administration of these drugs in patients with obstructive pulmonary diseases can induce significant respiratory depression, even at therapeutic doses. In such patients, therefore, it becomes crucial to control the occurrence of possible additive effects, following the simultaneous administration/intake of other drugs characterized by depressive action on the central nervous system. The additive Central Nervous System depression occurring when benzodiazepines are taken together with alcoholic beverages, analgesics, opioids, anticonvulsants, phenothiazines, and other sedative-hypnotics is well documented in the literature [?]. In particular, the simultaneous administration of morphine and sedative-hypnotics has the effect of strengthening the depression of the central nervous system, regarding the enhancement of respiratory depression [?]. In the case presented here, the patient had limited respiratory function following the extension of the neoplastic disease to the entire left hemithorax. Consequently, the administration of an active principle known to induce CNS depression required an adjusted dose to clinical conditions and the careful monitoring of the patient's clinical evolution and could only be justified to remedy a significant worsening of his painful symptoms.

Midazolam is classified as a "short-acting" drug, with a rapid onset of the pharmacological effects [?], further enhanced in the case presented here by the subcutaneous injection. Administration by intravenous injection bypasses the absorption phase, normally representing the slowest step directly determining the time required for the beginning of pharmacological effects. When administered intravenously, the clinical onset is determined exclusively by the time necessary for the drug to reach the brain through the bloodstream starting from the injection point and by the time required for the passive diffusion of the active principle across the blood–brain barrier: this process requires typically 15 s to 5 min, regardless of the intravenous access used, and *"depending on the size of the dose, the particular pharmacologic response, and the patient's sensitivity"* [?].

Toxicological findings showed the presence of midazolam in part A (yellow line) and part B solutions recovered from the central venous catheter present on the body, confirming the hypothesis of benzodiazepine administration through such a device. In view of its position on the body (under-right clavicular vein), the positivity found in all blood samples attests the effective midazolam distribution. In this regard, particularly relevant is the positivity of the blood sample from the portal vein: if the midazolam did not have time to distribute, such a sample would have been substantially negative. Moreover, considering the positivity of the brain homogenate sample, the drug had the opportunity to exert its pharmacological effects before the patient's death. Negative results obtained for bile, liver, and urine toward midazolam strongly supported the hypothesis of a strict correlation between drug administration and death. Such an aspect is of great relevance to assess the sanitary management, as discussed below.

In the case presented here, the midazolam administered dose, estimated by the empty ampoules (six of 5 mg and two of 15 mg) found in the deceased's bedroom, was about 60 mg by multiple intravenous injections performed in a short time sequence, therefore comparable to a single injection. Such an administered dose results as higher than dosages reported in the literature for palliative sedation of terminal cancer patients. In their revision of the literature, De Graeff and Dean reported the use of different drugs (both in terms of active principle and dosage) among countries, but, generally, midazolam is the sedative of choice, due to its several advantages, such as short half-life, few side effects, anxiolytic, antiepileptic, and muscle relaxant properties, apart from sedative effects [?]. The administered mean concentration in the literature reviewed by De Graeff and Dean varied in the range of (22–70) mg/24 h, while the median dose was within (30–45) mg/24 h [?]. In a 2011 retrospective cross-sectional study in a home cohort, Calvo-Espinos et al. [?] reported similar dosages: 35 patients treated at home were administered with a mean midazolam dose of 40 mg during the last day of life. Higher dosages were reported by Alonso-Babarro et al. [?] in a retrospective review on palliative therapies prescribed at home to terminal cancer patients between 2002 and 2004: 27 out of 29 patients received midazolam for palliative sedation, with a mean dosage in the last day of life of 74 mg; two patients required the administration of levomepromazine (mean dosage: 125 mg during the last 24 h). Porzio et al. [?] used a multi-step midazolam-based therapy to achieve sedation in patients presenting delirium (13 subjects) or dyspnea (3 subjects). Dosages of 1 mg/h were initially administered; in one third of treated patients, the dosage was doubled with the addition of chlorpromazine and promethazine to maintain a deep and effective sedation. Prommer recently published a review article on midazolam as an *essential palliative care* drug [?]: literature dosages varied in the range of (15–60) mg/day for the sedation of uncontrolled symptoms in a South Africa hospice [?], (23–58) mg/day in an Italian study on terminal cancer patients assisted at home [?], and up to 79 mg/day administered in an Israeli hospice [?]. As evident, all cited literature refers to therapies administered gradually during the 24 h, with a careful titration of the sedative dose *to the relief of symptoms and the distress it* causes [?]. Moreover, all changes in therapy—both in terms of the administered active principle and dosage increase—must be a consequence of a worsening in the patient's conditions, which must be well documented in the clinical care diary [?]. These recommendations were completely disregarded in the case presented here, as the physician proceeded with a 60 mg midazolam administration in a terminal cancer patient, presenting a well-documented reduction in lung function due to cancer extension (involving the entire left hemithorax and pleural surface and almost the entire left lung) and who was already on continuous morphine infusion therapy. Moreover, no indication of a worsening in patient's conditions that could justify and/or suggest the need for further sedation through benzodiazepine administration was reported on the clinical care diary. Finally, the physician left the patient's house immediately after midazolam administration, thus failing to comply with the obligation to monitor the evolution of his condition. Really, the positivity itself toward midazolam in a patient treated at home is of great concern. In Italy, such benzodiazepine is unavailable for extra hospital use, and its administration for palliative sedation of a terminal patient treated at home requires the authorization by hospital-home teams [?]. Such an authorization was not present, nor even required, in the case discussed here, thus representing the first critical aspect that negatively characterizes the healthcare professional's conduct. The sanitary personnel decided (i) to implement the therapy by adding midazolam, (ii) to administer a dose exceeding ranges normally applied in palliative therapies, (iii) to proceed without a clear and well-documented worsening of the patient's conditions; moreover, he moved away from the patient' house immediately after drug administration without any control of the patient clinical evolution: such actions configure precise profiles of severe negligence. Based on the results of toxicological analyses, and of the autopsy and pathological examination, the Prosecutor Office referred the physician who proceeded with midazolam administration for murder. Euthanasia is not allowed in Italy and the so-called "consented murder" can only be allowed if the terminally ill patient has clearly expressed the will to die and is unable, due to his infirmity, to commit suicide [?]. In fact, article 580 of the Code of Criminal Procedure (which punishes assisted suicide) has been declared not entirely compliant with constitutional principles [?]. In the case presented here, the act could not be configured as consented murder, as the young man had never expressed the will to end his life, wishing only relief from the pain he suffered.

6. Conclusions

Pharmacological management of palliative sedation must be carried out with particular care, as it is always recommended to: (i) draw up an adequate clinical diary to report the therapeutic responses and possible side-effects progressively evaluated; (ii) gradually increase the drug's dosages up to the desired sedation level; (iii) weigh the degree of sedation and any relative changes to therapy [? ?]. In general, sedation should be implemented at low initial doses, progressively increasing them until the degree of sedation is reached, aiming to control physical or mental symptoms. It is also necessary to safely conduct palliative sedation by monitoring its depth and symptom control, using tools such as recording vital parameters and measuring peripheral oxygen saturation. Of course, any variation in pharmacological therapy must take into account possible interactions with active principles already administered to the patient, as well as a pre-existing deficit and/or significative reduction in any function or organ that could be enhanced by the new drug, thereby compromising the patient's life.

Author Contributions: P.B.: formal analysis, conceptualization; P.G.: autopsy and medico-legal analysis; G.V.: medico-legal considerations, revision; A.S. (Angela Simonelli): formal analysis; R.G.: formal analysis; A.S. (Angela Silvestre): formal analysis; M.P.: conceptualization, writing—review and editing. All authors have read and agreed to the published version of the manuscript.

Funding: This research received no external funding.

Institutional Review Board Statement: The study was conducted according to the guidelines of the Declaration of Helsinki. Ethics review and approval were not required for this study, as all analyses described in the manuscript were asked by the Prosecutor Office as integral part of the investigations required to highlight the exact cause of the young man death. Relatives had been informed and agreed.We perform analyses strictly necessary to answer to the question posed by the Judicial Authority and none of them was aimed to research purposes. For this reason we were authorized by the Prosecutor Office to perform toxi-cological analyses, as well as autopsy and histological analyses, on biological matrices, and no further authorization was required.

Informed Consent Statement: Informed consent was obtained from all subjects involved in the study, since relatives of the young man had been informed by the Prosecutor Office of all requested analyses and had given their consent to the judicial authority.

Data Availability Statement: Not applicable.

Conflicts of Interest: The authors declare no conflict of interest.

Research Ethics: Research was carried out following the rules of the Declaration of Helsinki of 1975. Approval from the local institutional review board was not necessary, as all analyses were performed in accordance with Prosecutor Office requests.

References

1. Levy, M.H.; Cohen, S.D. Sedation for the relief of refractory symptoms in the imminently dying: A fine intentional line. *Semin. Oncol.* **2005**, *32*, 237–246. [CrossRef] [PubMed]
2. European Charter of Patient's Rights. 2002. Available online: https://ec.europa.eu/health/ph_overview/co_operation/mobility/docs/health_services_co108_en.pdf (accessed on 25 October 2021).
3. De Graeff, A.; Dean, M. Palliative sedation therapy in the last weeks of life: A literature review and recommendations for standards. *J. Pall. Med.* **2007**, *10*, 67–85. [CrossRef] [PubMed]
4. Italian Legislative decree No. 38, March 15th, 2010. National Official Gazette No. 65, March 19th, 2010, General Serie. 2010. Available online: https://www.gazzettaufficiale.it/eli/gu/2010/03/19/65/sg/pdf (accessed on 25 October 2021).
5. Corsi, C.D.; Turriziani, A.; Cavanna, L.; Morino, P.; Ribecco, A.S.; Ciaparrone, M.; Lanzetta, G.; Pinto, C.; Zagonel, V. Consensus document of the Italian Association of Medical Oncology and the Italian Society of Palliative Care on early palliative care. *Tumor. J.* **2019**, *105*, 103–112. [CrossRef] [PubMed]

6. Italian Committee for Bioethics. Deep and Continuous Palliative Sedation in the Imminence of Death. 2016. Available online: https://bioetica.governo.it/media/3211/p122_2016_palliative-sedation_en.pdf (accessed on 25 October 2021).
7. Arantzamendi, M.; Belar, A.; Payne, S.; Rijpstra, M.; Preston, N.; Menten, J.; Van der Elst, M.; Radbruch, M.; Hasselaar, J.; Genteno, C. Clinican aspects of palliative sedation in prospective studies. A systematic review. *J. Pain Symptom Manag.* **2021**, *61*, 831–844. [CrossRef] [PubMed]
8. De Lima, L. International Association for Hospice and Palliative Care list of essential medicines for palliative care. *Ann. Oncol.* **2007**, *18*, 395–399. [CrossRef]
9. Cheeti, S.; Budha, N.R.; Rajan, S.; Dresser, M.J.; Jin, J.Y. A physiologically based pharmacokinetic (PBPK) approach to evaluate pharmacokinetics in patients with cancer. *Biopharm. Drug Dispos.* **2013**, *34*, 141–154. [CrossRef] [PubMed]
10. Bruera, E.; Hui, D. Palliative care research: Lessons learned by our team over the last 25 years. *Palliat. Med.* **2013**, *27*, 939–951. [CrossRef]
11. Franken, L.G.; de Winter, B.C.; van Esch, H.J.; van Zuylen, L.; Baar, F.P.; Tibboel, D.; Mathôt, R.A.; van Gelder, T.; Koch, B.C. Pharmacokinetic considerations and recommendations in palliative care, with focus on morphine, midazolam and haloperidol. *Expert Opin. Drug Metab. Toxicol.* **2016**, *12*, 669–680. [CrossRef] [PubMed]
12. Horsfall, J.T.; Sprague, J.E. The Pharmacology and Toxicology of the 'Holy Trinity'. *Basic Clin. Pharmacol. Toxicol.* **2017**, *120*, 115–119. [CrossRef]
13. Zilg, B.; Thelander, G.; Giebe, B.; Druid, H. Postmortem blood sampling-Comparison of drug concentrations at different sample sites. *Forensic Sci. Int.* **2017**, *278*, 296–303. [CrossRef] [PubMed]
14. Basilicata, P.; Pieri, M.; Simonelli, A.; Faillace, D.; Niola, M.; Graziano, V. Application of a chemiluminescence immunoassay system and GC/MS for toxicological investigations on skeletonized human remains. *Forensic Sci. Int.* **2019**, *300*, 120–124. [PubMed]
15. Basilicata, P.; Pieri, M.; Settembre, V.; Galdiero, A.; Della Casa, E.; Acampora, A.; Miraglia, N. Screening of several drugs of abuse in Italian workplace drug testing: Performances comparison of an on-site screening tests and a Fluorescence Polarization ImmunoAssay-based device. *Anal. Chem.* **2011**, *83*, 8566–8574. [CrossRef] [PubMed]
16. Basilicata, P.; Silvestre, A.; Simonelli, A.; Guadagni, R.; Pieri, M. Il dato chimico-tossicologico post-mortale: Avvelenamento o non avvelenamento? *Riv. Ital. Med. Leg.* **2019**, *4*, 1509–1517.
17. Skopp, G. Postmortem toxicology. *Forensic Sci. Med. Pathol.* **2010**, *6*, 314–325. [CrossRef] [PubMed]
18. Nishiyama, T.; Hanaoka, K. Accidental overdose of midazolam as intramuscular premedication. *J. Clin. Anesth.* **2002**, *14*, 543–545. [CrossRef]
19. Flood, C.; Matthew, L.; Marsh, R.; Patel, B.; Mansaray, M.; Lamont, T. Reducing risk of overdose with midazolam injection in adults: An evaluation of change in clinical practice to improve patient safety in England. *J. Eval. Clin. Pract.* **2015**, *21*, 57–66. [CrossRef] [PubMed]
20. Wang, J.Z.; Wang, L. Revisit of a rare death by overdosed midazolam: A forensic pathological perspective. *J. Forensic Med.* **2018**, *3*, 121–124. [CrossRef]
21. Katzung, B.G.; Trevor, A.J.; Kruidering-Hall, M. *Basic and Clinical Pharmacology*, 13th ed.; McGraw-Hill: New Jersey, NJ, USA, 2014.
22. Greenblatt, D.J.; Shader, R.I.; Abernethy, D.R. Current status of benzodiazepines (first of two parts). *N. Engl. J. Med.* **1983**, *309*, 354–358. [PubMed]
23. Calvo-Espinos, C.; Ruiz De Gaona, E.; Gonzalez, C.; Ruiz De Galarreta, L.; Lopez, C. Palliative sedation for cancer patients included in a home care program: A retrospective study. *Pall. Supp. Care* **2015**, *13*, 619–624. [CrossRef] [PubMed]
24. Alonso-Babarro, A.; Varela-Cerdeira, M.; Torres-Vigil, I.; Rodriguez-Barrientos, R.; Bruera, E. At-home palliative sedation for end-of-life cancer patients. *Pall. Med.* **2010**, *24*, 486–492. [CrossRef] [PubMed]
25. Porzio, G.; Aielli, F.; Verna, L.; Micolucci, G.; Aloisi, P.; Ficorella, C. Efficacy and safety of deep, continuous palliative sedation at home: A retrospective, single-institution study. *Supp. Care Cancer* **2010**, *18*, 77–81. [CrossRef] [PubMed]
26. Prommer, E. Midazolam: An essential palliative care drug. *Palliat. Care Soc. Pract.* **2020**, *14*, 1–12. [CrossRef]
27. Fainsinger, R.L.; Landman, W.; Hoskings, M.; Bruera, E. Sedation for uncontrolled symptoms in a South African hospice. *J. Pain Symptom Manag.* **1988**, *16*, 145–152. [CrossRef]
28. Mercadante, S.; Porzio, G.; Valle, A.; Fusco, F.; Aielli, F.; Costanzo, V. Palliative sedation in patients with advanced cancer followed at home: A systematic review. *J. Pain Sym. Man.* **2011**, *41*, 754–760. [CrossRef] [PubMed]
29. Azoulay, D.; Shahal-Gassner, R.; Yehezkel, M.; Eliyahu, E.; Weigert, N.; Ein-Mor, E.; Jacobs, J.M. Palliative sedation at the end of life: Patterns of use in an Israeli hospice. *Am. J. Hosp. Palliat. Care* **2016**, *33*, 369–373. [CrossRef] [PubMed]
30. Italian Constitutional Court. Sentence No 249/2019. Available online: https://www.cortecostituzionale.it/actionSchedaPronuncia.do?anno=2019&numero=242 (accessed on 25 October 2021).
31. Cowan, J.D.; Palmer, T.W. Practical guide to palliative sedation. *Pall. Med.* **2002**, *4*, 242–249. [CrossRef] [PubMed]

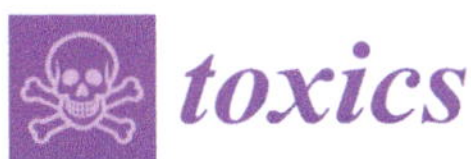 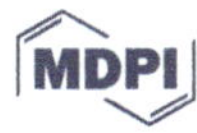

Brief Report

Detection of Morphine and Opioids in Fingernails: Immunohistochemical Analysis and Confirmation with Ultra-High-Performance Liquid Chromatography Coupled with High-Resolution Mass Spectrometry

Roberto Scendoni *, Emanuele Bury, Erika Buratti, Rino Froldi, Marta Cippitelli , Gianmario Mietti and Mariano Cingolani

Forensic Medicine Laboratory, Institute of Legal Medicine, University of Macerata, 62100 Macerata, Italy; emanuelebury92@gmail.com (E.B.); burattierika@gmail.com (E.B.); rino.froldi@unimc.it (R.F.); cippitelli.marta@gmail.com (M.C.); gianmario.mietti@gmail.com (G.M.); mariano.cingolani@unimc.it (M.C.)
* Correspondence: r.scendoni@unimc.it

Abstract: This study aimed to investigate the detection of morphine in fingernails from forensic autopsies using immunohistochemistry (IHC), with confirmation by ultra-high-performance liquid chromatography coupled with high-resolution mass spectrometry (UHPLC-HRMS). A primary antibody specific to morphine and a secondary antibody conjugated to horseradish peroxidase (HRP) was used. IHC on specimens of Subjects A and B (both drug addicts) resulted in the detection of morphine on a cell layer of the nail plate matrix. UHPLC-HRMS and GC-MS analysis showed that Subject A had a morphine concentration of 0.35 ng/mg in the fingernail and 472 ng/mL in the blood, while Subject B reached 1.23 ng/mg in the fingernail and 360 ng/ml in the blood. Most of those matrices were positive for codeine, methadone, EDDP, and 6-MAM. The use of IHC in Subject C (a former addict) showed no positivity for morphine in the fingernail, while the UHPLC-HRMS analysis confirmed its absence in the fingernail and blood. Additionally, an analysis of the scalp or pubic hair of the subjects was carried out using UHPLC-HRMS. The results suggest that IHC can be used to establish the site of accumulation of morphine in the nail matrix; for postmortem diagnosis; and that basic substances can be detected by UHPLC-HRMS. There are no previous studies on the use of IHC as a technique for forensic purposes in unconventional matrices, such as nails.

Keywords: morphine; opioids; fingernails; immunohistochemistry; ultra-high-performance liquid chromatography; high-resolution mass spectrometry; forensic toxicology; unconventional matrices

Citation: Scendoni, R.; Bury, E.; Buratti, E.; Froldi, R.; Cippitelli, M.; Mietti, G.; Cingolani, M. Detection of Morphine and Opioids in Fingernails: Immunohistochemical Analysis and Confirmation with Ultra-High-Performance Liquid Chromatography Coupled with High-Resolution Mass Spectrometry. *Toxics* **2022**, *10*, 420. https://doi.org/10.3390/toxics10080420

Academic Editor: Maria Pieri

Received: 5 July 2022
Accepted: 23 July 2022
Published: 26 July 2022

1. Introduction

Nails are made of keratin and fingernails grow at an average rate of 3 mm per month [1]. Unconventional matrices, such as nails, can provide important samples for clinical and forensic toxicology in the postmortem detection of drugs, but the mechanism of drug incorporation into nails is still unclear.

Studies suggest that drugs are primarily incorporated into nails by deposition into the matrix via the blood flow; other studies have demonstrated that certain drugs are incorporated via the nail bed [2]. In addition to the intake of drugs, exposure to environmental contamination and biological fluids are possible mechanisms of drug incorporation into nails, as is the case with the hair matrix [3]. The stability of drugs in nails makes their analysis very useful for postmortem investigations, especially when it is difficult to perform other tests (using other matrices) or when the material is too decomposed to produce reliable results.

Immunohistochemistry (IHC) is a technique that makes use of antigen-antibody binding to localize specific antigens in cells and tissue. IHC is not frequently used in forensic pathology. It has been applied in previous research to analyze forensic samples [4] or to study the morphine distribution in poisoning cases [5], using organs as the principal matrix. However, no study to date has applied this technique using unconventional matrices like nails. The nails, hair, and blood samples used for this study were obtained from autopsies of subjects with a suspected addiction to opioids.

2. Materials and Methods

2.1. Materials

2.1.1. Matrices

Analyses were performed on fingernail samples from the forensic autopsies of two drug addicts (Subjects A and B) and a former addict (Subject C). The entire index fingernail was removed postmortem, including the matrix portion. Subsequently, the fingernail of the same subject was cut in half so that two equal portions of the same sample could be used for both analytical methods. All three subjects were men. Subject A was 44 years old, Subject B was 57 years old, and Subject C was 38 years old.

2.1.2. Antibodies

Primary Antibody: Polyclonal anti-Morphine Antibody produced in Sheep (ARG23594, Arigo Biolaboratories, Hsinchu City 300 Taiwan, ROC).

Secondary Antibody: Monoclonal Anti-Goat/Sheep IgG-Peroxidase Antibody produced in Mouse (A9452, Sigma-Aldrich, Burlington, MA, USA).

2.1.3. Reagents for Immunohistochemistry

PBS: NaCl (Carlo Erba, Cornaredo, Italy), $NaH_2PO_4{\cdot}H_2O$ (J.T.Baker, Phillipsburg, NJ, USA), and $NaH_2PO_4{\cdot}2H_2O$ (Carlo Erba, Cornaredo, Italy).

3,3 Diamenobenzidine tablets (Sigma-Aldrich, Burlington, MA, USA), Bovine Serum Albumin (Sigma-Aldrich, Burlington, MA, USA), Gelatine (Carlo Erba, Cornaredo, Italy), Mayers Hematoxylin (Bio-Optica, Milano, Italy), Saponins (Carlo Erba, Cornaredo, Italy), and Triton X-100 (Carlo Erba, Cornaredo, Italy) were used.

2.1.4. Chemicals and Reagents for UHPLC Analysis

Nalorphine (internal standard (IS) for the analysis in GC-MS), proadifen (SKF) (internal standard (IS) for the analysis in UHPLC), and MSTFA (N-methyl-N-(trimethylsilyl)-trifluoroacetamide) were purchased from Sigma.

Standards of morphine, 6-monoacetylmorphine, methadone, EDDP, and codeine were purchased from Sigma. Methanol (MeOH) for analysis, water for analysis, dichloromethane, 2-propanol, ammonium hydroxide of reagent grade, methanol for HPLC, and ultrapure water for HPLC were obtained from Carlo Erba; Isolute HCX (130 ng/10 mL) from Biotage. All reagents were of analytical grade and stored according to the manufacturer's instructions.

2.2. Methods

2.2.1. Immunohistochemistry

Paraffin Embedding

Tissues were not fixed in formaldehyde to prevent the extraction of basic substances in the fixative fluid. Tissue dehydration was performed by incubation in solutions of increasing concentration of ethanol and left in xylene overnight. Tissues were transferred to liquid paraffin at 60 °C and allowed to cool. From the tissue blocks, sections of 2 um were cut on a rotating microtome then collected on SuperFrost Plus slides (Menzel Gläser) and left to dry at 60 °C for one hour.

Sections were deparaffinized with xylene for 20 min and then passed through 3 cycles of 10 min in 99% ethanol and 2 cycles of 10 min in 96% ethanol. Endogenous peroxidase activity was then blocked with 0.35% H_2O_2 in methanol for 30 min. Rehydration was completed by rinsing in 96% ethanol, 10 min in 70% ethanol, and triple rinsing in distilled water.

Antibody and Peroxidase Marking

The sections were washed three times in a blocking solution containing 10 mM PBS with 1% BSA, 0.2% gelatin, and 0.05% saponin. The antibodies were diluted in 10 mM PBS containing 0.1% BSA and 0.3% Triton X-100, and the sections were incubated with the primary antibodies for 1 h at room temperature and then at 4 °C overnight. The next day, once they reached room temperature, the sections were triple-rinsed in PBS containing 0.1% BSA, 0.2% gelatin, and 0.05% saponin, and incubated with secondary antibodies diluted in PBS with 0.1% BSA and 0.3% Triton X-100 for 1 h. After an additional 3 washes in a solution of PBS with 0.1% BSA, 0.2% gelatin, and 0.05% saponin, peroxidase activity was detected after 10 min of incubation using diaminobenzidine (3.3 Diamenobenzidine tablets, Sigma-Aldrich) at a concentration of 1 mg/mL. DAB tablets were thawed approximately 20 min before use and activated with 0.35% H_2O_2 just before use. Then, the sections were rinsed in PBS for 3 cycles of 10 min, twice in distilled water, and afterward were counterstained in Mayers Hematoxylin for 2 min and placed under cold running water for 20 min. Dehydration was performed by incubation for two 3 min cycles in 70%, 96%, and 99% ethanol, followed by three 5 min cycles in xylene before coverslips were finally mounted using Eukitt (ORSatec). The immunohistochemical protocol is inspired by the one developed by Paulsen, I.M et al. [6]. The semiquantitative evaluation of the immunohistochemical reaction was performed by expert histologists using the Nikon Eclipse E200 light microscope. The intensity of the DAB signal was measured using the free software ImageJ Fiji, as described by Crowe et al. [7].

2.2.2. Sample Preparation and Extraction

Extraction Procedure in Nail and Hair Matrices

The extraction procedure, specific to morphine, was carried out according to previous work [8]. Half of the nail was used for immunohistochemical analysis, the other half was used for UHPLC analysis (about 60 mg). Both the nail and hair (scalp or pubic) was washed with water, dried, and cut into small pieces.

The sample was extracted by adding 490 µL of distilled water with 0.1% of formic acid and 10 µL of methanol with 0.1% of formic acid. 20 ng of IS (SKF) were added. Hair samples were incubated for 24 h at 55 °C, while nail samples were incubated for 72 h at 55 °C. After incubation, the samples were centrifuged at 12.293× *g* in an ultracentrifuge. The supernatant was collected and evaporated; subsequently, the samples were resuspended with 50 µL of phase B (Methanol + 1% formic acid) for chromatographic injection.

Acid Hydrolysis and Extraction Procedure in Blood Matrix

The acid hydrolysis and extraction procedure were carried out according to previous work [9]. Morphine is found in the blood as 3-glucuronide and 6-glucuronide forms after administration, so it was extracted by acid hydrolysis, detaching glucuronides to reveal the total amount of free morphine [10]. A total of 2 mL of blood was added with 200 µL of chloridric acid and 250 ng of IS. The samples were incubated for 24 h at 55 °C.

The solid-phase extraction procedure followed the method used in our laboratory described in previous work [11].

Derivatization

The eluted samples were completely evaporated and then derivatized with 20 µL of MSTFA at 60 °C for 20 min. One microliter of the derivatized sample was injected into the GC-MS.

2.2.3. Hr-LC and GC-MS Parameters

Hair and Nail Analysis and Quantification by UHPLC-HRMS

The Thermo Scientific Dionex Ultimate 3000 chromatographic system (UHPLC) coupled with Thermo Exactive Plus Orbitrap (HR-MS) was used for hair and nail analysis. The conditions applied for chromatographic analysis were as follows: the column used was Kinetex Biphenyl 2.6 µm (50 × 2.1 mm) by Phenomenex; column flow was set at 0.4 mL/min. Phase A used H_2O + 0.1% formic acid; Phase B used MeOH + 0.1% formic acid. The column temperature was set to 25 °C. The elution gradient is shown in Table 1.

Table 1. UHPLC elution gradient.

TIME	PHASE A (%)	PHASE B (%)
0–0.5	98	2
0.5–10	0	100
10–12	0	100
12–13	98	2
13–15	98	2

Scheme 60: For the identification of analytes, exact mass (EM) obtained from In Source Collision Induced Dissociation (50 eV) (In source CID), with an acceptance range of ±5 ppm, and production (PI) were used. The values monitored for analytes were as follows: 286.14377 (EM) (PI: 201.09101, 229.08592, 183.08044) for morphine; 328.15433 (EM) (PI: 211.07540, 183.08040, 193.06480) for 6-MAM; 300.15942 (EM) (PI 215.10666, 243.10157, 199.07536) for codeine; 310.21654 (EM) (PI: 105.03349, 219.11683, 195.11683) for methadone; 287.19033 (EM) (PI: 234.12773, 249.15120, 186.12773) for EDDP; and 354.24276 (EM) (PI: 167.08553, 91.05423, 105.06988) for SKF (IS).

Blood Analysis and Quantification by GC-MS

The GC-MS Polaris-Q was used for blood analysis. Analytical conditions were as follows: a capillary column (ZB 5 MS 30 m × 0.25 mm × 0.25 µm); helium as a carrier gas at a flow rate of 1.5 mL/min; a temperature program that started at 100 °C for 1 min and was increased first to 220 °C at 30 °C/min for 1 min, and then to 320 °C at 20 °C/min for 6 min (total run time of 17 min); an injection volume that was 1 µL in splitless mode; Full Scan mode, and a mass spectra range of 70–500. Subsequently, the specific SIM layout for morphine, 6-MAM, codeine, methadone, and EDDP was applied. The ion values monitored for analytes were as follows: m/z 429 414 324 for morphine-TMS, m/z 399 340 287 for 6-MAM-TMS, m/z 371 178 196 for codeine-TMS, m/z 72 294 223 for methadone, m/z 276 277 262 for EDDP, and m/z 455 414 440 324 for nalorphine-TMS (IS).

2.2.4. Validation

The method was validated for linearity, quantitation limits (limit of detection (LOD) and limit of quantitation (LOQ)), according to the Scientific Working Group for Forensic Toxicology guidelines (SWCTOX) [12].

Standard curves for morphine and 6-MAM were obtained from previously checked blank samples (hair, nails, and blood) spiked with six concentration points with three replicates for each. Concentrations ranging from 0.05 to 5 ng/mg were prepared for hair and nail HR-LC analysis and concentrations ranging from 0.2 to 10 ng/mg were prepared for blood GC-MS analysis.

The area (analyte)/area (IS) was plotted against the known concentrations of the standard solutions to establish calibration equations. A linear regression equation was calculated using the least-squares method. LOD was determined according to the standard deviation of y-intercepts and the average slope of regression lines $[(3.3{\cdot}s_y)/Avg_m]$. The LOQ value was the lowest concentration showing acceptable values of bias (±20%) and precision (CV ≤ 20%); for details, see Table 2.

Table 2. Summary of validation results.

		Hair	
Substances	**Linearity Range**	**R2**	**LOQ(LOD)**
Morphine	0.05–5 (ng/mg)	0.9933	0.05 (0.02) (ng/mg)
MAM	0.05–5 (ng/mg)	0.9897	0.05 (0.02) (ng/mg)
		Nail	
Morphine	0.05–5(ng/mg)	0.9942	0.05 (0.02) (ng/mg)
MAM	0.05–5 (ng/mg)	0.9853	0.05 (0.02) (ng/mg)
		Blood	
Morphine	0.5–500 (ng/mL)	0.9959	0.5 (0.2) (ng/mL)

3. Results

The semiquantitative evaluation of the immunohistochemical reaction, performed by expert histologists using the Nikon Eclipse E200 light microscope, suggested an accumulation of morphine on the cytoplasm of the epithelial cells, at the level of the nail plate matrix, located in the germinal matrix section of the nail in drug-addicted subjects (Figures 1 and 2). "Subject A" and "Subject B" were drug addicts, while "Subject C" was a former addict.

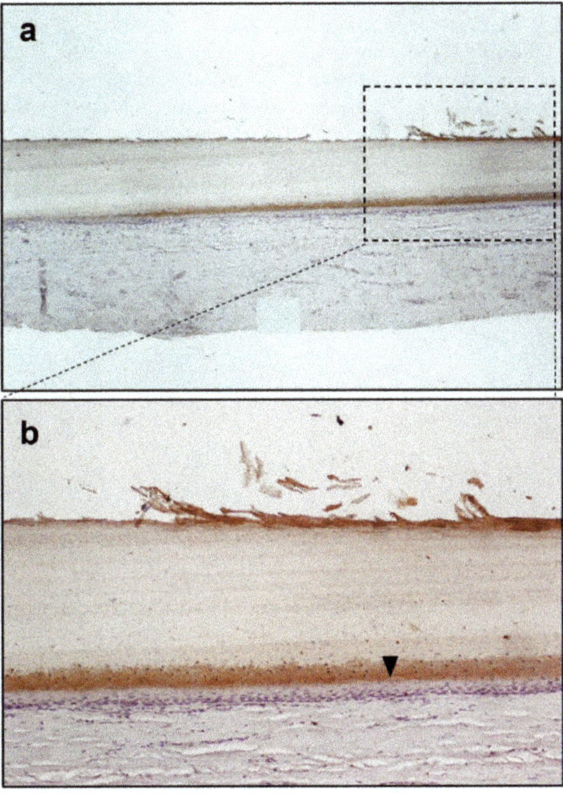

Figure 1. Immunoperoxidase staining for Sheep Anti-Morphine in the fingernail of Subject A. FigPicture (**a**) shows the 4× magnification, while picture (**b**) shows the 10× magnification. The figure shows the cytoplasmic staining of nail matrix cells of Subject A, indicating morphine positivity, shown in particular by a black arrow on the 10× picture.

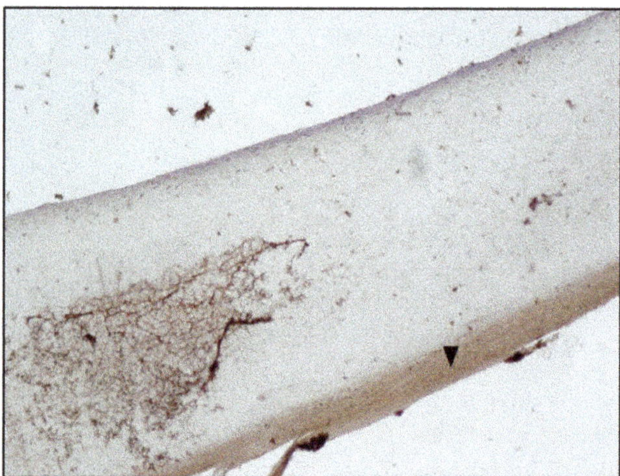

Figure 2. Immunoperoxidase staining for Sheep Anti-Morphine in the fingernail of Subject B, 10× magnification; the picture shows the peroxidase reaction across the nail matrix cells of Subject B, indicating morphine positivity, shown in particular by a black arrow.

The no-primary antibody and no-secondary antibody controls were performed to determine if those antibodies were binding non-specifically to cellular components that did not contain the biomarker or protein of interest. It was applied to the fingernail of Subject A and was successful, showing no staining at all (Figures 3 and 4). Both antibodies were used on the fingernail of the former addict (Subject C), as a negative control, with no reaction detected in any cell of the tissue (Figures 5 and 6). The results of the DAB intensity measure using ImageJ Fiji are shown in Table 3, where "Area" gives the size of the IHC image, and "Mean grey value" represents the quantified signal. These data confirm the positive staining given by the peroxidase to the fingernail of the drug-addicted subjects and its absence in the formerly addicted subject.

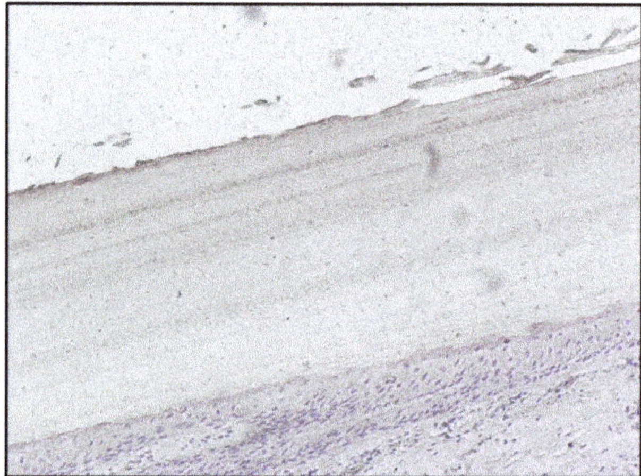

Figure 3. Immunoperoxidase staining for Sheep Anti-Morphine in the fingernail of Subject A, 10× magnification. The immunohistochemistry protocol has been modified to observe the presence of any non-specific reaction; in this figure the primary antibody has been used, while the secondary antibody conjugated to the peroxidase enzyme has not been used.

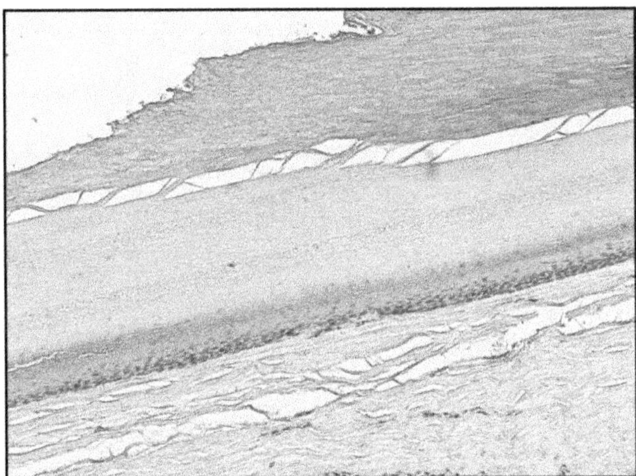

Figure 4. Immunoperoxidase staining for Sheep Anti-Morphine in the fingernail of Subject A, 10× magnification. The immunohistochemistry protocol has been modified to observe the presence of any non-specific reaction; in this figure the primary antibody has not been used, while the secondary antibody conjugated to the peroxidase enzyme has been used.

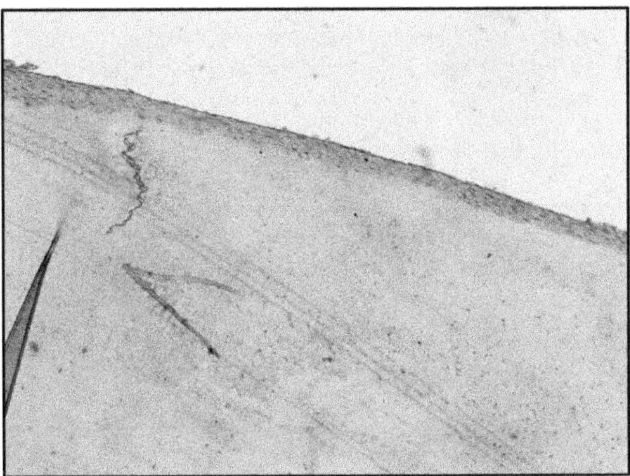

Figure 5. Immunoperoxidase staining for Sheep Anti-Morphine in the fingernail of Subject C, 10× magnification. The pictures show an absence of positivity for morphine in the nail matrix cells. Counterstaining with hematoxylin. Primary Ab: Polyclonal anti-Morphine Antibody produced in Sheep, dil. 1:100. Secondary Ab: Monoclonal Anti-Goat/Sheep IgG-Peroxidase Antibody produced in Mouse, dil. 1:100, original magnification: 10×.

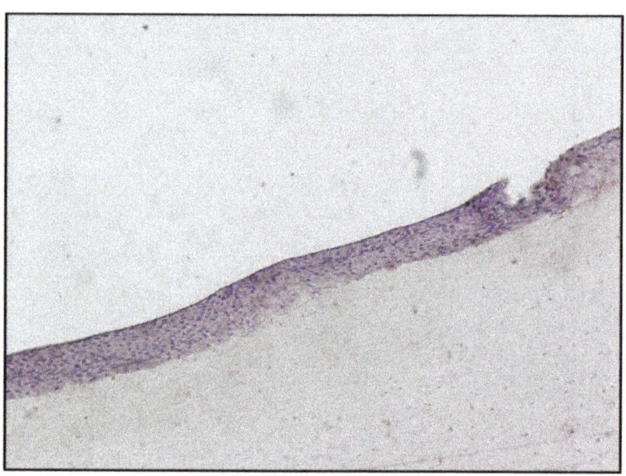

Figure 6. Immunoperoxidase staining for Sheep Anti-Morphine in the fingernail of Subject C, 10× magnification. The pictures show an absence of positivity for morphine in the nail matrix cells. Counterstaining with hematoxylin. Primary Ab: Polyclonal anti-Morphine Antibody produced in Sheep, dil. 1:100. Secondary Ab: Monoclonal Anti-Goat/Sheep IgG-Peroxidase Antibody produced in Mouse, dil. 1:100, original magnification: 10×.

Table 3. ImageJ Fiji DAB intensity measure.

Fingernail matrix	Area	Mean
Subject A (Figure 1)	1,228,800	19.695
Subject B (Figure 2)	1,228,800	26.049
Subject C (Figure 5)	1,228,800	2.252

The primary antibody is specific for morphine and exhibits negligible cross-reaction with codeine. Over the years, numerous works have been carried out to find an antibody with no cross-reaction with other opioids [13]. Even if cross-reactions do not seem to affect the reliability of the results, UHPLC confirmation is important to be able to classify the similar molecules found in the sample, morphine, and codeine in this case. UHPLC analysis was able to distinguish several substances and their respective metabolites, as shown in Table 4. The quantitative analysis of morphine in Subject A showed a morphine concentration of 0.35 ng/mg in the fingernail, 3.64 ng/mg in scalp hair, and 472 ng/mL in blood, while 6-MAM concentrations were 0.43 ng/mg in the fingernail, 1.42 ng/mg in scalp hair, and negative in blood. The morphine in Subject B reached 1.23 ng/mg in the fingernail, 1.60 ng/mg in pubic hair, and 360 ng/mL in blood, while 6-MAM concentrations were 1.18 ng/mg in the fingernail, 0.44 ng/mg in pubic hair, and negative in blood. All these matrices were positive for codeine, methadone, and EDDP in both subjects. The use of immunohistochemistry in the case of the former addict (Subject C) led us to infer an absence of positivity for morphine in the fingernail; the UHPLC-HRMS analysis confirmed its absence in the fingernail and blood. On the other hand, the fingernail of this subject presented 1.03 ng/mg of 6-MAM, while the concentration of morphine in the pubic hair matrix was 2.2 ng/mg, with 4.43 ng/mg of 6-MAM and codeine, methadone, and EDDP positivity.

Table 4. UHPLC and GC-MS analysis results for morphine and opioids concentrations.

Subject A matrix	**Instrument**	**Morphine**	**6-MAM**	**Codeine**	**Methadone**	**EDDP**
Blood	GC-MS	472 ng/ml	Negative	Positive	Positive	Positive
Scalp hair	UHPLC	3.64 ng/mg	1.42 ng/mg	Positive	Positive	Positive
Fingernail	UHPLC	0.35 ng/mg	0.43 ng/mg	Positive	Positive	Positive
Subject B matrix	**Instrument**	**Morphine**	**6-MAM**	**Codeine**	**Methadone**	**EDDP**
Blood	GC-MS	360 ng/ml	Negative	Positive	Positive	Positive
Pubic hair	UHPLC	1.60 ng/mg	0.44 ng/mg	Positive	Positive	Positive
Fingernail	UHPLC	1.23 ng/mg	1.18 ng/mg	Positive	Positive	Positive
Subject C matrix	**Instrument**	**Morphine**	**6-MAM**	**Codeine**	**Methadone**	**EDDP**
Blood	GC-MS	Negative	Negative	Negative	Negative	Negative
Pubic hair	UHPLC	2.2 ng/mg	4.43 ng/mg	Positive	Positive	Positive
Fingernail	UHPLC	Negative	1.03 ng/mg	Negative	Negative	Negative

4. Discussion

In the field of forensic toxicology, it is well-known that the detection of drugs in the blood is the most relevant way of determining the cause of death, given short-term information related to drug addiction. Long-term drug history can be traced by hair analysis [14,15]. A scalp hair matrix can be used to derive a chronological history of drug use, with an extended detection window of approximately 1 month per half-inch of hair, while pubic hair grows more slowly [16,17]. On the other hand, studies suggest that pubic hair can offer an alternative way of proving previous drug use, but it should be avoided when estimating drug use history, and higher quantitative results in pubic hair do not represent heavier drug use [18]. Furthermore, pubic hair does not grow continually like scalp hair; it has a longer resting phase and a different anagen to telogen ratio [19]. This could explain why the accumulation of substances in pubic hair can be higher than in scalp hair.

Over the past few decades, nails (fingernails and toenails) have become a useful specimen type for the detection of drug use and abuse [20]. The innovation of our study was not only to have introduced a new technique for identifying morphine in nails with an accurate stratification of substance accumulation but also to have made a comparison with other biological matrices, particularly hair and pubic hair as well as blood.

Regarding the results obtained from our samples, the UHPLC-HRMS analysis for Subjects B and C showed the presence of morphine and its metabolite in pubic hair. We believe that even if the fingernail has a keratinous matrix similar to hair, pubic hair shows a more long-term and more contaminated drug accumulation in comparison to the nail. The presence of 6-MAM in the fingernail sample of Subject C, analyzed by UHPLC-HRMS, demonstrates that there was no cross-reaction between 6-MAM and morphine during the immunohistochemical analysis.

Histologically, the nail matrix is composed of a thick stratified squamous epithelium that lacks a granular layer. Matrix cells divide, move distally, and cornify, forming the nail plate that slides over the nail bed. When forming the nail plate, matrical keratinocytes flatten and lose their nuclei; this occurs in the eosinophilic keratogenous zone. Below the keratogenous zone is the prekeratogenous zone and below that lies the basal layer. The prekeratogenous zone is made of polygonal cells with clear cytoplasm and oval nuclei arranged parallel to the nail plate and the reaction to the morphine antigen is located in the cytoplasm of those cells [21]. The nail root produces most of the volume of the nail plate and the nail bed. It can be assumed that morphine is transported by blood vessels and deposed in the cells of the nail germinal matrix. As the nail grows, those cells slide distally toward the nail-free margin, pushed by the newer cells of the nail matrix. Proceeding in this direction, the peroxidase reaction stops in the proximity of the nail bed, which extends from the edge of the nail root to the hyponychium [22].

Regarding the distribution of morphine, based on our results, we can assume that the drug is less incorporated via the nail bed and that the main mechanism of distribution is deposition into the nail matrix cells, transported by the blood flow.

The staining located in the cytoplasm of not yet keratinized cells can lead to speculations about the drug metabolism; its accumulation is probably correlated to its binding with other molecules like proteins and phospholipids. A hair matrix, composed of dead keratinized cells, could be the right comparison to better understand the exact location of where the drugs can be incorporated and accumulated [23]. For instance, drugs such as nicotine, morphine, cocaine, and amphetamine are weak bases and they bind to the melanin with electrostatic bonding, because it is acidic [24]. The dead keratinized cells of the hair shaft medulla contain a high level of melanin. On the other hand, in the proximal nail matrix, melanocytes typically lie dormant where the nail originates, leading to a lower level of melanin production in the nail plate compared to the hair shaft [25]. Further studies are needed to better understand the kinetics of weak bases such as morphine inside the nail cells and hair shaft.

The absence of peroxidase reaction in the narrow-keratinized cells of the nail plate could be explained by the differential staining properties of the nail plate [26–29].

The search for exogenous substances on nail material is an ongoing subject of study and more research is required to better understand its characteristics. Further studies are needed to determine if the period of substance intake can influence the specific location of the morphine-accumulating cell layer in the nail matrix or on the nail bed; this could potentially be used as a method to study the addiction history of heroin addicts.

5. Conclusions

The detection of a drug of abuse in the nails indicates an intake in an antecedent period, which can vary from a few weeks up to several months. This matrix certainly represents a new frontier of research in the medico-legal field and, above all, in the forensic toxicology field. There is a need to carry out studies aimed at defining the temporal determination of the intake, due to the double path of blood flow to the nails from the root and the bed, and due to the double growth mechanism [30]. On the other hand, nails are still a valid alternative to hair, especially if we consider characteristics such as the absence of ethnic differences in the composition of the nail and the fact that it is more difficult to alter nail samples compared to hair.

Immunohistochemistry represents an innovative technique in the forensic toxicology field. This work demonstrates that immunohistochemical analysis can be applied for forensic purposes in unconventional matrices, such as nails, which can be successfully used to establish the site of accumulation of substances such as morphine, and for postmortem diagnosis in autopsy specimens of alternative matrices. This study aimed to enrich our scientific knowledge about the use of unconventional matrices and to investigate how a substance can accumulate in this kind of material. The research has also shown that substances such as morphine, 6-MAM, codeine, methadone, and EDDP can be detected in nails using UHPLC-HRMS, with the ability to distinguish changes in intake over time, based on the distribution of the substance in the matrix and on quantitative assessments.

Author Contributions: Conceptualization and investigation, E.B. (Emanuele Bury) and E.B. (Erika Buratti); methodology, R.S.; writing—original draft preparation, E.B. (Emanuele Bury) and R.S.; software and data Curation, M.C. (Marta Cippitelli) and G.M.; validation, R.F. and M.C. (Mariano Cingolani); supervision, M.C. (Mariano Cingolani). All authors have read and agreed to the published version of the manuscript.

Funding: This study was supported by For.Med.Lab., Forensic Medicine and Laboratory S.R.L. of Macerata. Funds have been arranged by deliberation number 3 of 13 May 2021.

Institutional Review Board Statement: Not applicable.

Informed Consent Statement: Not applicable.

Data Availability Statement: All data are contained in the manuscript.

Acknowledgments: Thanks to Jemma Dunnill for proofreading the manuscript.

Conflicts of Interest: The authors declare no conflict of interest.

References

1. Baumgartner, M.R. Nails: An adequate alternative matrix in forensic toxicology for drug analysis? *Bioanalysis* **2014**, *6*, 2189–2191. [CrossRef] [PubMed]
2. Palmeri, A.; Pichini, S.; Pacifici, R.; Zuccaro, P.; Lopez, A. Drugs in nails: Physiology, pharmacokinetics and forensic toxicology. *Clin. Pharmacokinet.* **2000**, *38*, 95–110. [CrossRef] [PubMed]
3. Shu, I.; Jones, J.; Jones, M.; Lewis, D.; Negrusz, A. Detection of Drugs in Nails: Three Year Experience. *J. Anal. Toxicol.* **2015**, *39*, 624–628. [CrossRef] [PubMed]
4. Lesnikova, I.; Schreckenbach, M.N.; Kristensen, M.P.; Papanikolaou, L.L.; Hamilton-Dutoit, S. Usability of Immunohistochemistry in Forensic Samples with Varying Decomposition. *Am. J. Forensic Med. Pathol.* **2018**, *39*, 185–191. [CrossRef] [PubMed]
5. Shan, Y.M.; Hao, C.Y.; Wang, L. An immunohistochemical study on the distribution in organs in cases with morphine poisoning. *Fa Yi Xue Za Zhi* **2002**, *18*, 9–11.
6. Paulsen, I.M.; Dimke, H.; Frische, S. A single simple procedure for dewaxing, hydration and heat-induced epitope retrieval (HIER) for immunohistochemistry in formalin fixed paraffin-embedded tissue. *Eur. J. Histochem.* **2015**, *59*, 2532. [CrossRef]
7. Crowe, A.R.; Yue, W. Semi-quantitative Determination of Protein Expression using Immunohistochemistry Staining and Analysis: An Integrated Protocol. *Bio-Protocol* **2019**, *9*, e3465. [CrossRef]
8. Kronstrand, R.; Forsman, M.; Roman, M. Quantitative analysis of drugs in hair by UHPLC high resolution mass spectrometry. *Forensic Sci. Int.* **2018**, *283*, 9–15. [CrossRef]
9. Tassoni, G.; Cacaci, C.; Zampi, M.; Froldi, R. Bile analysis in heroin overdose. *J. Forensic Sci.* **2007**, *52*, 1405–1407. [CrossRef]
10. Moffat, A.C.; Osselton, M.D.; Widdop, B.; Watts, J. *Clarke's Analysis of Drugs and Poisons*, IV ed.; Pharmaceutical Press: London, UK, 2011; Volume II, pp. 1734–1735.
11. Cippitelli, M.; Mirtella, D.; Ottaviani, G.; Tassoni, G.; Froldi, R.; Cingolani, M. Toxicological Analysis of Opiates from Alternative Matrices Collected from an Exhumed Body. *J. Forensic Sci.* **2018**, *63*, 640–643. [CrossRef]
12. Scientific Working Group for Forensic Toxicology. Scientific Working Group for Forensic Toxicology (SWGTOX) standard practices for method validation in forensic toxicology. *J. Anal. Toxicol.* **2013**, *37*, 452–474. [CrossRef] [PubMed]
13. Usagawa, T.; Itoh, Y.; Hifumi, E.; Takeyasu, A.; Nakahara, Y.; Uda, T. Characterization of morphine-specific monoclonal antibodies showing minimal cross-reactivity with codeine. *J. Immunol. Methods* **1993**, *157*, 143–148. [CrossRef]
14. Tassoni, G.; Mirtella, D.; Zampi, M.; Ferrante, L.; Cippitelli, M.; Cognigni, E.; Froldi, R.; Cingolani, M. Hair analysis in order to evaluate drug abuse in driver's license regranting procedures. *Forensic Sci. Int.* **2014**, *244*, 16–19. [CrossRef] [PubMed]
15. Boumba, V.A.; Ziavrou, K.S.; Vougiouklakis, T. Hair as a biological indicator of drug use, drug abuse or chronic exposure to environmental toxicants. *Int. J. Toxicol.* **2006**, *25*, 143–163. [CrossRef]
16. Gryczynski, J.; Schwartz, R.P.; Mitchell, S.G.; O'Grady, K.E.; Ondersma, S.J. Hair drug testing results and self-reported drug use among primary care patients with moderate-risk illicit drug use. *Drug Alcohol Depend.* **2014**, *141*, 44–50. [CrossRef]
17. Harkey, M.R. Anatomy and physiology of hair. *Forensic Sci. Int.* **1993**, *63*, 9–18. [CrossRef]
18. Lee, S.; Han, E.; In, S.; Choi, H.; Chung, H.; Chung, K.H. Analysis of pubic hair as an alternative specimen to scalp hair: A contamination issue. *Forensic Sci. Int.* **2011**, *206*, 19–21. [CrossRef]
19. Han, E.; Yang, W.; Lee, J.; Park, Y.; Kim, E.; Lim, M.; Chung, H. Correlation of methamphetamine results and concentrations between head, axillary, and pubic hair. *Forensic Sci. Int.* **2005**, *147*, 21–24. [CrossRef]
20. Cappelle, D.; Yegles, M.; Neels, H.; van Nuijs, A.L.N.; De Doncker, M.; Maudens, K.; Covaci, A.; Crunelle, C.L. Nail analysis for the detection of drugs of abuse and pharmaceuticals: A review. *Forensic Toxicol.* **2015**, *33*, 12–36. [CrossRef]
21. Brahs, A.B.; Bolla, S.R. Histology, Nail. In *StatPearls 2021*; StatPearls Publishing Copyright© 2021; StatPearls Publishing LLC.: Treasure Island, FL, USA, 2021.
22. Lin, M.H.; Kopan, R. Long-range, nonautonomous effects of activated Notch1 on tissue homeostasis in the nail. *Dev. Biol.* **2003**, *263*, 343–359. [CrossRef]
23. Kalasinsky, K.S.; Magluilo, J., Jr.; Schaefer, T. Study of drug distribution in hair by infrared microscopy visualization. *J. Anal. Toxicol.* **1994**, *18*, 337–341. [CrossRef] [PubMed]
24. Gygi, S.P.; Joseph, R.E., Jr.; Cone, E.J.; Wilkins, D.G.; Rollins, D.E. Incorporation of codeine and metabolites into hair. Role of pigmentation. *Drug Metab. Dispos.* **1996**, *24*, 495–501. [PubMed]
25. Perrin, C.; Michiels, J.F.; Boyer, J.; Ambrosetti, D. Melanocytes Pattern in the Normal Nail, With Special Reference to Nail Bed Melanocytes. *Am. J. Dermatopathol.* **2018**, *40*, 180–184. [CrossRef] [PubMed]

26. Perrin, C.; Langbein, L.; Schweizer, J. Expression of hair keratins in the adult nail unit: An immunohistochemical analysis of the onychogenesis in the proximal nail fold, matrix and nail bed. *Br. J. Dermatol.* **2004**, *151*, 362–371. [CrossRef]
27. Achten, G.; André, J.; Laporte, M. Nails in light and electron microscopy. *Semin. Dermatol.* **1991**, *10*, 54–64.
28. Jarrett, A.; Spearman, R.I. The histochemistry of the human nail. *Arch. Dermatol.* **1966**, *94*, 652–657. [CrossRef]
29. Jarrett, A.; Spearman, R.I.; Hardy, J.A. The histochemistry of keratinization. *Br. J. Dermatol.* **1959**, *71*, 277–295. [CrossRef]
30. Kintz, P.; Raul, J.S.; Ameline, A. The use of multiple keratinous matrices (head hair, axillary hair, and toenail clippings) can help narrowing a period of drug exposure: Experience with a criminal case involving 25I-NBOMe and 4-MMC. *Int. J. Leg. Med.* **2021**, *135*, 1461–1465. [CrossRef]

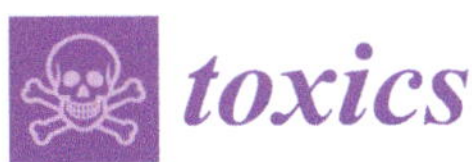

MDPI

Case Report

Forensic Aspects of a Fatal Intoxication Involving Acetaminophen, Citalopram and Trazodone: A Case Report

Giulio Mannocchi [1,†], Roberta Tittarelli [2,†], Flaminia Pantano [3], Francesca Vernich [2], Margherita Pallocci [2,*], Pierluigi Passalacqua [2], Michele Treglia [2] and Luigi Tonino Marsella [2]

1 School of Law, University of Camerino, Piazza Cavour 19/f, 62032 Camerino, Italy
2 Section of Legal Medicine, Social Security and Forensic Toxicology, Department of Biomedicine and Prevention, University of Rome Tor Vergata, Via Montpellier 1, 00133 Rome, Italy
3 Independent Researcher, Via della Divisione Torino 69, 00143 Rome, Italy
* Correspondence: margherita.pallocci@gmail.com
† These authors contributed equally to this work.

Abstract: We report the case of a young man, a former heroin addict, found dead at home by the Police Forces in an advanced state of decomposition. Numerous blisters and unpacked tablets of medications were found all over the bed and on the floor of the room. Multiple injuries to the face, left arm and neck of the deceased were noted. The latter damages were attributed to post-mortem dog bites, since no indications of a possible defense against the animal were observed. The autopsy findings were unremarkable. Toxicological investigations performed on peripheral blood and urine by gas chromatography-mass spectrometry (GC-MS) technique showed the presence of acetaminophen, citalopram and trazodone. Combined drug intoxication was proposed as the cause of death since acetaminophen and trazodone concentrations were comparable with the ones found in fatal cases. Moreover, citalopram concentration in peripheral blood was above the toxic range and in accordance with levels found in fatalities due to poly-drug intoxication.

Keywords: acetaminophen; citalopram; trazodone; poly-drug intoxication; dog attack; gas chromatography-mass spectrometry

Citation: Mannocchi, G.; Tittarelli, R.; Pantano, F.; Vernich, F.; Pallocci, M.; Passalacqua, P.; Treglia, M.; Marsella, L.T. Forensic Aspects of a Fatal Intoxication Involving Acetaminophen, Citalopram and Trazodone: A Case Report. *Toxics* **2022**, *10*, 486. https://doi.org/10.3390/toxics10080486

Academic Editor: Maria Pieri

Received: 18 July 2022
Accepted: 19 August 2022
Published: 22 August 2022

Publisher's Note: MDPI stays neutral with regard to jurisdictional claims in published maps and institutional affiliations.

1. Introduction

1.1. Acetaminophen

Acetaminophen, also known as paracetamol, is a common pain reliever and antipyretic used since 1955 for the management of several pathological conditions such as headache, osteoarthritis, chronic backache and postoperative pain as part of a multimodal approach [1]. It is commercially available alone or in combination with other drugs [2]. In Italy, paracetamol in specific formulations and only at certain dosages can be sold as an over-the-counter drug (without a prescription). Paracetamol is a safe drug when administered at therapeutic doses; however, several fatal cases related to the onset of hepatotoxicity consequent to the administration of single or repeated high doses and chronic ingestion were reported, starting from the mid-1980s [3]. Adverse reactions commonly related to paracetamol intoxication are acute liver failure (ALF), centrilobular hepatic necrosis, hypoglycaemic coma and renal tubular necrosis [4,5]. Liver damage is caused by the excessive production of its toxic breakdown metabolite, N-acetyl-p-benzoquinone imine (NAPQI). At therapeutic doses, approximately 5–9% of acetaminophen is converted by Cytochrome P 450 (CYP 2E1, CYP1A2 and CYP 3A4) to NAPQI [6]. Normally, it is inactivated in conjugation with the sulphydryl groups of glutathione, but in overdose cases, glutathione is depleted, and NAPQI is not detoxified. The exact mechanism by which toxicity occurs is not known, but it has been proposed that in the case of GSH depletion, NAPQI causes toxicity by binding to cellular macromolecules. Treatment for acetaminophen intoxication is based on the administration of N-acetylcysteine, which is associated with mortality reduction of less than 30% [6].

Paracetamol overdoses are frequently related to suicide intents, but cumulative or accidental ingestion is also reported. Recently, unconventional uses of paracetamol for the treatment of sleep disorders, to enhance athletic performances and mixed with drinks, waterpipe and illicit drugs were reported by Bloukh et al., especially among patients with a history of substance use, parents of young children or athletes [7].

Several acetaminophen intoxications are due to the co-products contained in paracetamol formulations, such as caffeine, dextromethorphan, codeine, oxycodone, antihistamines, acetylsalicylic acid and propoxyphene [8]. Furthermore, several contributing factors could be implicated in the induction of paracetamol hepatotoxicity even at therapeutic doses: malnutrition, alcohol abuse and liver impairment [9]. Therapeutic blood concentrations range from 10 to 25 mg/L, whereas toxic and lethal values range from 100 to 150 mg/L and 200 to 300 mg/L, respectively [10]. However, paracetamol hepatotoxicity is known to be dose-dependent, different from the toxic liver damage induced by the use of other drugs or herbs, which can be idiosyncratic [11,12].

1.2. Citalopram

Citalopram is an antidepressant drug, only available by prescription, belonging to the selective serotonin reuptake inhibitor (SSRI) class, approved for the treatment of major depression and panic disorders with or without agoraphobia with minimal effects on norepinephrine and dopamine reuptake [13]. In the case of therapeutic use, it is rarely associated with severe side effects and serotonin syndrome (SS), characterized by specific symptoms such as mental status changes, autonomic hyperactivity and neuromuscular abnormalities, occurs only in a few cases, often related to alterations in cytochrome P450 (CYP)-mediated metabolism [14]. Recreational uses of citalopram are not currently reported in the literature. Fatalities attributed either to citalopram alone or in combination with other drugs have been reported in the scientific literature [13–18]. Therapeutic oral doses range from 20 to 40 mg per day, with a maximum daily dose of 60 mg, and therapeutic concentrations in the blood range from 0.02 to 0.2 mg/L. The lethal concentration is 0.5 mg/L [19]. Other authors suggest the following therapeutic, toxic and comatose/fatal values: 0.05–0.11 mg/L, from 0.22 mg/L and from 5–6 mg/L, respectively [10].

1.3. Trazodone

Trazodone is a psychoactive substance, purchasable by prescription only and belonging to the piperazines class, approved by the Food and Drug Administration (FDA) for the treatment of depression [20]. However, several off-label uses of this compound are reported. This drug is also prescribed for the treatment of insomnia, bulimia, anxiety disorders, alcohol and benzodiazepine dependence, degenerative diseases of the central nervous system, fibromyalgia, sexual dysfunction, chronic pain and schizophrenia [21]. Its mechanism of action includes serotonin (5-HT-5-hydroxytryptamine) uptake inhibition, but the strongest effect develops through antagonism towards 5-HT2/1C receptors [22]. Some fatality reports due to trazodone intake, alone or in combination with other substances, have been described in the literature [23–26]. Therapeutic and toxic concentrations in the blood range from 0.7 to 1 mg/L and from 1.2 to 3–4 mg/L, respectively, whereas the comatose–fatal concentration has been suggested to be 12–15 mg/L [10].

Recreational use of trazodone is increasing. Trazodone is sold in the illicit market under the street name "sleepeasy" for its relaxing and calming effects: this drug is commonly taken by snorting or smoking the crushed tablets mixed with marijuana or by adding trazodone powder to alcohol. Concomitant use of trazodone with other substances, such as alcohol, ecstasy or methamphetamine, enhances its effects. These routes of administration expose users to a high risk of overdose and other harmful side effects. In cases of misuse, dependency and addiction can also occur.

2. Case Report

2.1. Scene of Death Inspection

We report the case of a Caucasian man, 32 years old, found dead in the bedroom of his flat by the Police Forces. The intervention of law enforcement was requested by the father of the deceased, as he had not heard from him for about 15–20 days. He was initially unconcerned about his silence because of a previous family quarrel, but due to the unanswered doorbell and insistent barking of the dog from the apartment, the relatives alerted the fire department. The apartment door was locked from the inside, with a key stuck in the lock. Criminal evidence of violence was missing.

The victim was found in the bedroom, dressed in his shoes and with the upper half of the body tucked under the left side of the bed. From the information provided by law enforcement officers who attended the scene, the deceased was a former heroin user. His doctor was unaware of his addiction history, and it is not known whether the drugs found in his apartment had been illegally obtained.

Numerous blisters and unpacked tablets of medications were found all over the bed and on the floor of the room. The forensic pathologist who was called at the scene excluded criminal action as the cause of death since there were no signs of forced entry and no evidence to suggest pre-fatal external injurious action. Multiple injuries to the face, left arm and neck were noted. In particular, the soft tissues of the face and neck were completely absent, exposing the underlying bone structures. (Figure 1). The latter damages were attributed to post-mortem dog bites since no indications of a possible defence against the animal were observed. The dog that was found in the flat of the deceased had torn and fed on the soft parts of the dead body. The rest of the body was clothed and the right arm, covered by a blanket, was not ripped.

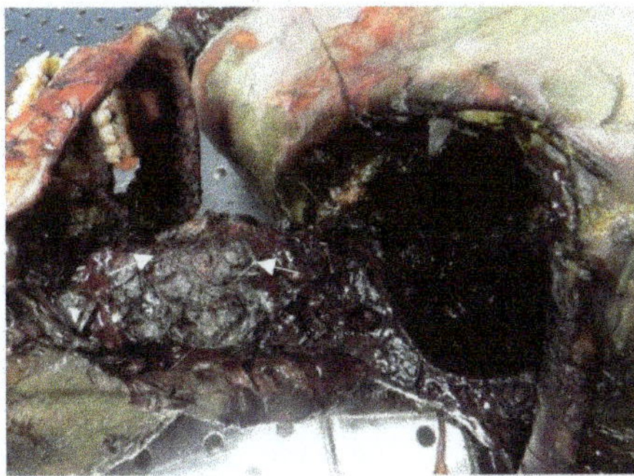

Figure 1. Skeletonized skull and cervical spine tract. Dog hair is noticeable on the neck (white arrows).

2.2. Autopsy Findings

The deceased was an Italian male in an advanced state of decomposition. Because of the alterations caused by putrefactive phenomena, the forensic pathologist estimated that the post-mortem interval ranged from 10 to 15 days. External examination revealed nothing remarkable. The head and the neck were completely skeletonized without fractures. The left arm consisted exclusively of the humerus. A part of the forearm and elbow soft tissues and the fingers of his left hand were missing due to the dog's action. Another injury was noticed in the poster lateral trunk, also caused by the dog. There was no trauma to the lower extremities. The internal examination showed congestion signs in the examined organs. There were no fractures to the skull base, and there was no evidence of hemorrhage involving the brain and the soft tissues of the chest. The internal organs were removed from the chest cavity due to the dog's action. The organs of the abdominal cavity, though in an advanced state of putrefaction, did not show any traumatic injury. There was no pre-existing disease that could cause the death. Moreover, since the deceased was known to be a former heroin user, as reported by the victim's relatives to the Police Forces, peripheral blood and urine specimens were collected for toxicological analysis.

2.3. Histological Findings

Sections of splenic, hepatic, encephalic and renal tissues were investigated to determine the presence of morphological and functional alterations. All the slides were analyzed with the hematoxylin and eosin (H&E) staining technique. The histological examination performed on splenic tissue showed the presence of thanatological changes due to the advanced state of decomposition. The capsule was regular; in splenic tissue, macrophages with pigmented cytoplasmic granules were detected. A preserved lobular architecture was observed in the liver section. Hepatocytes were poorly preserved because of post-mortem alterations. Chronic cholestatic liver disease and mild fibrosis (L1) in the portal area were noticed (Figure 2). Encephalic slides revealed the presence of cerebral edema, particularly in perivascular spaces, without traumatic signs. Histological observation of kidney sections showed serious thanatological modifications with glomerular and tubular shadows.

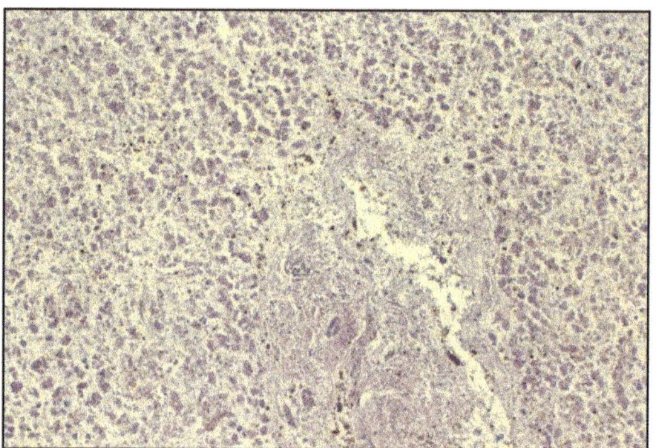

Figure 2. Histological examination of hepatic tissue. Magnification 40×. Hematoxylin and eosin stain.

3. Materials and Methods

3.1. Samples

Toxicological analyses were performed on unpreserved peripheral blood (35 mL) and urine (40 mL), collected during the autopsy and stored at −20 °C until the analysis.

3.2. Chemical and Reagents

Reference standards for paracetamol, paracetamol-*d4* (IS), citalopram, trazodone and methadone-*d9* (IS) were purchased from Cerilliant® (Round Rock, TX, USA). Ethyl-acetate from Carlo Erba® (Milan, Italy) and BSTFA (with 1% TMCS) were purchased from Sigma-Aldrich (Milan, Italy). Ultrapure deionized water was homemade (Millipore® Helix 70).

3.3. Qualitative Analysis

Immunochemical screening (ILab 650, Instrumentation Laboratory, Milan, Italy) was performed on the urine sample with a positive result for amphetamines and MDMA (3,4-methylenedioxymethamphetamine). The toxicological screening performed on urine was negative for opiates, methadone, cannabinoids, cocaine, benzodiazepines and alcohol. The positive amphetamines and MDMA immunoassay results were not confirmed by the analysis in gas chromatography coupled with mass spectrometry (GC/MS). The false positive results were probably related to the presence of trazodone [27]. As part of routine investigation, aliquots of non-diluted peripheral blood and urine were analyzed using a screening method in GC-MS (Figure 3). Samples were extracted at pH 8.0 (adding 50 mg of solid HCO3-/CO3– buffer) with 4 mL of ethyl acetate after 15 min stirring. After centrifugation (4000 rpm, 3 min), the organic layer was evaporated to dryness under a gentle stream of nitrogen. The residues were reconstituted in 50 μL of ethyl acetate (Figure 3).

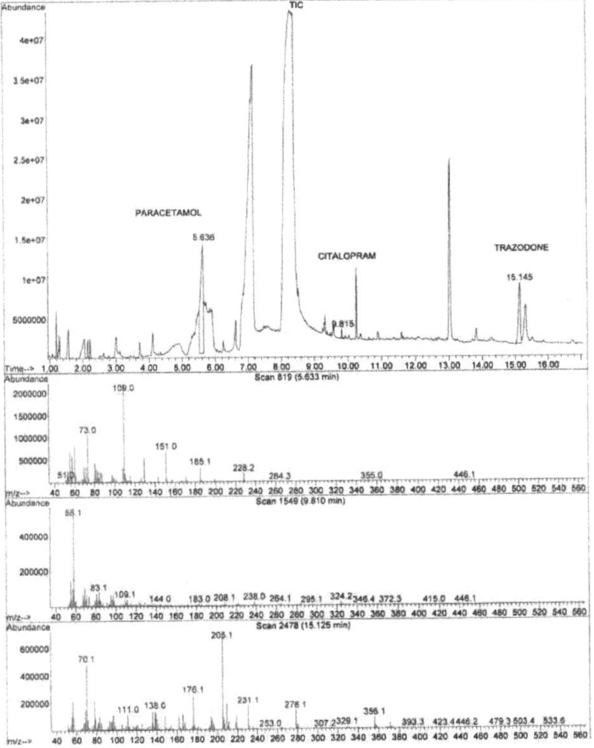

Figure 3. Full scan mode chromatogram and mass spectra obtained from peripheral blood analysis.

3.4. Quantitative Analysis of Acetaminophen

To 100 μL of diluted (1:100) fortified blank urine, peripheral blood and samples, 200 ng of paracetamol-d_4 were added. Samples were then extracted at pH 4.0 (adding 500 μL of acetate buffer) with 4 mL of ethyl acetate after 15 min stirring. After centrifugation (4000 rpm, 3 min), the organic layer was collected and evaporated to dryness under a gentle stream of nitrogen. The residues were derivatized using 50 μL of BSTFA+1% TMCS and put in a heating block for 30 min at 70 °C.

3.5. Quantitative Analysis of Citalopram and Trazodone

To 100 μL of diluted (1:100) fortified blank urine, peripheral blood and samples, 100 ng of methadone-*d9* were added. Samples were extracted at pH 8.0 (adding 50 mg of solid HCO3−/CO3− buffer) with 4 mL of ethyl acetate after 15 min stirring. After centrifugation (4000 rpm, 3 min), the organic layer was evaporated to dryness under a gentle stream of nitrogen. The residue was reconstituted in 50 μL of ethyl acetate.

3.6. Instrumentation and Conditions

GC analysis was carried out on a gas chromatography instrument Agilent HP 7028A GC coupled with an Agilent MSD 5975. The capillary column used was an HP-5MS (17 m × 0.25 mm I.D coated with a 0.25 μm film). The GC conditions were as follows: the column temperature was programmed from 120 °C to 290 °C with an increase of 15 °C/min; the injection port and the transfer line temperature was 270 °C; helium was used as carrier gas at a flow rate of 1ml/min; split ratio 10:1. The mass analyzer was operated by electron impact (70 eV) in full scan mode for qualitative analysis (mass range 40–500 *m*/*z*).

For quantitative analysis, the mass analyzer was operated by electron impact (70 eV) in selected ion monitoring (SIM). Quantitative analysis of paracetamol was carried out recording ions *m*/*z* 206-280-295 for paracetamol and *m/z* 299 for paracetamol-*d4*. The underlined ions were used for quantitative analysis (target/qualifier). Quantitative analysis of trazodone and citalopram was performed, recording ions *m*/*z* 205-278-356 for trazodone, *m*/*z* 58-324-238 for citalopram and *m*/*z* 78-229-303 for methadone-*d9*.

Validation of new analytical methods to be used in a single case study or for the analysis of rare analytes was performed for blood and urine, in accordance with updated established international criteria [28].

The following parameters were evaluated for a quantitative method: selectivity, linearity, accuracy, precision, the limit of detection (LOD) and lower limit of quantification (LLOQ). Selectivity was evaluated by checking the interfering signals of blank matrices and interfering signals of paracetamol-d_4 and methadone-d_9 through zero samples. The standard acetaminophen, citalopram and trazodone calibration curves were obtained by fortification of blank human blood (5 levels) and blank human urine (5 levels) with an appropriate amount of pure standards in a range of concentration from 50 to 800 µg/mL for acetaminophen and trazodone and from 2.5 to 40 µg/mL for citalopram.

Blood and urine methods were linear for all the analytes, with a determination coefficient (R2) ranging from 0.991 to 0.997. The precision for all the analytes was always lower than 15% (CV%), while bias never exceeded ±15%.

The limit of detection (LOD) for peripheral blood was 4.80 µg/mL for acetaminophen, 0.34 µg/mL for citalopram and 0.28 µg/mL for trazodone with a signal-to-noise ratio (S/N) of 3. The latter values fit the purpose of the current case.

LOD and LLOQ evaluated for blood and urine are reported in Table 1.

Table 1. LOD and LLOQ for acetaminophen, trazodone and citalopram in blood and urine.

	Blood		Urine	
Compound	**LOD (µg/mL)**	**LLOQ (µg/mL)**	**LOD (µg/mL)**	**LLOQ (µg/mL)**
Acetaminophen	4.80	15.00	2.50	8.10
Citalopram	0.34	1.10	0.10	0.32
Trazodone	0.28	0.90	0.18	0.60

4. Results

Acetaminophen, citalopram and trazodone were detected in peripheral blood and urine using a non-targeted analysis performed by GC-MS. Blood alcohol and volatile compounds determination were carried out by gas chromatography with a head-space FID detector (HS-GC-FID), and alcohol was detected at 0.47 g/L. The alcohol concentration found in peripheral blood, may be related with the advanced state of decomposition of the body. Several authors correlate an increase in the alcohol concentration with post-mortem production due to the action of different species of bacteria. In most of the cases in which the production of post-mortem ethanol was observed, the concentration was not higher than 0.3 g/L [29–32]. In Table 2, the analyte concentrations found in peripheral blood and urine are reported. To date, it is not known to what extent the advanced state of decomposition affected the concentration of the three analytes detected.

Table 2. Analytical results in biological matrices.

Samples	Acetaminophen (μg/mL)	Citalopram (μg /mL)	Trazodone (μg/mL)
Peripheral Blood	328	2.7	21
Urine	155	50	109

5. Discussion

To the best of our knowledge, a fatal case involving all three of the substances found here has not been described before in the literature. Nevertheless, fatalities attributed to intoxication by acetaminophen together with citalopram are documented. Moore et al. reported a fatal case due to metaxalone and gabapentin intoxication, in which acetaminophen and citalopram were detected together with the latter compounds in heart blood at the concentrations of 97 mg/L and 0.4 mg/L, respectively [16]. Seetohul et al. presented a post-mortem case involving citalopram and acetaminophen, among other substances: nefopam, nicotine, caffeine, amitriptyline, gabapentin and diazepam. The death was attributed to atherosclerotic coronary artery disease and therapeutic drug toxicity. Citalopram was quantified at 0.7 mg/L and 0.9 mg/L in unpreserved femoral and cardiac blood, respectively, whereas acetaminophen concentrations were not provided [33]. Acetaminophen and citalopram are among the 10 most frequently detected drugs in hanging and drug poisoning (intoxication) suicides. Moreover, poly-drug use was found to be more common in intoxication suicides, 3.6 drugs/case compared with 1.8 drugs/case in hanging cases. Acetaminophen and citalopram were detected in femoral blood in 652 and 345 out of 2468 intoxication suicides at the median concentration of 20 and 0.7 mg/L, respectively. Similarly, citalopram and acetaminophen were found at the median concentration of 0.3 and 5 mg/L in 428 and 396 out of 4551 hanging suicide cases [34]. Therapeutic, toxic and fatal blood concentrations, as presented by Schulz et al. for the three substances detected in the presented case, are reported in Table 3 [10].

Table 3. Therapeutic, toxic and fatal blood concentrations as provided by Schulz et al. [10].

Substance	Blood-Plasma Concentration (μg/mL)		
	Therapeutic ("Normal")	Toxic (From)	Comatose-Fatal (From)
Acetaminophen	(5-)10–25	100–150	200–300
Citalopram	0.05–0.11	0.22	5–6
Trazodone	0.7–1	1.2; 3–4	12–15

In relation to trazodone toxicity, a few cases of attributable deaths have been reported in the literature, with both cardiovascular and liver toxicity occurring. In the latter cases, both an idiosyncratic reaction [35] and mediated by mechanisms of acute cytotoxicity and cholestasis have been shown. In a study carried out to test the molecular mechanisms underlying trazodone toxicity, it was shown that exposure to the drug results in increased lipid peroxidation with increased production of ROS (Reactive Oxygen Species), as well as reduced cellular GSH content [36].

With reference to the case under investigation, from a pathophysiological point of view, it is possible that a negative synergistic action between trazodone and acetaminophen occurred; in this context, trazodone caused, among other effects, an increase in cellular ROS production and a reduction in GSH reserves, thus exacerbating the toxicity of NAPQI, which, in cases of GSH depletion, is not inactivated, making its toxicity particularly evident, especially in the liver. Concerning the interaction between trazodone and other psychoactive drugs, in a study conducted in Italy in 2020 on 97 patients with depressive syndrome, the interaction between trazodone, citalopram and fluoxetine was studied over a period of 1 year. The results of this study showed that the use of citalopram and fluoxetine in combination with trazodone did not have a significant impact on serum trazodone concentrations; furthermore, no cases of headache, daytime sedation, fatigue or serotonergic syndrome were reported during the study [37].

In relation to the stability of the investigated substances in biological samples collected from decomposed corpses, there are notmuch data available in the literature.

Karinen et al. measured concentrations of acetaminophen in forensic blood specimens after long-term storage (16–18 years) at −20 °C. The authors reanalyzed 13 blood samples, and in 10 of these, the results were within ±30% of the initial concentrations, and they concluded that generally, the results decreased slightly than to those reported by other authors [38,39].

Citalopram stability was studied by Moretti et al. in dried blood spots (DBSs) stored at room temperature for three months. DBSs were analyzed in triplicate immediately after collection, within the following 3 weeks and after 3 months. The long-term stability (3 months) was also tested in blood specimens stored at −20 °C. The authors observed that citalopram stability in DBSs was about 2–3 weeks, and there was also degradation in blood specimens by more than 50% after 3 months of storage [40]. Their findings were comparable to those previously reported by other authors: Lewis et al. reported stability of 5 days for citalopram in whole blood specimens stored at 4 °C, whereas Karinen et al. reported a stability up to 1 year in post-mortem blood samples after storage at −20 °C [41].

Martin et al. studied the tissue distribution and post-mortem redistribution of trazodone in two fatalities, and they observed that trazodone had low potential for post-mortem redistribution lacking significant solid organ deposits of the drug. The authors also reported that trazodone concentrations were relatively stable in post-mortem blood samples, with a lower increase than 40% observed 60 h after the death and a less than two-fold change during early putrefaction. For peripheral blood samples, they observed marked stability with no significant change [42].

McIntyre et al. compared trazodone concentrations in liver, peripheral blood and central blood in 19 medical examiner cases stored up to eight months. The authors observed a minor degradation of trazodone in post-mortem blood samples stored at 4 °C and about a 20% decrease in samples stored up to eight months. The data collected by the authors demonstrated that trazodone was unlikely to show significant redistribution [43].

6. Conclusions

Combined drug intoxication was proposed as a cause of death since acetaminophen and trazodone concentrations were comparable with the ones found in fatal cases. Moreover, citalopram concentration in peripheral blood was above the toxic range and in accordance with levels found in fatalities due to poly-drug intoxication. From a pathophysiological point of view, based on the results of the toxicological and autopsy examinations performed (particularly histological ones), it is possible to ascribe the death to acute liver failure due to a synergistic action between drugs (acetaminophen and trazodone in particular).

Author Contributions: Conceptualization, G.M. and F.P.; methodology, R.T.; formal analysis, G.M., F.P. and R.T.; investigation, M.T. writing—original draft preparation, F.V.; writing—review and editing, M.P. and P.P.; supervision, L.T.M. All authors have read and agreed to the published version of the manuscript.

Funding: This research received no external funding.

Institutional Review Board Statement: The approval of the ethics committee was not necessary as all the procedures carried out are set by legislation as essential to ascertain the causes of death.

Informed Consent Statement: Not applicable.

Data Availability Statement: Not applicable.

Conflicts of Interest: The authors declare no conflict of interest.

References

1. Gupta, A.; Bah, M. NSAIDs in the Treatment of Postoperative Pain. *Curr. Pain Headache Rep.* **2016**, *20*, 62. [CrossRef] [PubMed]
2. Sheen, C.L.; Dillon, J.F.; Bateman, D.N.; Simpson, K.J.; MacDonald, T.M. Paracetamol-related deaths in Scotland, 1994–2000. *Br. J. Clin. Pharmacol.* **2002**, *54*, 430–432. [CrossRef] [PubMed]
3. Tittarelli, R.; Pellegrini, M.; Scarpellini, M.G.; Marinelli, E.; Bruti, V.; di Luca, N.M.; Busardo, F.P.; Zaami, S. Hepatotoxicity of paracetamol and related fatalities. *Eur. Rev. Med. Pharmacol. Sci.* **2017**, *21* (Suppl. 1), 95–101. [PubMed]
4. Lancaster, E.M.; Hiatt, J.R.; Zarrinpar, A. Acetaminophen hepatotoxicity: An updated review. *Arch. Toxicol.* **2015**, *89*, 193–199. [CrossRef] [PubMed]
5. De-Giorgio, F.; Lodise, M.; Chiarotti, M.; D'Aloja, E.; Carbone, A.; Valerio, L. Possible Fatal Acetaminophen Intoxication with Atypical Clinical Presentation. *J. Forensic Sci.* **2013**, *58*, 1397–1400. [CrossRef]
6. Moyer, A.M.; Fridley, B.L.; Jenkins, G.D.; Batzler, A.J.; Pelleymounter, L.L.; Kalari, K.R.; Ji, Y.; Chai, Y.; Nordgren, K.K.; Weinshilboum, R.M. Acetaminophen-NAPQI hepatotoxicity: A cell line model system genome-wide association study. *Toxicol. Sci.* **2011**, *120*, 33–41. [CrossRef]
7. Bloukh, S.; Wazaify, M.; Matheson, C. Paracetamol: Unconventional uses of a well-known drug. *Int. J. Pharm. Pract.* **2021**, *29*, 527–540. [CrossRef]
8. Doyon, S.; Klein-Schwartz, W.; Lee, S.; Beuhler, M.C. Fatalities involving acetaminophen combination products reported to United States poison centers. *Clin. Toxicol.* **2013**, *51*, 941–948. [CrossRef]
9. Yoon, E.; Babar, A.; Choudhary, M.; Kutner, M.; Pyrsopoulos, N. Acetaminophen-Induced Hepatotoxicity: A Comprehensive Update. *J. Clin. Transl. Hepatol.* **2016**, *4*, 131–142. [CrossRef]
10. Schulz, M.; Schmoldt, A.; Andresen-Streichert, H.; Iwersen-Bergmann, S. Revisited: Therapeutic and toxic blood concentrations of more than 1100 drugs and other xenobiotics. *Crit. Care* **2020**, *24*, 195. [CrossRef]
11. Pantano, F.; Tittarelli, R.; Mannocchi, G.; Zaami, S.; Ricci, S.; Giorgetti, R.; Terranova, D.; Busardo, F.P.; Marinelli, E. Hepatotoxicity Induced by "the 3Ks": Kava, Kratom and Khat. *Int. J. Mol. Sci.* **2016**, *17*, 580. [CrossRef] [PubMed]
12. Danan, G.; Teschke, R. RUCAM in Drug and Herb Induced Liver Injury: The Update. *Int. J. Mol. Sci.* **2016**, *17*, 14. [CrossRef] [PubMed]
13. Luchini, D.; Morabito, G.; Centini, F. Case Report of a Fatal Intoxication by Citalopram. *Am. J. Forensic Med. Pathol.* **2005**, *26*, 352–354. [CrossRef] [PubMed]
14. Schult, R.F.; Morris, A.J.; Picard, L.; Wiegand, T.J. Citalopram overdose and severe serotonin syndrome in an intermediate metabolizing patient. *Am. J. Emerg. Med.* **2019**, *37*, 1993.e5–1993.e6. [CrossRef] [PubMed]
15. Gruszecki, A.C.; Kloda, S.; Simmons, G.T.; Daly, T.M.; Hardy, R.W.; Robinson, C.A. Polydrug fatality involving metaxalone. *J. Forensic Sci.* **2003**, *48*, 432–434. [CrossRef] [PubMed]
16. Moore, K.A.; Levine, B.; Fowler, D. A fatality involving metaxalone. *Forensic Sci. Int.* **2005**, *149*, 249–251. [CrossRef]
17. Kraai, E.P.; Seifert, S.A. Citalopram Overdose: A Fatal Case. *J. Med. Toxicol.* **2015**, *11*, 232–236. [CrossRef]
18. Hargrove, V.; Molina, D.K. A Fatality Due to Cyproheptadine and Citalopram. *J. Anal. Toxicol.* **2009**, *33*, 564–567. [CrossRef]
19. Moffat, A.C.; Osselton, D.M.; Widdop, B. *Clarke's Analysis of Drugs and Poisons in Pharmaceuticals, Body Fluids and Postmortem Material*, 4th ed.; Pharmaceutical Press: London, UK, 2011.
20. Khouzam, H.R. A review of trazodone use in psychiatric and medical conditions. *Postgrad. Med.* **2017**, *129*, 140–148. [CrossRef]
21. Bossini, L.; Casolaro, I.; Koukouna, D.; Cecchini, F.; Fagiolini, A. Off-label uses of trazodone: A review. *Expert Opin. Pharmacother.* **2012**, *13*, 1707–1717. [CrossRef]
22. Marek, G.J.; McDougle, C.J.; Price, L.H.; Seiden, L.S. A comparison of trazodone and fluoxetine: Implications for a serotonergic mechanis of antidepressant action. *Psychopharmacology* **1992**, *109*, 2–11. [CrossRef] [PubMed]
23. Martínez, M.A.; Ballesteros, S.; Sánchez de la Torre, C.; Almarza, E. Investigation of a Fatality Due to Trazodone Poisoning: Case Report and Literature Review. *J. Anal. Toxicol.* **2005**, *29*, 262–268. [CrossRef] [PubMed]
24. de Meester, A.; Carbutti, G.; Gabriel, L.; Jacques, J. Fatal overdose with trazodone: Case report and literature review. *Acta Clin. Belg.* **2001**, *56*, 258–261. [CrossRef] [PubMed]
25. Soe, K.K.; Lee, M.Y. Arrhythmias in Severe Trazodone Overdose. *Am. J. Case Rep.* **2019**, *20*, 1949–1955. [CrossRef]
26. Adson, D.E.; Erickson-Birkedahl, S.; Kotlyar, M. An Unusual Presentation of Sertraline and Trazodone Overdose. *Ann. Pharmacother.* **2001**, *35*, 1375–1377. [CrossRef]
27. Saitman, A.; Park, H.-D.; Fitzgerald, R.L. False-Positive Interferences of Common Urine Drug Screen Immunoassays: A Review. *J. Anal. Toxicol.* **2014**, *38*, 387–396. [CrossRef]
28. Peters, F.T.; Drummer, O.H.; Musshoff, F. Validation of new methods. *Forensic Sci. Int.* **2007**, *165*, 216–224. [CrossRef]
29. Ferrari, L.A.; Triszcz, J.M.; Giannuzzi, L. Kinetics of ethanol degradation in forensic blood samples. *Forensic Sci. Int.* **2006**, *161*, 144–150. [CrossRef]
30. O'Neal, C.L.; Poklis, A. Postmortem Production of Ethanol and Factors that Influence Interpretation. *Am. J. Forensic Med. Pathol.* **1996**, *17*, 8–20. [CrossRef]
31. Boumba, V.A. Modeling Postmortem Ethanol Production/Insights into the Origin of Higher Alcohols. *Molecules* **2022**, *27*, 700. [CrossRef]
32. Lin, Z.; Wang, H.; Jones, A.W.; Wang, F.; Zhang, Y.; Rao, Y. Evaluation and review of ways to differentiate sources of ethanol in postmortem blood. *Int. J. Leg. Med.* **2020**, *134*, 2081–2093. [CrossRef] [PubMed]

33. Seetohul, L.N.; De Paoli, G.; Drummond, G.; Maskell, P.D. Nefopam Hydrochloride: A Fatal Overdose. *J. Anal. Toxicol.* **2015**, *39*, 486–489. [CrossRef] [PubMed]
34. Jones, A.W.; Holmgren, A.; Ahlner, J. Toxicology findings in suicides: Concentrations of ethanol and other drugs in femoral blood in victims of hanging and poisoning in relation to age and gender of the deceased. *J. Forensic Leg. Med.* **2013**, *20*, 842. [CrossRef]
35. Fernandes, N.F.; Martin, R.R.; Schenker, S. Trazodone-induced hepatotoxicity: A case report with comments on drug-induced hepatotoxicity. *Am. J. Gastroenterol.* **2000**, *95*, 532–535. [CrossRef] [PubMed]
36. Taziki, S.; Sattari, M.R.; Eghbal, M.A. Mechanisms of trazodone-induced cytotoxicity and the protective effects of melatonin and/or taurine toward freshly isolated rat hepatocytes. *J. Biochem. Mol. Toxicol.* **2013**, *27*, 457–462. [CrossRef]
37. Incalzi, R.A.; Caraci, F.; Cuomo, A.; Fagiolini, A.; Ferini Strambi, L. Trattamento Personalizzato dei Fenotipi di Depressione: Ruolo del Trazodone nella Depressione con Insonnia. *Riv. Psichiatr.* **2020**, *55*, 371–379. Available online: https://www.rivistadipsichiatria.it/archivio/3503/articoli/34896/ (accessed on 3 August 2022).
38. Karinen, R.; Andresen, W.; Smith-Kielland, A.; Morland, J. Long-term storage of authentic postmortem forensic blood samples at −20 degrees C: Measured concentrations of benzodiazepines, central stimulants, opioids and certain medicinal drugs before and after storage for 16–18 years. *J. Anal. Toxicol.* **2014**, *38*, 686–695. [CrossRef]
39. Holmgren, P.; Druid, H.; Holmgren, A.; Ahlner, J. Stability of drugs in stored postmortem femoral blood and vitreous humor. *J. Forensic Sci.* **2004**, *49*, 820–825. [CrossRef]
40. Moretti, M.; Freni, F.; Valentini, B.; Vignali, C.; Groppi, A.; Visonà, S.D.; Osculati, A.M.M.; Morini, L. Determination of Antidepressants and Antipsychotics in Dried Blood Spots (DBSs) Collected from Post-Mortem Samples and Evaluation of the Stability over a Three-Month Period. *Molecules* **2019**, *24*, 3636. [CrossRef]
41. Lewis, R.J.; Angier, M.K.; Johnson, R.D.; Rains, B.M.; Nepal, S. *Analysis of Citalopram and Desmethylcitalopram in Postmortem Fluids and Tissues Using Liquid Chromatography-Mass Spectrometry*; Technical Report for Federal Aviation Administration Oklahoma City OK Civil Aerospace Medical Institute; Civil Aerospace Medical Institute, Federal Aviation Administration: Oklahoma City, OK, USA, 2011; p. 11.
42. Martin, A.; Pounder, D.J. Post-mortem toxico-kinetics of trazodone. *Forensic Sci. Int.* **1992**, *56*, 201–207. [CrossRef]
43. McIntyre, I.M.; Mallett, P.; Stabley, R. Postmortem distribution of trazodone concentrations. *Forensic Sci. Int.* **2015**, *251*, 195–201. [CrossRef] [PubMed]

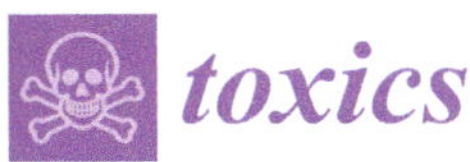 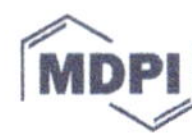

Systematic Review

Hofmann vs. Paracelsus: Do Psychedelics Defy the Basics of Toxicology?—A Systematic Review of the Main Ergolamines, Simple Tryptamines, and Phenylethylamines

Luis Alberto Henríquez-Hernández [1,2,*], Jaime Rojas-Hernández [2,3], Domingo J. Quintana-Hernández [2,4] and Lucas F. Borkel [2]

1 Unit of Toxicology, Clinical Science Department, Universidad de Las Palmas de Gran Canaria, Paseo Blas Cabrera Felipe s/n, CP 35016 Canary Islands, Spain
2 Asociación Científica Psicodélica, CP 35300 Canary Islands, Spain
3 Asociación Canaria para el Desarrollo de la Salud a través de la Atención, CP 35007 Canary Islands, Spain
4 Faculty of Psychology, Universidad del Atlántico Medio, CP 35017 Canary Islands, Spain
* Correspondence: luis.henriquez@ulpgc.es

Abstract: Psychedelics are experiencing a strong renaissance and will soon be incorporated into clinical practice. However, there is uncertainty about how much harm they can cause at what doses. This review aimed to collect information on the health-hazardous doses of psychedelic substances, to be aware of the risks to which patients may be subjected. We focused on ergolamines, simple tryptamines, and phenylethylamines. We reviewed articles published in major medical and scientific databases. Studies reporting toxic or lethal doses in humans and animals were included. We followed PRISMA criteria for revisions. We identified 3032 manuscripts for inclusion. Of these, 33 were ultimately useful and gave relevant information about effects associated with high psychedelics doses. Despite having different molecular structures and different mechanisms of action, psychedelics are effective at very low doses, are not addictive, and are harmful at extremely high doses. For LSD and psilocybin, no dose has been established above which the lives of users are endangered. In contrast, MDMA appears to be the most dangerous substance, although reports are biased by recreational missuses. It seems that it is not only the dose that makes the poison. In the case of psychedelics, the set and setting make the poison.

Keywords: psychedelics; LSD; MDMA; mescaline; psilocybin; lethal dose; overdose; toxicology

Citation: Henríquez-Hernández, L.A.; Rojas-Hernández, J.; Quintana-Hernández, D.J.; Borkel, L.F. Hofmann vs. Paracelsus: Do Psychedelics Defy the Basics of Toxicology?—A Systematic Review of the Main Ergolamines, Simple Tryptamines, and Phenylethylamines. *Toxics* **2023**, *11*, 148. https://doi.org/10.3390/toxics11020148

Academic Editor: Maria Pieri

Received: 15 January 2023
Revised: 30 January 2023
Accepted: 31 January 2023
Published: 3 February 2023

1. Introduction

Today, psychedelics are back in the spotlight, at a very important time for public health due to the rising incidence of mental illness [1]. Governments now seem to accept the scientific evidence [2] and it appears that science will have the opportunity to resume research. However, much time has been wasted and research needs to be effectively focused. On the basis of the available information, it appears that psychedelic substances defy classic pharmacological models, calling into question even Paracelsus' universal postulate that the dose makes the poison. Thus, basic research on psychedelics is needed, as well as translational and clinical research, which constitutes the main body of knowledge on these substances. In fact, little is known about the mechanism of action of many of these substances, as well as their metabolic pathways, all of which are necessary for the safe use of these potent chemicals.

In general terms, the toxicity of a drug can be defined as the specific ratio between the active dose and the lethal dose [3]. This gives rise to various indices that can be calculated mathematically, with the lethal dose 50 (LD_{50}) being the most important. LD_{50} is the amount of a substance that kills 50% of the individuals subjected to that substance, by a specific route of administration and for a defined species. The relationship between effectiveness and toxicity must be well studied in order to understand the risks and benefits of a medicine (Figure 1). In classical pharmacological and toxicological models, the effects observed in a population follow a normal distribution. Thus, 66% of the population will have an expected effect around the mean dose ± standard deviation (SD); 95% of the population will have an expected effect around the mean dose ± 2SD; and 99.8% of the population will have an expected effect around the mean dose ± 3SD, with sensitive individuals at the left extreme of the curve experiencing a high effect at low doses, and resistant individuals at the right extreme experiencing no effect even at high doses [4].

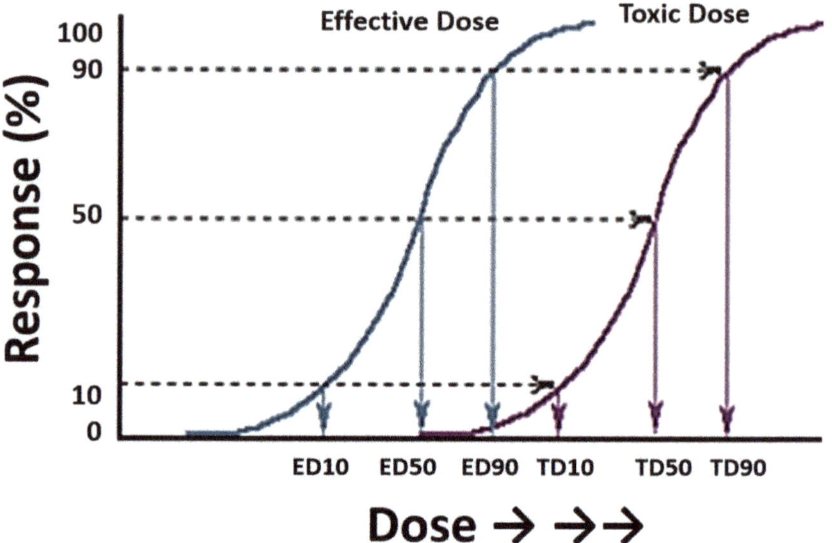

Figure 1. Typical sigmoid curves representing the dose of a drug and its response (measured as a percentage) in a group of individuals. The plot includes two curves relating to effective doses (left) and toxic doses (right). Extrapolation of the response gives the effective and toxic doses (ED and TD, respectively) for 10, 50, and 90% of the individuals exposed to these doses. Figure modified from the Toxicology Teaching Manual of the University of Las Palmas de Gran Canaria with the authors' permission.

In the evaluation of dose response, pharmacogenetics—an area of pharmacology that is used to determine in advance what will be the best medicine or dose for an individual—is a key element. In that context, it is necessary to determine the main metabolization pathways of different substances, and it is important to determine how certain genetic variations affect the functioning and efficiency of these metabolization pathways (e.g., single-nucleotide polymorphisms (SNPs) or methylation status in cytochrome P450 family and other enzymes). Pharmacogenetics constitute an important tool for the interpretation of toxicological data, and can be crucial for determining the cause and modality of drug-related deaths [5], especially in cases of non-overdose of drugs of abuse [6]. Forensic pharmacogenetics is a field of toxicology not fully understood in general terms and almost unknown in the case of psychedelics.

Psychedelics had their golden age in the 1950s and the first half of the 1960s, when promising effects were observed in relation to the treatment of addictions and the resolution of psychological and psychiatric problems [7,8]. Despite this, their use was banned by the Richard Nixon administration in mid-1970s. These substances were stigmatized, giving rise to a period we have called the "Acid Panic". During that period, many publications demonstrating the therapeutic power of psychedelic substances were censored, and even false or scientifically unsound articles were published [9]. As a consequence, society was imbued with a fear to psychedelics that has lasted for 50 years. Fortunately, scientific studies have continued, helping to dispel many of the myths surrounding these substances. Since the late 1980s, the use of psychedelics in the clinic has seen a renaissance, timid at first and very strong in recent years [10]. At present, there has been a translational evolution from the bench to the bedside, with phase 2 and 3 trials and/or evidence synthesis in particular. However, basic research (pharmacological and toxicological), which may not have been updated for decades, has taken a back seat. Thus, while the therapeutic potential of these substances—and their enormous potency—is well known, the reality is that the toxic/lethal doses of many of these substances are currently unknown [11]. Referring to mushrooms and LSD, "it's virtually impossible to die from an overdose of them; they cause no physical harm; and if anything they are anti-addictive, as they cause a sudden tolerance which means that if you immediately take another dose it will probably have very little effect" [12,13]. Thus, do these substances defy the basic law of toxicology that says that the dose makes the poison?

The aim of the present review is to understand the potentially lethal doses of three groups of psychedelics (ergolamines, simple tryptamines, and phenylethylamines), in order to determine the safety of these substances and to understand their very special nature.

2. Materials and Methods

The search for articles was carried out in major medical and scientific databases from the early years of the 20th century to 31 August 2022, using the following search terms and Medical Subject Headings (MeSHs): psychedelic overdose, LSD overdose, MDMA overdose, LD_{50} LSD, LD_{50} MDMA, LD_{50} mescaline, LD_{50} psilocybin, psychedelic poisoning, death by LSD, death by MDMA, death by psychedelics, dosing psychedelics, and acute toxicity by psychedelics. The inclusion criteria were: (1) Original Article, (2) Case Report, (3) Review, (4) Articles in English, and (4) In vivo studies. Exclusion criteria were (1) In vitro studies, (2) abstract, (3) poster, and (4) communications at conferences. Two articles were written in a language other than English. In these cases, the abstract was translated to extract the most relevant information for this review. It should be noted that many of the clinical case reports were published in the 1960s and 1970s, when analytical methods were less developed. Articles that did not contain sufficient information to discern the role of psychedelic substances in the individual's clinic were discarded.

Once the search was conducted, studies reporting toxic or lethal doses related to psychedelics were included. We identified 3032 manuscripts for inclusion. The initial quality assessment was made evaluating the title and the abstract. We excluded articles referred to other psychedelic and psychoactive substances. After a screening and evaluation of the whole text, a total of 67 manuscripts were eligible: 33 gave relevant information about effects associated to high doses of psychedelics and 34 were included in the text to complete the discussion. Articles reporting experimental data on lethal doses in animals were also included. Characteristics of eligible studies are summarized in Figure 2. The revision was made according to PRISMA 2020 guidelines. The search was conducted between 1 July and 31 July 2022.

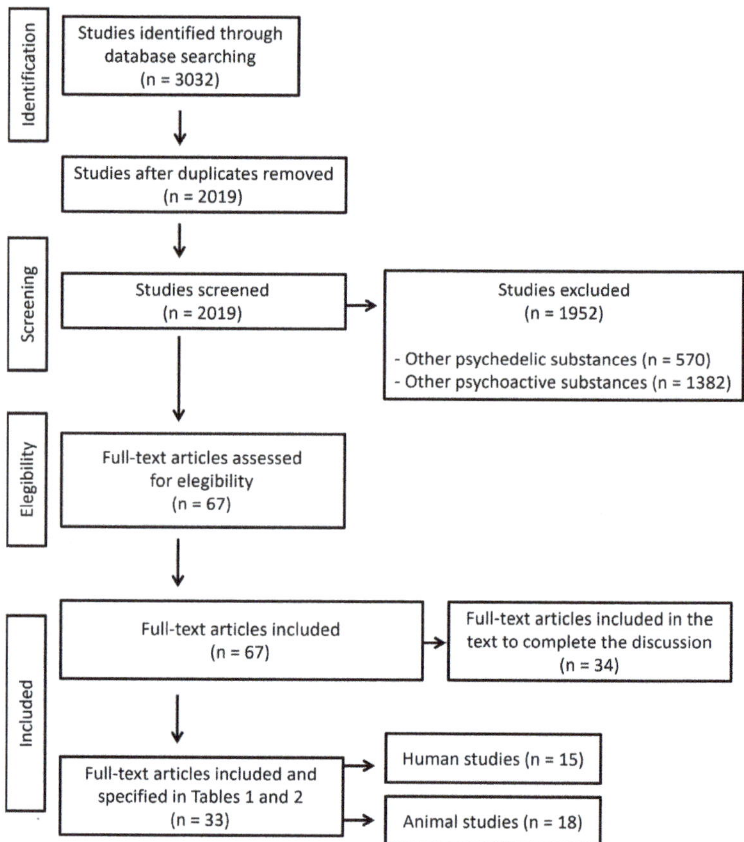

Figure 2. Flow diagram illustrating included and excluded studies in this systematic review. Articles reporting dosage are included in Tables 1 and 2 (n = 33), while articles reporting information that may explain clinical outcome are included in the text to complete the discussion (n = 34).

3. Results and Discussion

A total of 67 articles were included in this review. Of them, 33 gave relevant information about high/lethal doses of psychedelics. Eighteen studies (54.5%) were referred to high/lethal doses of psychedelics in animals and 15 (45.5%) were publications related to high/lethal doses of psychedelics in humans. Of them, 2 studies were experiments conducted directly on humans, 4 were reviews of clinical cases, and 9 were case reports. Additionally, 34 articles were included for being useful in the discussion of the main results.

3.1. Ergolamines: Does LSD Defy the Basics of Toxicology?

Lysergic acid diethylamide (LSD) is a semi-synthetic natural product created by Albert Hofmann at Sandoz Laboratories (Switzerland) in 1938. From the early days, studies were initiated to determine the toxicity of a product that was striking for its potency, achieving intense effects at very low doses. Despite being used by psychologists and psychiatrists, LSD was classified as an 'experimental drug', which prevented its use in clinical trials, in 1962 [14]. In 1965, its illegal production and sale were criminalized; in April 1966, Sandoz Laboratories stopped marketing LSD, and in 1968, possession and sale became a criminal offence [14]. In 1971, it was classified as a psychotropic drug under the Vienna Convention and banned. The period we have called "Acid Panic" began, during which an enormous effort was made to prove that LSD was harmful and highly toxic, mainly based on clinical cases reported in the scientific literature.

Table 1 summarizes experiments related to high/lethal doses of psychedelics in animals. The elephant was found to be the most sensitive animal, as administration of 0.06 mg/kg caused the death of one of these animals in 1962 [15]. However, the experiment was repeated years later, in 1984, without any consequence [16]. The LD_{50} in mice was 50–60 mg/kg; 16.5 mg/kg in rats; 0.3 mg/kg in rabbits [9,17,18]. In all cases, LSD was administered intramuscular or intravenously. Although there are important inter-species differences, LSD appeared to be a very potent substance when administered in this way, which is not the route of administration for humans. LSD has been tested in other species (i.e., Guinea pig or wild birds), at different doses and by different routes of administration, but no reliable conclusion has been reached as to a dose above which it is lethal [19,20]. Given that the effective dose in humans is 0.001–0.003 mg/kg, it can be inferred that the LD_{50} for our species could be 300–600 times that of the rabbit and up to 50,000–100,000 times that of the mouse [9]. It was deduced that LSD was remarkably well tolerated by humans, on whom it nevertheless exerted intense effects at very low doses.

Table 1. Description of experiments related to high/lethal doses of psychedelics in animals.

Substance	Year	Species	Dose/[Blood]	Route	LD/LD_{50} (mg/kg)	Author
LSD	1957	Rabbit	0.3 mg/kg	iv		Rothlin
	1959	Rat	17 mg/kg	iv		Gable **
	1959	Mouse	46 mg/kg	iv	100 *	Gable **
	1962	Elephant	297 mg	iv	14 *	West et al.
	1962	Guinea pig	16 mg/kg	sc		De Jonge
	1972	Bird	1.8 mg/kg	oral		Schafer
	1984	Elephant	0.003–0.10 mg/kg	oral		Siegel
MDMA	1973	Mouse		ip	97	Hardman et al.
		Rat		ip	49	
		Guinea pig		ip	98	
		Dog		iv	14	
		Monkey		iv	22	
	1985	Rat		oral	325	Goad
	1997	Rat	20–360 mg/kg	oral	160	De Souza
Mescaline	1934	Guinea pig		sc	500	Grace
		Frog		p	750	
	1961	Mouse (50)		oral	880	Greenblatt et al.
	1962	Mouse		sc	534	Hoshikawa
	1968	Mouse		iv	157	Horibe
	1968	Mouse		NA	261	Walters et al.
	1973	Mice (40)		ip	212	Hardman et al.
		Rat (28)		ip	13	
		Guinea pig (32)		ip	328	
		Dog (16)		iv	54	
		Monkey (17)		iv	130	
	1985	Rat		sc	534	Becker
		Rat		iv	15	
		Rat		im	330	
	2004	Mouse		oral	880	Gable
Psilocybin	1968	Mouse		ip	420	Horibe
		Mouse		iv	275	
	1972	Rabbit		iv	13	Usdin
		Rat		iv	280	
	2015	Mouse	200–450 mg/kg	ip	316.9 ☨	Zhuk et al.

Abbreviations: M, male; F, female; iv, intravenous; sc, subcutaneous; ip, intraperitoneal; p, parenteral; im, intramuscular; NA, not available. * Estimated value from the experiment (mg). ** Details of the original manuscript were obtained from Gable, 2004. ☨ For *Psilocybe semilanceata*. LD_{50} for *Psilocybe cyanopus* was 316.9 mg/kg. LD_{50} for psilocin was 293.1 mg/kg.

Table 2 summarizes clinical reports related to high/lethal doses of psychedelics in humans. In 1973, the first article on LSD overdose was published [21]. It concerned eight patients (four men and four women), aged between 19 and 39 years. Of these, four were tested for LSD in their blood, showing concentrations between 0.0021 and 0.026 µg/mL. Two individuals—not tested for blood—had LSD in their gastric contents, and reported having snorted the substance. Half of the patients were also positive for ethanol and/or cocaine. This heterogeneity makes it difficult to determine what role LSD may have played in the individual's medical history. In addition, it is necessary to relate the concentration detected in blood to the dose of LSD taken.

The first pharmacokinetic study of LSD dates back to 1972. After oral administration of 160 µg of LSD, the blood concentration of the substance was observed to be 4.16 ng/mL two hours later [22]. Similar results were obtained later [23,24], allowing an approximation of the maximum amount taken of more than 1.5 mg. For the eight reported patients in 1972, this is 7 times the maximum effective dose (250 µg [25]), which would presuppose moderate-severe intoxication. However, all patients survived with no adverse health consequences.

Four years later, a case of death from LSD overdose was reported in which 31.2 µg/mL of LSD was quantified in the liver of the deceased. The authors inferred, on the basis of cat studies, that the deceased must have received an extrapolated dose of 320 mg intravenously (1600 times the recommended dose) [26]. This particular death is one of two probable cases of death by LSD overdose [17]. The other case was reported in 1985 as follows. Under the title "A fatal poisoning with LSD", the authors reported the death of a 25-year-old male who died, allegedly, from the action of the substance [27]. Analyses were performed by radioimmunoassay, a semi-quantitative technique with limited expert value, giving a concentration of 14.8 and 4.8 ng/mL before and after death. High-performance liquid chromatography analysis, considered the gold standard, gave a result of 8 ng/mL before the individual's death. According to pharmacokinetic studies, this may result in an exposure to about 500 µg of LSD, slightly more than twice the maximum recommended effective oral dose. Although, for some substances, doubling or tripling the effective dose may pose an undisputed health risk (i.e., hypoglycemics, cytostatics, or anticoagulants), for LSD, numerous cases of massive overdose without health consequences have been reported [11]. One of the most extreme cases is that of a 46-year-old woman who snorted 55,000 µg of LSD—275 to 550 times the maximum recommended effective dose—mistaking it for cocaine. The incident had no adverse health consequences. Moreover, she overcame an opiate addiction shortly afterward [28].

The literature is full of studies reporting LSD intoxications, with hundreds of individuals included [29–31] and no serious cases with fatal outcome reported. However, the message given during the "Acid Panic" era was that LSD was extremely dangerous and should remain banned. Since then, the scientific community has published cases and studies in the opposite direction: LSD is not only a safe molecule, due to its wide margin of safety, but also showed no addiction potential [32]. In 1993, the LD_{50} was set as 14,000 µg [32], which was then raised to 100,000 µg in 2004 [17], which is 400 times the maximum dose commonly used in the therapeutic setting, without empirical evidence. Even taking this theoretical value for granted, it is difficult to think of drugs or medicines that, when administered 100 or 200 times their therapeutic dose, do not cause serious damage to the health of the individual.

While it is true that there have been reported cases of deaths where LSD was present, they are all related to violent incidents—police intervention and aggressive restraint measures—where the victims had made missuses of the substance, not because of the substance, but because of the experience: inappropriate places and inappropriate circumstances [11]. The scientific community now recognizes that LSD is an extremely safe substance when used in moderate doses (50–250 µg) in controlled settings and orally, with only modest elevations in blood pressure, heart rate, and body temperature [33,34].

Dosing brings up an all-important question that applies to any substance under scrutiny: pharmacologically speaking, what is the drug's toxicity? Hofmann himself knew that the substance was effective at very low doses. Substances that are effective at low doses usually have very narrow safety margins. Interestingly, in the case of LSD, not only are there no adverse health effects, reported incidents at very high doses have had no serious or irreversible consequences, and these facts call into question Paracelsus' toxicological principle that the dose makes the poison.

3.2. *Phenylethylamines*

3.2.1. Does MDMA Defy the Basics of Toxicology?

3,4-methylenedioxy-methamphetamine (MDMA) was synthesized by the E. Merck pharmaceutical firm in Darmstadt (Germany) in 1912. The patent was registered on 24 December of that year and came into force on 16 May 1914 (number 274350) [35]. It was included as an experimental drug by the US government in its 'truth serum' mind control program [36] and was the subject of research by psychiatrists, led by Alexander Shulgin [37]. However, although clinical trials showed promising results [38,39], MDMA was banned by the Federal Drug Administration (FDA) in July 1985.

MDMA has a number of particularities that mean it needs to be treated specifically. First, it has non-linear kinetics, which means that there is no linear correspondence between the dose ingested, the amount of MDMA in blood, and the physiological effects [40]. Second, the metabolites generated in the metabolization of the drug cause an inhibition of CYP2D6, which is the main MDMA-metabolizing enzyme, exposing the individual to drug intoxication and overdose of MDMA itself, in the case of repeated ingestions [40]. The effective oral dose in humans is 1–2 mg/kg [17,25]. Even at moderate doses, there are a number of potential health risks including cerebral hyperthermia, hyponatremia, or disseminated intravascular coagulation. However, the wide variety of adverse effects it can produce leads experts to believe that there must be factors other than the substance itself that explain these effects: environmental conditions in places where the substance is taken recreationally, the quality of the synthesis in home laboratories, or impurities added to maximize the benefits [41]. In addition, the metabolization of MDMA is carried out mainly by CYP2D6, whose genetic polymorphisms condition the efficiency of metabolization. Although the role of these polymorphisms is not entirely clear, they may have an important influence on a fatal outcome, although it is likely that several factors are required concomitantly [42].

MDMA can be injected, smoked, or snorted, but is usually ingested orally. The LD_{50} of MDMA via intraperitoneal administration has been reported as 97, 49, and 98 mg/kg for the mouse, rat, and guinea pig, respectively (Table 1). The LD_{50} of MDMA via intravenous administration has been reported as 22, and 14 mg/kg for the monkey and dog, respectively [43]. The LD_{50} of MDMA via oral administration has been reported with a range from 160 mg/kg [44] to 325 mg/kg [45] among rats.

There are many case reviews of MDMA-overdose-related deaths in the scientific literature [46], although no clear conclusions can be drawn: (i) in most publications, it was not possible to definitively know the role of the substance in the death; (ii) the concentrations of MDMA in the deceased were unknown; (iii) when available, it is difficult to infer the dose taken because the time between intake and death was unknown [42]. In a series of 392 cases reported in Australia between 2000 and 2018, an average of 0.45 mg/L of MDMA was detected [47]. In a series of 142 cases reported in Norway between 2000 and 2019, an average of 0.73 mg/L of MDMA was detected, although 36% of the cases had other drugs besides MDMA [48]. The lethal concentration found in 27 MDMA-related deaths was 3 mg/L, reporting a high influence of environmental factors [17]. A reasonable estimate of the acute LD_{50} of MDMA for a healthy 70 kg person would appear to be approximately 2 g, or about 15–16 times a single recreational oral dose of 125 mg/kg [49].

Table 2. Description of clinical reports related to high/lethal doses of psychedelics in humans.

Substance	Year	N	Gender	Type of publication	Dose/[Blood]	Route	Outcome	LD/LD_{50}	Author
LSD	1943	1	M	Sandoz Laboratory	0.25 mg	oral	Survive		Hofmann
	1974	7	M/F	Recreational use	0.026 µg/mL	in	Survive		Klock et al.
	1977	1	NA	Case report	31.2 µg/mL *	oral	Death	320 (mg)	Griggs et al.
	1985	1	M	Case report	0.008 µg/mL	NA	Death	0.6 (mg)	Fysh et al.
	1993	NA	M/F	Clinical case reviews		oral	Survive	14 (mg)	Gable
	2020	1	F	Recreational use	0.5 mg	oral	Survive		Haden et al.
		1	F	Recreational use	1.2 mg	oral	Survive		
		1	F	Recreational use	55 mg	in	Survive		
MDMA	2004	27	M/F	Clinical case reviews	3 mg/L	oral			Gable
	2020	392	M/F	Clinical case reviews	0.45 mg/L	oral			Roxburg et al.
	2022	142	M/F	Clinical case reviews	0.37–0.73 mg/L	oral			Jamt et al.
Mescaline	1962	10	M	Experiment	2.5 mg/kg	im	Survive		Wolbach et al.
	1985	1	NA	Case report		NA	Death	9.7 (mg/L)	Reynolds et al.
	1993	NA	M/F	Clinical case reviews		oral	Survive	6000 (mg)	Gable
	1999	1	M	Case report		oral	Death	0.48 (mg/L)	Nolte et al.
Psilocybin	1960	16	NA	Experiment	60 µg/kg	oral	Survive		Hollister et al.
		16	NA	Experiment	37 µg/kg	ip	Survive		
	1962	10	M	Experiment	75 µg/kg	im	Survive		Wolbach et. al
	1993	NA	M/F	Clinical case reviews		oral	Survive	14,000 (mg)	Gable
	1996	1	M	Case report	6000 mg	oral	Death	4 (mg/L)	Gerault et al.
	2012	1	F	Case report		oral	Death	30 (µg/L)	Lim et al.

Abbreviations: M, male; F, female; in, intranasal; im, intramuscular; ip, intraperitoneal; NA, not available. * Found in liver.

MDMA is a drug with low addictive power but with certain risks, essentially linked to the way it is taken [32]. Despite its massive and uncontrolled use, a fatal incident risk of 0.003% (1 in 33,000 pills) has been estimated, lower than other illegal drugs of abuse consumed in the same context [50], which makes it a very safe drug. To maximize its therapeutic benefits, it is not only the dosage that must be appropriate, but also the circumstances and setting of the treatment. In this scenario, no significant adverse effects or deaths have been reported in individuals who have taken the substance in the context of guided therapy. MDMA is, however, a strange case for two reasons. First, despite being more harmful to health than other psychedelics, it is, along with ketamine, among the substances that are closest to being approved for clinical use. It has to be taken into account that MDMA, together with ketamine and ibogaine, are distinguished from classic psychedelics, both in their effects and in their pharmacology [51]. Secondly, although there is a large literature on MDMA-related deaths, the lethal dose orally administered under controlled conditions is unknown.

3.2.2. Does Mescaline Defy the Basics of Toxicology?

Natural psychedelics such as mescaline or psilocybin are found in plants considered sacred since ancient times. In the case of mescaline (trimethoxyphenethylamine), it is found in San Pedro (*Echinopsis pachanoi*) and Peyote (*Lophophora williamsii*) cacti. Although they have been used by indigenous tribes for centuries, they reappeared in Europe and the United States in the mid-1950s [52]. In any case, mescaline was already being investigated by the American government years before its immersion in the society of that time [36].

Mescaline is the least toxic of the methoxyamphetamines tested in animal models [53], and is 2500–4000 times less potent than LSD [54]. The toxic effects of trimethoxyphenethylamine were investigated for the first time in 1934, reporting an LDL_0 (Lethal Dose Low) of 500 and 750 mg/kg in the Guinea pig and frog, respectively [55]. In the 1960s, several studies were published in mice, reporting an LD_{50} between 157 and 880 mg/kg depending on the route of administration [56–59] (Table 1). While for the rat, the reported LD_{50} was 15 mg/kg, among monkeys, the dose reached 130 mg/kg, which is 8.6 times more [43,60]. The LD_{50} via the oral route—the main route of administration in humans—in animals reaches almost 1 g/kg [17]. In any case, none of these values can be extrapolated to the human species, mainly because the animal studies use trimethoxyphenethylamine and the intake in humans is a preparation of the cactus, which implies the intake of many other substances with the interactions inherent to it.

The first study in humans began in 1921 and ran for several years. Sixty subjects (90% males) were injected with 200, 400, 500, and 600 mg of pure mescaline. The results were published in an extensive document entitled Der Meskalinrausch (Mescaline intoxication) by Kurt Beringer in 1927 [61]. Physical and psychological reactions were described as "mescal psychosis", with no relevant adverse effects or deaths reported. The TDL_0 was set at 2.5 mg/kg (intramuscular administration), according to Wolbach in 1962. The experiment was made in 10 males who were morphine addicts serving sentences for violations of the U.S. national narcotic laws. The authors concluded that reactions induced by LSD, mescaline, and psilocybin were qualitatively similar, with no relevant adverse effects or deaths reported [62].

Two case reports were published in 1985 and 1999 with fatal outcome. The first one was a subject who fell from a cliff while they were under the influence of mescaline. Concentrations of the drug were 9.7, 70.8, and 1163 μg/mL or μg/g in the blood, liver, and urine, respectively [63]. Concentrations in the blood and the actions described by eyewitnesses presuppose that the deceased was suffering from the hallucinogenic effects of mescaline, whose hallucinogenic effects are acquired at doses of 200–500 mg of the salt [63]. The second one was a 32-year-old Native American man with a history of alcoholism who died from bronchial aspiration of vomit during a Peyote ceremony [64]. Antemortem blood concentration was 0.48 mg/L (Table 2). Mescaline has potent emetic effects [65]; therefore, it should be used with caution if there are esophageal or respiratory pathologies or concomitant use of central nervous system depressants (i.e., alcohol). To our knowledge, no further cases of mescaline-associated death have been reported.

From these two cases, it cannot be inferred a dose from which the consumer's life is in danger, especially if the consumption is performed in a controlled environment [66]. The usual effective dose (and range) for non-medical purposes is 350 mg (200–450) [17]. Although mescaline is assigned a lower safety ratio than other classical psychedelics [17], it has pharmacokinetic properties that make it especially safe. The plasma half-life of mescaline is approximately 6 h [67]. Its low lipid solubility means that it crosses the blood–brain barrier more slowly, is stored temporarily in the liver, and is released slowly, reducing its potential adverse effects [67]. Thus, the peak of psychological effects, which occurs 2 h after ingestion, does not coincide with the peak of mescaline concentration in the brain. In general terms, mescaline is very poorly absorbed orally. It is estimated that 60% of the substance consumed is eliminated unchanged in urine one hour after ingestion [68]. Unlike other psychedelics, the mechanism of action of mescaline is not known. Hallucinogenic effects are believed to be due to stimulation of serotonin and dopamine receptors in the central nervous system.

If we add to all this the way it is taken—preparations and cooking of the cactus—where many other alkaloids interact, mescaline should be taken with caution. Even so, it is a substance that has been used for centuries and that, even today, is an elemental part of the culture of some tribes. However, no serious cases with fatal endings have been reported [54,69], which again brings into question the basic principle of toxicology.

3.3. *Tryptamines: Does Psilocybin Defy the Basics of Toxicology?*

Natural psychedelics such as psilocybin ([3-[2-(dimethylamino)ethyl]-1H-indol-4-yl] dihydrogen phosphate) is found in so-called magic mushrooms (Psilocybe semilanceata, P. cubensis or Pholiotina cuanopus). It is a substance that has been used since ancient times and was reintroduced into Western culture in the mid-1950s after the publication, in *Life Magazine*, of R.G. Wasson's psychedelic experiences with magic mushrooms, in Mexico, guided by María Sabina in 1957 [70].

Some of the most potent psychedelics belong to the group of tryptamines (i.e., N,N-dimethyltryptamine (DMT) or N,N-dimethyl-5-methoxytryptamine (5-MeO-DMT)) and, curiously, they are among those with the greatest margin of safety [17]. Regarding psilocybin, studies in animal models show a high tolerance up to 400 mg/kg, with the substance proving highly toxic at higher concentrations [71]. In 1968, the LD_{50} in mice was established at 275 and 420 mg/kg intravenously and intraperitoneally, respectively [59]. Similar results were reported later [71]. The rabbit was shown to be the most sensitive species, in which the LD_{50} intravenously was 13 mg/kg, while for the rat, it was 280 [72] (Table 1).

For the human species, 30–40 mg is considered to be a high dose of psilocybin [25], which, in comparison with the data reported in animals, suggests that we are a particularly sensitive species. the TDL_0 was established at 60 and 37 µg/kg orally and intraperitoneally, respectively, in a group of 16 volunteer subjects tested in 1960 [73]. By the intramuscular route, the TDL_0 was 75 µg/kg (Table 2), highlighting that reactions induced by LSD, mescaline, psilocin, and psilocybin are qualitatively similar [62].

Two case reports were published in 1996 and 2012 with fatal outcome. The first one report a case that occurred in France in 1993 [74]. A quantity of 4 ng/mL of psilocybin was found in the blood. However, the work appears to be invalidated by numerous methodological deficiencies and contradictions [75], and was highly controversial and criticized by some sectors of French society. The second one is a fatal case of magic mushroom ingestion in a heart transplant recipient, who collapsed 2–3 h after the intake [76]. Plasma toxicology revealed a psilocin level of 30 mg/L and a tetrahydrocannabinol level of 4 mg/L. No alcohol or other common drugs of abuse were detected. The cause of death was determined to be psilocin toxicity. The toxicity of psilocybin is low (LD_{50} = 280 mg/kg in rats); a 60 kg person would need to ingest up to 17 kg of fresh mushrooms to reach this dose. However, psilocybin toxicity includes cardiovascular toxicity; therefore, beyond the dosage, it must be taken into account that the individuals have a good health and body condition before ingestion. There is a third publication reporting a death associated to psilocybin, but details are scanty [77]. There are other deaths reported as a result of accidents or self-harm following mushroom ingestion [78], which are beyond the scope of this review.

In the United States, approximately over one million people have used mushrooms without fatalities [79]. Similar outcomes have been reported in Europe [80], which makes magic mushrooms a safe substance at different doses, from micro-doses to so-called heroic doses [78]. Under controlled circumstances, psilocybin has a wide margin of safety. Although the dose makes the poison, in order for these potent transformative substances to be dangerous to humans, Paracelsus' own principle is called into question.

3.4. Limitations of the Study

Although this systematic review was made according to PRISMA 2020 guidelines, some limitations were present. First, many studies published in non-indexed journals were not included; second, many studies published in non-selected databases were not included; third, no statistical analysis was performed; fourth, the biological reasons behind the particular behavior of these substances can only be hypothesized.

With respect to the latter, is important to highlight the role of pharmacogenetics studies in drug-related overdoses and deaths [5], especially in the case of MDMA, the most risky psychedelic among those included in this review, whose complex metabolism is linked to CYP2D6. Thus, determining the presence of cytochrome inducing or suppressing mutations can provide answers in cases of death related to a suspected drug overdose. This is especially relevant if we take into account that these substances are not only used in assisted therapies but, increasingly, for personal growth mainly due to its neuroenhancement effects [81]. Although there are conflicting opinions regarding their actual functioning and benefit [82], it seems that psychedelics report benefits even in microdoses [83]. In any case, the effects that these practices may have when receiving higher doses of psychedelics in relation to tolerance, metabolization efficiency, and other parameters related to the pharmacokinetics of the substances are not known.

4. Conclusions

Despite their therapeutic potential in psychology and psychiatry, psychedelics have been subjected to severe scrutiny that led to their prohibition in the 1960s and 1970s. They are currently undergoing what is called a 'psychedelic renaissance', being the subject of extensive research—especially clinical research—and are close to legalization in many parts of the world (e.g., the State of Oregon, USA). Despite their high potency—they are capable of very potent actions at very low doses—they have very low addiction rates and very high safety rates, especially the classic psychedelics (LSD, mescaline, or psilocybes). In some cases, a 100-fold increase in the effective dose does not cause harmful effects on the health of individuals, which defies the basic principle of toxicology. Perhaps with the exception of MDMA, historically reported deaths do not appear to be the sole responsibility of the substance, but rather related to the environment and circumstances of intake. In order to understand this unique behavior, pharmacogenetics may be crucial. In view of the current situation regarding psychedelics, there is a need to invest in basic research, which clarifies the pharmacokinetics of these substances as well as their mechanism of action.

In view of the results shown in this review, it seems that it is not only the dose that makes the poison; in the case of psychedelics, the set and setting also make the poison.

Author Contributions: Conceptualization, L.A.H.-H. and L.F.B.; methodology, L.A.H.-H. and D.J.Q.-H.; investigation, L.A.H.-H. and J.R.-H.; writing—original draft preparation, L.A.H.-H.; writing—review and editing, J.R.-H. and D.J.Q.-H.; supervision, L.F.B. All authors have read and agreed to the published version of the manuscript.

Funding: This research received no external funding.

Institutional Review Board Statement: Not applicable.

Informed Consent Statement: Not applicable.

Data Availability Statement: Not applicable.

Conflicts of Interest: The authors declare no conflict of interest.

References

1. WHO. Depression. 2021. Available online: https://www.who.int/news-room/fact-sheets/detail/depression (accessed on 9 December 2022).
2. SAMHSA. *Response to Task Force*; Department of Health & Human Services; Substance Abuse and Mental Health Services Administration: Rockville, MD, USA, 2022.
3. Escohotado, A. *Historia de las Drogas*; Alianza Editorial: Madrid, Spain, 1998; Volume 1.
4. Luzardo, O.P.; Almeida-González, M.; Zumbado, M.; Ruíz-Suárez, N.; Henríquez-Hernández, L.A.; Boada, L.D. Manual Docente de Toxicología Veterinaria [Manual docente] 2012. p. 70. Available online: https://spdc.ulpgc.es/libro/manual-docente-de-toxicologia-veterinaria_50717/(accessed on 9 November 2022).
5. Di Nunno, N.; Esposito, M.; Argo, A.; Salerno, M.; Sessa, F. Pharmacogenetics and Forensic Toxicology: A New Step towards a Multidisciplinary Approach. *Toxics* **2021**, *9*, 292. [CrossRef]
6. Bertol, E.; Trignano, C. Poisoning Caused by Medicines and Drugs of Abuse. *Toxics* **2022**, *10*, 515. [CrossRef] [PubMed]
7. Smith, C.M. A new adjunct to the treatment of alcoholism: The hallucinogenic drugs. *Q. J. Stud. Alcohol.* **1958**, *19*, 406–417. [CrossRef] [PubMed]
8. Maclean, J.R.; Macdonald, D.C.; Byrne, U.P.; Hubbard, A.M. The use of LSD-25 in the treatment of alcoholism and other psychiatric problems. *Q. J. Stud. Alcohol.* **1961**, *22*, 34–45. [CrossRef] [PubMed]
9. Hofmann, A. *LSD: Cómo Descubrí el Ácido y qué pasó Después en el Mundo*; Editorial Arpa Ideas: Barcelona, Spain, 2018.
10. Solmi, M.; Chen, C.; Daure, C.; Buot, A.; Ljuslin, M.; Verroust, V.; Mallet, L.; Khazaal, Y.; Rothen, S.; Thorens, G.; et al. A century of research on psychedelics: A scientometric analysis on trends and knowledge maps of hallucinogens, entactogens, entheogens and dissociative drugs. *Eur. Neuropsychopharmacol.* **2022**, *64*, 44–60. [CrossRef]
11. Nichols, D.E.; Grob, C.S. Is LSD toxic? *Forensic Sci. Int.* **2018**, *284*, 141–145. [CrossRef]
12. Liechti, M.E. Modern Clinical Research on LSD. *Neuropsychopharmacology* **2017**, *42*, 2114–2127. [CrossRef]
13. Nutt, D. *Drugs without the Hot Air: Minimising the Harms of Legal and Illegal Drugs*, 1st ed.; UIT Cambridge Ltd.: Cambridge, UK, 2012; p. 368.
14. Lee, M.A.; Shlaim, B. *Historia Social del LSD: La CIA, los Sesenta y todo lo Demás*; Castellarte: Barcelona, Spain, 2002.
15. West, L.J.; Pierce, C.M.; Thomas, W.D. Lysergic Acid Diethylamide: Its Effects on a Male Asiatic Elephant. *Science* **1962**, *138*, 1100–1103. [CrossRef]

16. Siegen, R.K. LSD-induced effects in elephants: Comparisons with musth behavior. *Bull. Psychon. Soc.* **1984**, *22*, 53–56. [CrossRef]
17. Gable, R.S. Comparison of acute lethal toxicity of commonly abused psychoactive substances. *Addiction* **2004**, *99*, 686–696. [CrossRef]
18. Rothlin, E. Lysergic acid diethylamide and related substances. *Ann. N. Y. Acad. Sci.* **1957**, *66*, 668–676. [CrossRef] [PubMed]
19. de Jonge, M.; Funcke, A.B. Sinistrotorsion in guinea pigs as a method of screening central anticholinergic activity. *Arch. Int. Pharmacodyn. Ther.* **1962**, *137*, 375–382.
20. Schafer, E.W. The acute oral toxicity of 369 pesticidal, pharmaceutical and other chemicals to wild birds. *Toxicol. Appl. Pharmacol.* **1972**, *21*, 315–330. [CrossRef] [PubMed]
21. Klock, J.C.; Boerner, U.; Becker, C.E. Coma, hyperthermia and bleeding associated with massive LSD overdose. A report of eight cases. *West. J. Med.* **1974**, *120*, 183–188. [CrossRef]
22. Upshall, D.G.; Wailling, D.G. The determination of LSD in human plasma following oral administration. *Clin. Chim. Acta* **1972**, *36*, 67–73. [CrossRef] [PubMed]
23. Dolder, P.C.; Schmid, Y.; Haschke, M.; Rentsch, K.M.; Liechti, M.E. Pharmacokinetics and Concentration-Effect Relationship of Oral LSD in Humans. *Int. J. Neuropsychopharmacol.* **2015**, *19*, pyv072. [CrossRef]
24. Dolder, P.C.; Schmid, Y.; Steuer, A.E.; Kraemer, T.; Rentsch, K.M.; Hammann, F.; Liechti, M.E. Pharmacokinetics and Pharmacodynamics of Lysergic Acid Diethylamide in Healthy Subjects. *Clin. Pharmacokinet.* **2017**, *56*, 1219–1230. [CrossRef] [PubMed]
25. Liechti, M.E.; Holze, F. Dosing Psychedelics and MDMA. *Curr. Top. Behav. Neurosci.* **2021**, *56*, 3–21. [CrossRef]
26. Griggs, E.A.; Ward, M. LSD toxicity: A suspected cause of death. *J. Ky. Med. Assoc.* **1977**, *75*, 172–173.
27. Fysh, R.R.; Oon, M.C.; Robinson, K.N.; Smith, R.N.; White, P.C.; Whitehouse, M.J. A fatal poisoning with LSD. *Forensic Sci. Int.* **1985**, *28*, 109–113. [CrossRef]
28. Haden, M.; Woods, B. LSD Overdoses: Three Case Reports. *J. Stud. Alcohol Drugs* **2020**, *81*, 115–118. [CrossRef] [PubMed]
29. Shick, J.F.; Smith, D.E.; Meyers, F.H. Patterns of drug use in the Haight-Ashbury neighborhood. *Clin. Toxicol.* **1970**, *3*, 19–56. [CrossRef] [PubMed]
30. Smith, D.E. Use of LSD in the Haight-Ashbury. Observations at a neighborhood clinic. *Calif. Med.* **1969**, *110*, 472–476.
31. Smith, D.E.; Rose, A.J. The use and abuse of LSD in Haight-Ashbury (observations by the Haight-Ashbury Medical Clinic). *Clin. Pediatr.* **1968**, *7*, 317–322. [CrossRef]
32. Gable, R.S. Toward a comparative overview of dependence potential and acute toxicity of psychoactive substances used nonmedically. *Am. J. Drug Alcohol Abuse* **1993**, *19*, 263–281. [CrossRef]
33. Holze, F.; Caluori, T.V.; Vizeli, P.; Liechti, M.E. Safety pharmacology of acute LSD administration in healthy subjects. *Psychopharmacology* **2022**, *239*, 1893–1905. [CrossRef] [PubMed]
34. Holze, F.; Vizeli, P.; Ley, L.; Muller, F.; Dolder, P.; Stocker, M.; Duthaler, U.; Varghese, N.; Eckert, A.; Borgwardt, S.; et al. Acute dose-dependent effects of lysergic acid diethylamide in a double-blind placebo-controlled study in healthy subjects. *Neuropsychopharmacology* **2021**, *46*, 537–544. [CrossRef]
35. Henry, J.A.; Rella, J.G. Medical risks associated with MDMA use. In *Ecstasy: The Complete Guide*; Julie Holland, M.D., Ed.; Park Street Press: Rochester, VT, USA, 2001; pp. 71–86.
36. Passie, T.; Benzenhofer, U. MDA, MDMA, and other "mescaline-like" substances in the US military's search for a truth drug (1940s to 1960s). *Drug Test. Anal.* **2018**, *10*, 72–80. [CrossRef]
37. Shulgin, A.T. The background and chemistry of MDMA. *J. Psychoact. Drugs* **1986**, *18*, 291–304. [CrossRef] [PubMed]
38. Greer, G.; Tolbert, R. Subjective reports of the effects of MDMA in a clinical setting. *J. Psychoact. Drugs* **1986**, *18*, 319–327. [CrossRef]
39. Liester, M.B.; Grob, C.S.; Bravo, G.L.; Walsh, R.N. Phenomenology and sequelae of 3,4-methylenedioxymethamphetamine use. *J. Nerv. Ment. Dis.* **1992**, *180*, 345–352, discussion 353–344. [CrossRef] [PubMed]
40. Oña, G. Farmacocinética y farmacodinamia de las drogas psicodélicas. In *Tu Cerebro con Psicodélicos*; Argonowta: Madrid, Spain, 2022; pp. 155–156.
41. Rochester, J.A.; Kirchner, J.T. Ecstasy (3,4-methylenedioxymethamphetamine): History, neurochemistry, and toxicology. *J. Am. Board Fam. Pract.* **1999**, *12*, 137–142. [CrossRef]
42. Pardo-Lozano, R.; Farre, M.; Yubero-Lahoz, S.; O'Mathuna, B.; Torrens, M.; Mustata, C.; Perez-Mana, C.; Langohr, K.; Cuyas, E.; Carbo, M.; et al. Clinical pharmacology of 3,4-methylenedioxymethamphetamine (MDMA, "ecstasy"): The influence of gender and genetics (CYP2D6, COMT, 5-HTT). *PLoS ONE* **2012**, *7*, e47599. [CrossRef] [PubMed]
43. Hardman, H.F.; Haavik, C.O.; Seevers, M.H. Relationship of the structure of mescaline and seven analogs to toxicity and behavior in five species of laboratory animals. *Toxicol. Appl. Pharmacol.* **1973**, *25*, 299–309. [CrossRef] [PubMed]
44. De Souza, I.; Kelly, J.P.; Harkin, A.J.; Leonard, B.E. An appraisal of the pharmacological and toxicological effects of a single oral administration of 3,4-methylenedioxymethamphetamine (MDMA) in the rat. *Pharmacol. Toxicol.* **1997**, *80*, 207–210. [CrossRef] [PubMed]
45. Goad, P.T. *Acute and Subacute Oral Toxicity of Methylenedioxymethamphetamine in Rats*; Intox Laboatories: Redfield, AK, USA, 1985.
46. Roxburgh, A.; Sam, B.; Kriikku, P.; Mounteney, J.; Castanera, A.; Dias, M.; Giraudon, I. Trends in MDMA-related mortality across four countries. *Addiction* **2021**, *116*, 3094–3103. [CrossRef]
47. Roxburgh, A.; Lappin, J. MDMA-related deaths in Australia 2000 to 2018. *Int. J. Drug Policy* **2020**, *76*, 102630. [CrossRef]

48. Jamt, R.E.G.; Edvardsen, H.M.E.; Middelkoop, G.; Kallevik, A.S.; Bogstrand, S.T.; Vevelstad, M.S.; Vindenes, V. Deaths associated with MDMA in the period 2000–2019. *Tidsskr Nor Laegeforen* **2022**, *142*. [CrossRef]
49. Gable, R.S. Acute toxic effects of club drugs. *J. Psychoact. Drugs* **2004**, *36*, 303–313. [CrossRef]
50. van Amsterdam, J.; Pennings, E.; van den Brink, W. Fatal and non-fatal health incidents related to recreational ecstasy use. *J. Psychopharmacol.* **2020**, *34*, 591–599. [CrossRef]
51. Schlag, A.K.; Aday, J.; Salam, I.; Neill, J.C.; Nutt, D.J. Adverse effects of psychedelics: From anecdotes and misinformation to systematic science. *J. Psychopharmacol.* **2022**, *36*, 258–272. [CrossRef] [PubMed]
52. Huxley, A. *The Doors of Perception*; Harper & Row: New York City, NY, USA, 1954.
53. Davis, W.M.; Bedford, J.A.; Buelke, J.L.; Guinn, M.M.; Hatoum, H.T.; Waters, I.W.; Wilson, M.C.; Braude, M.C. Acute toxicity and gross behavioral effects of amphetamine, four methoxyamphetamines, and mescaline in rodents, dogs, and monkeys. *Toxicol. Appl. Pharmacol.* **1978**, *45*, 49–62. [CrossRef] [PubMed]
54. Halpern, J.H.; Sherwood, A.R.; Hudson, J.I.; Yurgelun-Todd, D.; Pope, H.G., Jr. Psychological and cognitive effects of long-term peyote use among Native Americans. *Biol. Psychiatry* **2005**, *58*, 624–631. [CrossRef] [PubMed]
55. Grace, G.S. The action of mescaline and some related compounds. *J. Pharmacol. Exp. Ther.* **1934**, *50*, 359–372.
56. Greenblatt, E.N.; Osterberg, A.C. Correlations of activating and lethal effects of excitatory drugs in grouped and isolated mice. *J. Pharmacol. Exp. Ther.* **1961**, *131*, 115–119.
57. Hoshikawa, E. Pharmacological studies on hallucinogens. I. 2. Investigation of the general pharmacological action of mescaline. *Nihon Yakurigaku Zasshi* **1962**, *58*, 261–274. [CrossRef] [PubMed]
58. Walters, G.C.; Cooper, P.D. Alicyclic analogue of mescaline. *Nature* **1968**, *218*, 298–300. [CrossRef] [PubMed]
59. Horibe, M. Pharmacological studies of hallucinogens. Report 3. II. Pharmacological studies of influence of psilocybin on the central nervous system. *Nihon Yakurigaku Zasshi* **1968**, *64*, 159–185.
60. Becker, H. Constituents of the cactus Lophophora williamsii. *Pharm. Unserer. Zeit.* **1985**, *14*, 129–137. [CrossRef]
61. Beringer, K. *Der Meskalinrausch*, 1st ed.; Springer: Berlin/Heidelberg, Germany, 1927. [CrossRef]
62. Wolbach, A.B., Jr.; Miner, E.J.; Isbell, H. Comparison of psilocin with psilocybin, mescaline and LSD-25. *Psychopharmacologia* **1962**, *3*, 219–223. [CrossRef]
63. Reynolds, P.C.; Jindrich, E.J. A mescaline associated fatality. *J. Anal. Toxicol.* **1985**, *9*, 183–184. [CrossRef] [PubMed]
64. Nolte, K.B.; Zumwalt, R.E. Fatal peyote ingestion associated with Mallory-Weiss lacerations. *West. J. Med.* **1999**, *170*, 328. [PubMed]
65. Kapadia, G.J.; Fayez, M.B. Peyote constituents: Chemistry, biogenesis, and biological effects. *J. Pharm. Sci.* **1970**, *59*, 1699–1727. [CrossRef] [PubMed]
66. Henry, J.L.; Epley, J.; Rohrig, T.P. The analysis and distribution of mescaline in postmortem tissues. *J. Anal. Toxicol.* **2003**, *27*, 381–382. [CrossRef]
67. Dasgupta, A. (Ed.) Abuse of Magic Mushroom, Peyote Cactus, LSD, Khat, and Volatiles. In *Critical Issues in Alcohol and Drugs of Abuse Testing*; Academic Press: Cambridge, MA, USA, 2019; pp. 477–494.
68. Dart, R.C. Natural Toxins. In *Medical Toxicology*, 3rd ed.; Dart, R.C., Ed.; Lippincott Williams & Wilkins: Philadelphia, PA, USA, 2004; p. 1706.
69. Carstairs, S.D.; Cantrell, F.L. Peyote and mescaline exposures: A 12-year review of a statewide poison center database. *Clin. Toxicol.* **2010**, *48*, 350–353. [CrossRef]
70. Wasson, R.G. Seeking the Magic Mushroom. In *LIFE Magazine*; Clair Maxwell: New York City, NY, USA, 1957.
71. Zhuk, O.; Jasicka-Misiak, I.; Poliwoda, A.; Kazakova, A.; Godovan, V.V.; Halama, M.; Wieczorek, P.P. Research on acute toxicity and the behavioral effects of methanolic extract from psilocybin mushrooms and psilocin in mice. *Toxins* **2015**, *7*, 1018–1029. [CrossRef]
72. Usdin, E. *Psychotropic Drugs and Related Compounds*; Usdin, E., Efron, D.H., Eds.; National Institute of Mental Health: Washington, DC, USA, 1972; p. 791.
73. Hollister, L.E.; Prusmack, J.J.; Paulsen, A.; Rosenquist, N. Comparison of three psychotropic drugs (psilocybin, JB-329, and IT-290) in volunteer subjects. *J. Nerv. Ment. Dis.* **1960**, *131*, 428–434. [CrossRef]
74. Gerault, A.; Picart, D. Fatal poisoning after a group of people voluntarily consumed hallucinogenic mushrooms. *Le Bulletin de la Societe Mycologique de France* **1996**, *112*, 1–14.
75. Gartz, J.; Samorini, G.; Festi, F. On the presumed French case of fatality caused by ingestion of Liberty Caps. *Eleusis* **1996**, *6*, 40–41.
76. Lim, T.H.; Wasywich, C.A.; Ruygrok, P.N. A fatal case of 'magic mushroom' ingestion in a heart transplant recipient. *Intern. Med. J.* **2012**, *42*, 1268–1269. [CrossRef]
77. Buck, R.W. Mushroom poisoning since 1924 in United States. *Mycologia* **1961**, *53*, 537–538. [CrossRef]
78. van Amsterdam, J.; Opperhuizen, A.; van den Brink, W. Harm potential of magic mushroom use: A review. *Regul. Toxicol. Pharmacol.* **2011**, *59*, 423–429. [CrossRef] [PubMed]
79. Barbee, G.; Berry-Caban, C.; Barry, J.; Borys, D.; Ward, J.; Salyer, S. Analysis of mushroom exposures in Texas requiring hospitalization, 2005–2006. *J. Med. Toxicol.* **2009**, *5*, 59–62. [CrossRef]
80. Samorini, G.; Festi, F. Le micotossicosi psicotrope volontarie in Europa. *Annali del Museo Civico di Rovereto* **1989**, *4*, 251–258.
81. Vargo, E.J.; Petroczi, A. "It Was Me on a Good Day": Exploring the Smart Drug Use Phenomenon in England. *Front. Psychol.* **2016**, *7*, 779. [CrossRef] [PubMed]

82. Esposito, M.; Cocimano, G.; Ministrieri, F.; Rosi, G.L.; Nunno, N.D.; Messina, G.; Sessa, F.; Salerno, M. Smart drugs and neuroenhancement: What do we know? *Front. Biosci. (Landmark. Ed.)* **2021**, *26*, 347–359. [CrossRef]
83. Rootman, J.M.; Kiraga, M.; Kryskow, P.; Harvey, K.; Stamets, P.; Santos-Brault, E.; Kuypers, K.P.C.; Walsh, Z. Psilocybin microdosers demonstrate greater observed improvements in mood and mental health at one month relative to non-microdosing controls. *Sci. Rep.* **2022**, *12*, 11091. [CrossRef]

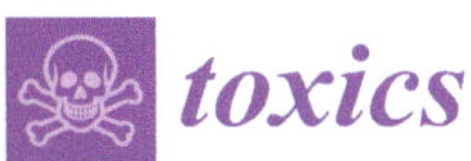

Review

Intrauterine and Neonatal Exposure to Opioids: Toxicological, Clinical, and Medico-Legal Issues

Giuseppe Davide Albano *,†, Corinne La Spina †, Walter Pitingaro, Vanessa Milazzo, Valentina Triolo, Antonina Argo, Ginevra Malta and Stefania Zerbo

Section of Legal Medicine, Department of Health Promotion, Mother and Child Care, Internal Medicine and Medical Specialties, University of Palermo, 90129 Palermo, Italy

* Correspondence: giuseppedavide.albano@unipa.it

† These authors contributed equally to this work.

Abstract: Opioids have a rapid transplacental passage (i.e., less than 60 min); furthermore, symptoms characterize the maternal and fetal withdrawal syndrome. Opioid withdrawal significantly impacts the fetus, inducing worse outcomes and a risk of mortality. Moreover, neonatal abstinence syndrome (NAS) follows the delivery, lasts up to 10 weeks, and requires intensive management. Therefore, the prevention and adequate management of NAS are relevant public health issues. This review aims to summarize the most updated evidence in the literature regarding toxicological, clinical, and forensic issues of intrauterine exposure to opioids to provide a multidisciplinary, evidence-based approach for managing such issues. Further research is required to standardize testing and to better understand the distribution of opioid derivatives in each specimen type, as well as the clinically relevant cutoff concentrations in quantitative testing results. A multidisciplinary approach is required, with obstetricians, pediatricians, nurses, forensic doctors and toxicologists, social workers, addiction specialists, and politicians all working together to implement social welfare and social services for the baby when needed. The healthcare system should encourage multidisciplinary activity in this field and direct suspected maternal and neonatal opioid intoxication cases to local referral centers.

Keywords: intrauterine; neonatal; opioids; exposure; forensic toxicology; medico-legal issues

Citation: Albano, G.D.; La Spina, C.; Pitingaro, W.; Milazzo, V.; Triolo, V.; Argo, A.; Malta, G.; Zerbo, S. Intrauterine and Neonatal Exposure to Opioids: Toxicological, Clinical, and Medico-Legal Issues. *Toxics* **2023**, *11*, 62. https://doi.org/10.3390/toxics11010062

Academic Editor: Maria Pieri

Received: 25 November 2022
Revised: 27 December 2022
Accepted: 5 January 2023
Published: 9 January 2023

1. Introduction

Heroin and methadone are the opioids most frequently used by pregnant women. It is estimated that approximately 7000 opiate-exposed births occur annually [1]. The degree of intrauterine exposure to drugs largely depends on the substance's molecular structures and the pregnancy physiology. Drugs cross the placenta more via passive diffusion and less via active transport and pinocytosis. The placenta can metabolize drugs; furthermore, it expresses enzymes, such as cytochrome P450. The fetus also metabolizes certain drugs, especially in the final stages of pregnancy. Opioids have a rapid transplacental passage (less than 60 min), and several symptoms characterize maternal and fetal withdrawal syndrome. Opioid withdrawal significantly impacts the fetus, inducing worse outcomes and a higher risk of mortality [1,2].

Moreover, neonatal abstinence syndrome (NAS) follows delivery, lasts up to 10 weeks, and requires intensive management [3]. NAS leads to irritability, tremulousness, and temperature dysregulation, as well as to a disorganized and subsequent failure to thrive. Therefore, the prevention of NAS and its adequate management are relevant public health issues [3]. Indeed, neonatal opioid intoxication requires cooperation between the public health system, social services, and the judicial system to guarantee the health of both the mother and the baby, as well as to better implement the neonatal welfare system [3,4]. This narrative review aims to summarize the most updated evidence in the literature regarding the toxicological, clinical, and medico-legal issues of intrauterine exposure to opioids. This is conducted to suggest an evidence-based, multidisciplinary approach when dealing with such cases.

2. Biological Matrices

Different matrices of maternal and fetal origin are utilized to identify uterine exposure to drugs. Monitoring drug usage during pregnancy has also been done using maternal blood, oral secretions, and sweat. However, there are no standardized tests to monitor drug use with these biological matrices, which are also not widely available. Another disadvantage for these matrices, which is due to the quick elimination of most drugs, is the reduced ability to detect remote drug intakes [5]. The detection window is narrow in the case of urine, blood, oral fluids, and sweat, rendering these matrices to be not helpful in identifying sporadic use [5–9]. As such, testing a biological matrix with a long detection window would provide a better opportunity to identify drug exposure. The ideal situation would be to identify all drugs used during pregnancy with a single sample that is easy to collect. However, this is currently impossible.

The presence of drugs in the maternal biological matrices is not always correlated to the intrauterine exposure of the fetus to these substances because of the different degrees of placental transport of drugs. Since the uterine exposure of the fetus to drugs is not directly correlated to the presence of drugs in the biological matrices of maternal origin, due to the different degrees of placental transport of these toxic substances, it is preferable to use matrices to identify any fetal exposure to drugs in biological products from the newborn [5]. Comparing the results obtained from different biological matrices allows for improvement in interpreting the results regarding drug exposure during pregnancy. Furthermore, these matrices could be used to correlate the history of drug exposure and the potential impact on the newborn's health [5]. However, in practical work, there are often differences between drug test results achieved by analyzing various biological matrices.

It must be noted that there are two methods of identifying drug users: self-reports or biological sample testing. Although no single approach can accurately determine the presence and quantity of drugs used during pregnancy, combining the toxicological examination with a structured interview could improve the identification of drug exposure [5,7,9,10]. Medical history derived from a self-report is a practical method for the purposes of identifying antenatal drug exposure. The only available way by which such information is obtained relates to the history of use during pregnancy and the quantity administered [5–7].

Unfortunately, self-reports suffer from problems resulting from a lack of information and accuracy; furthermore, pregnant women tend to underestimate or deny drug use out of fear of the consequences and the stigma associated with drug use during pregnancy [5,7]. Furthermore, an accurate history of the drugs exposure and other details are difficult to remember, thus negatively affecting the accuracy of the self-report [5–8]. The collection and the choice of the specimen in the case of a suspected intrauterine, as well as perinatal exposure to opioids, is an essential topic in forensic toxicology. Each matrix has its characteristics, advantages, and limitations, which need to be considered. Moreover, the pathologist needs to know the pharmacodynamics and pharmacokinetics of opioids to deal with a suspected case of intrauterine and neonatal opioid intoxication. In recent years, numerous authors have analyzed the best biological matrix of maternal origin, of the fetus and the newborn, in detecting intrauterine exposure to opioids. Several experimental studies have shown that the umbilical cord is an excellent matrix for the isolation of opioids, with the identification of codeine, morphine, and 6 AM. However, at the same time, they have not found identification of some synthetic opioids [9–12]. Another experimental study conducted by Colmenero et al. used different biological matrices, such as maternal hair, meconium, the umbilical cord, and the placenta, to research opioids and other drugs. Different matrices made it possible to analyze the frequency of drug use throughout the pregnancy. Maternal hair was the matrix that identified the highest number of cases and possessed the largest detection window, followed by meconium [13]. Two other scientific studies, both published in 2017, analyzed the ability of meconium, urine, and umbilical cord blood to detect intrauterine opioid exposure [14,15]; these clear findings may assist clinicians in selecting the most appropriate test to confirm a suspicion of intrauterine opioid exposure. In the following section, the properties of biological matrices are discussed.

2.1. Maternal Biological Matrices

2.1.1. Urine

Urine is the most universally used biological matrix for the purposes of drug testing on adults. This is the case because of the non-invasiveness of sample collection and the availability of standardized tests [7,16,17]. Urine can identify recent drug use within days of the sample collection. Urine is an excellent way to identify nicotine, opiates, cocaine, and amphetamines [7,18]. On this note, screening and confirmation testing are the two main types of urine drug tests. The presence of a drug or drug class is determined from screening tests when it is higher than a predefined cutoff value. When compared to confirmation tests, screening tests typically have less sensitive and specific measurements [18,19]. Definitive testing includes gas chromatography–mass spectrometry (GC-MS), liquid chromatography–mass spectrometry (LC-MS), and liquid chromatography–tandem mass spectrometry (LC-MS/MS). Although the definitive tests possess higher sensitivity and are often more expensive than the presumptive urine drug tests, the results are more accurate and trustworthy [19]. Urine is a biological matrix used to identify fetal exposure to opioids; furthermore, methadone can be detected in the urine up to 2 weeks after the last intake, and heroin up to 72 h. In addition, morphine and codeine can also be isolated in this matrix. The main disadvantage of urine is the short detection window, as it only allows the identification of drug use in the days before collection [1,16,20–22].

2.1.2. Hair

Maternal hair is the most sensitive biological sample in respect to detecting certain drugs during pregnancy, exposure to substances such alcohol, smoke, cocaine, opioids, cannabinoids, barbiturates, benzodiazepines, and methamphetamines, as well as to therapeutic drugs and common chemical compounds [8,20,21]. Adults' hair grows at a rate of about 1 cm each month; thus, this must be considered when analyzing the data. Maternal hair collected during delivery may not show drug use in the days or weeks before delivery. As such, it would be advisable to postpone the collection of maternal hair to 1 month after birth. Based on the length of the hair, the specimen should be analyzed in different portions to assess the history of drug abuse [7]. However, the biases that can be derived from the adult hair test are manifold, from the color of the hair to its texture, as well as the possible inclusion of cosmetic treatments [20].

2.1.3. Nails

The germinal matrix of the nail or the nail root under the epidermis creates layers of closely packed keratinized cells that form the nail. The newly formed keratin cells push the older cells through the cuticle, where they are differentiated (i.e., flatten and harden) to form the nail plate [5]. Adult fingernails and toenails grow distally at around 0.1 mm/d and 0.03–0.04 mm/d, respectively. However, age, sex, health status, season, environment, and exercise all affect how quickly nails can develop [5]. Maternal nail testing, based on the length of the nail that may be tested, suggests chronic exposure that may have occurred over months or weeks.

2.1.4. Breast Milk

Licit and illicit drugs can range from maternal to milk circulation through to passive diffusion or carrier-mediated drug transport. The rate of drug excretion into breast milk is determined by the physicochemical properties of the drugs (such as ionizability, lipophilicity, molecular weight, volume of distribution, lipid solubility, maternal plasma protein, and lipid binding), as well as by blood flow and circulation in the mammary glands [7,22]. Drug concentrations in breast milk are influenced by the dosage, length of use, daily milk production, genotype, which may impact how medications are metabolized, and maternal health. Several scientific studies have highlighted the presence of opioids, such as morphine, codeine, and 6-AM [22], in breast milk. Breastfeeding is advised if medicines are not concentrated in the breast milk or if the exposure is not anticipated to damage the child. The Academy of Breastfeeding Medicine Clinical Protocol#21 [23] has provided breastfeeding guidelines regarding when the use of drugs is known. In respect to mothers who are receiving methadone or buprenorphine treatment, for instance, nursing is advised because of the low levels of these medicines in breast milk. Mothers who are consuming codeine should avoid breastfeeding because of the ultrarapid metabolizers that may unintentionally expose the nursing child to extremely high levels of morphine [5,20–22].

2.1.5. Blood

Maternal blood was one of the earliest forms of biological matrix to be examined for the purposes of drug detection. For quantitative data and acute poisoning, blood is currently the best option. However, the narrow detection window and the intrusive nature of the sample collection limit the efficacy of blood tests for the long-term use of illicit drugs [8,22].

2.1.6. Sweat

Sweat is a secretion, the production of which is stimulated by the sympathetic nervous system. This system possesses the critical task of maintaining a constant body temperature. Several mechanisms are involved in respect of the deposition of drugs in sweat, such as passive diffusion and transdermal migration. There are two ways to perform a drug test with sweat: the first involves the identification of drugs taken in the last 24 h of collection, while the second method consists of applying a dermal patch in which sweat will be collected for a period of the time variable, which is usually less than one week. Sweat is a matrix that can be quickly and easily collected. Still, it is difficult to quantify the volume of sweat expelled, thereby making this matrix useful only for qualitative tests. Several scientific studies have dealt with isolating drugs such as cocaine, cannabis, and opiates in sweat [24–26].

2.1.7. Oral Fluid

Oral fluid is a compound tissue primarily formed by saliva. It is also where mixed gingival and buccal fluids, mucosal transudates, cellular debris, bacteria, and undigested food residues reside. The peculiarity of the oral fluid is that it better isolates the drug inside of it, instead of its metabolites [8,21]. Several factors influence the concentration of drugs in oral fluid [8,21]. The collection of oral fluid, even if it is easy to perform and not invasive, is often inadequate or insufficient. As such, there needs to be a standardized protocol. The detection window ranges from 30 min to 36 h, depending on the substance studied. Moreover, the scientific community has highlighted the presence of cocaine, cannabis, and even opiate in oral fluids [27–29].

The characteristics of maternal biological matrices are summarized in Table 1.

Table 1. The properties of maternal biological matrices summarized.

Maternal Biological Matrices	Advantages	Disadvantages	Detection Window
URINE	Represents the most-used matrix; The collection is easy and non-invasive.	Restricted detection window; Easily adulterate.	Few days.
HAIR	The collection is not invasive and is easy to carry out; It is a very stable matrix (even for years); It has turned out to be more sensitive than the other matrices.	Unable to detect recent drug use; Possible biases derived from the color of the hair; The detection of drugs depends on the length of the hair.	One year maximum.
NAIL	The collection is simple and non-invasive; Long detection window;	Sebum and sweat can contaminate the sample; The detection of drugs depends on their length.	Few weeks.

Table 1. *Cont.*

Maternal Biological Matrices	Advantages	Disadvantages	Detection Window
BREAST MILK	The collection is easy and non-invasive; Reflects postpartum exposure.	The collection can be performed only in women who are breastfeeding; High variability of proteins and lipids, which makes interpretation of results difficult; It is a matrix that changes during breastfeeding.	Few days.
BLOOD	It is one of the most commonly used matrices;	The collection is invasive and requires qualified personnel.	Few days.
SWEAT	The collection is easy and non-invasive; Longer urine detection window;	Harvesting can cause skin irritation; Individual variations within sweat production; Estimating the volume of sweat produced is complicated.	Few days.
ORAL FLUID	Sample collection is simple, fast, and non-invasive; Availability of devices as collection points;	It is common to collect an inadequate sample volume; The collection procedure is not standardized; Possible unintentional contamination.	Few days.

2.2. Neonatal Biological Matrices

2.2.1. Urine

Neonatal urine is usually the matrix of choice for newborn drug testing [6,8,21,30]. The first void is frequently missed because the newborn may urinate during or immediately after delivery. Furthermore, the collection is complex, and the value of collecting and testing later voids is diminished because they are less indicative of intrauterine drug exposure [5,6,21]. However, collecting urine from newborns has produced a poor yield for the purposes of detecting drug exposure. Moreover, it only reveals maternal drug use history up to a few days before the testing. In addition, there have also been reports of analytical difficulties in regard to the different distribution of drug analytes and the composition of newborn urine from adult urine [1].

2.2.2. Meconium

Meconium is a complicated, viscous substance with a dark green appearance full of metabolic waste products. It is a good choice for the purposes of determining utero drug exposures because it can potentially contain other substances to which the fetus was exposed [5,7,21,31,32]. Around the 12th week of pregnancy, meconium forms when the swallowing reflex matures; drugs go into fetal circulation directly through placental transfer and amniotic fluid ingestion, such that they are deposited in the meconium [5,6,8,20,32]. Meconium typically passes within the first one to three days of life, but in premature infants defecation may take longer [8,21]. Third-trimester exposures are more easily recognized because meconium production is nonlinear. Indeed, more than two-thirds of the meconium develops during the last eight weeks of pregnancy [5,7,8,16,20,30,32]. Meconium passage frequently takes place over several days. Meconium testing sample volumes are frequently insufficient, especially in preterm births. Additionally, the collection is often difficult because meconium is removed from a newborn's diaper. As such, the medical practitioner must be careful not to remove milk stools or urine [5,21,32]. Numerous investigations have found that meconium possesses higher drug concentrations than other matrices, probably because drugs and their metabolites build up in meconium. Gray et al. demonstrated that an increase in the proportion of opioid-positive maternal urine samples throughout the third trimester of pregnancy was associated with opioids in the meconium, notably morphine [33]. Meconium has been proven to be more sensitive than the cord tissue or the placenta in regard to detecting buprenorphine and its metabolites in babies who have been born to women receiving buprenorphine therapy. Additionally, it is better capable of detecting cocaine or opiate re-exposure [5,7,31,34]. Although meconium has been used extensively to identify utero drug exposures, collecting the specimen is time consuming and has numerous drawbacks. Generally, drug concentrations in meconium remain stable when stored at 20 °C. The high rate of false-positive results in screening procedures, particularly immunoassay approaches, is another drawback of meconium analysis [21,31,32].

During pregnancy, the umbilical cord is a lifeline connecting the growing embryo or fetus to the placenta. It possesses two umbilical arteries and one umbilical vein, which serve as conduits for oxygen, nutrients, and waste products—such as carbon dioxide—and are shielded and protected within the Wharton jelly. It is approximately 50–70 cm (20 inches) long and 2 cm (0.75 inches) in diameter at full term. In addition, the umbilical cord is formed by the fifth week of development. Similar to meconium, this naturally complex matrix necessitates effective sample preparation techniques to reduce matrix interference [5]. The weight of tissue tested, the handling and storage of the material, the quality of the specimen submitted for testing, the recovery of drug analytes from cord tissue, and the analytical sensitivity of the methods utilized can all impact the detection window for drugs in the umbilical cord. Similar to meconium, tissue also forms nonlinearly, with the third trimester serving as the time when most of the tissue is formed. As a result, there is almost no probability that first- and second-trimester maternal drug use will be discovered [5]. The umbilical cord was studied to detect the possible fetal exposure to opioids. These studies have highlighted the presence of many opioids, such as morphine and methadone [35–37].

2.2.3. Hair

Neonatal hair begins to grow from around 20 weeks of pregnancy and emerges on the scalp after about 3 weeks. It reflects exposure during the final trimester of a full-term pregnancy because it retains medications found in the fetal blood and amniotic fluid. The inability to identify medicines used during labor and delivery is a significant benefit of neonatal hair. However, because the neonate may have little to no hair, it is frequently impossible to gather enough material [5,9,21]. Several studies have focused on the detection of opioids in neonatal hair. Most molecules belonging to this class have been identified, such as morphine, codeine, m6g, 6-monoacetylmorphine, and methadone [38–40].

2.2.4. Nails

Nails start to develop around 10weeks into pregnancy, and at the end of the eighth month of pregnancy (the last trimester), the neonate's nails have grown to the tips of the fingers and toes. The neonate nail taken from the newborn represents exposure during the second and third trimesters. The disadvantages include the fact that it may be challenging to obtain enough nail samples from small newborns and that such testing is not widely available [5,21].

2.2.5. Placenta

The placenta develops at about four weeks and provides the exchange of oxygen, nutrients, and waste materials between the mother and fetus [5,8]. Most pharmaceutical drugs passively diffuse across the placenta; in addition, the amount that reaches the fetal bloodstream depends on the physicochemical characteristics of the medications and their metabolites, as well as the affinity of the drug analytes for placental drug transporters. According to animal experiments with morphine, methadone, and meperidine, opiates readily penetrate the placenta and reach their peak blood levels in the fetus soon after intravenous injection [5,8,22,41–44]. Based on its high level of lipid solubility, heroin has a high index of prenatal exposure, since it easily crosses both the blood–brain barrier and the placenta. De Castro et al. created a technique in 2009 for the purposes of measuring heroin metabolites in the placenta. Morphine was discovered, when analyzing the placentas of five pregnant opioid-dependent women, in one sample at a concentration of 41.3 ng/mg. However, 6-AM was not found, thereby rendering it impossible to detect heroin use [45]. In pregnant women receiving buprenorphine maintenance treatment, buprenorphine glucuronide concentrations in the placenta were significantly correlated with the maternal daily dose, according to Concheiro et al. [46]. The maximal NAS score and the length of the infant were both positively and adversely linked with the norbu-prenorphine/norbuprenorphine glucuronide ratio. Placenta norbuprenorphine glucuronide concentrations were also positively correlated with the time to NAS onset and negatively correlated with the duration of NAS. Moreover, buprenorphine was less accurate at predicting neonatal outcomes than was norbuprenorphine glucuronide at higher concentrations [46,47].

2.2.6. Vernix

The creamy-white film that covers the baby's skin throughout the last trimester of pregnancy and is often present on the newborn's skin at birth is known as the vernix caseosa, which is made up of a mixture of water (80.5%), protein (10%), and a fat (10%) called vernix. Although the quantity of samples available for testing varies, it is easily collected from a newborn's skin following delivery by swabbing it with gauze [5,21].

2.2.7. Amniotic Fluid

The amniotic fluid in the early stages of pregnancy comprises a filtrate of fetal cells and maternal blood. Furthermore, as the fetus grows, it gradually changes with gestational age. The fluid is similar to the fetal plasma that is found between weeks 10 and 20 of gestation; in addition, toward the second half of pregnancy, it is primarily made up of fetal secretions, such as lung fluids and urine. An amniocentesis operation is used to collect amniotic fluid; this method is intrusive and may harm the unborn child [5,8,21]. The amniotic fluid is continuously swallowed, such that the fetus may again be exposed to medicines passed on through the urine [5,8,21]. The properties of neonatal biological matrices are summarized in Table 2.

Table 2. The properties of neonatal biological matrices summarized.

Neonatal Biological Matrices	Advantages	Disadvantages	Detection Window
URINE	Specimen of choice for the purposes of newborn drug testing.	The first void is frequently missed.	Few days.
MECONIUM	The collection is not invasive; Detects drug exposure for the second and third trimesters.	This matrix is only available a few days after delivery; Easily contaminated by urine or milk stool; Identifies drugs administered during labor and delivery; Prolonged storage can alter the stability of the drugs.	Second and third trimester of pregnancy.
UMBILICAL CORD (tissue or blood)	The collection is easily carried out and done so in a single time; It does not identify the drugs taken after birth.	Identifies the medications taken during labor and delivery; Maternal blood can contaminate this matrix.	Third trimester of pregnancy.
HAIR	The sample can be stored at environmental temperature; It reflects drug exposure in the third trimester of pregnancy; Avoids the detection of drugs administered during labor and delivery.	It may be difficult or impossible to obtain; Inability to detect recent drug use; The detection of drugs depends on the length of the hair.	Few months.
NAIL	Neonatal nail collected at birth accounts for second and third trimester exposure; Avoids the detection of drugs administered after birth.	It may be challenging to obtain enough nail samples from small newborns; The test is not widely available.	Few weeks.

Table 2. *Cont.*

Neonatal Biological Matrices	Advantages	Disadvantages	Detection Window
PLACENTA	Easy and noninvasive collection; Avoids the detection of drugs administered after birth.	Requires additional sample preparation and efficient cleanup; The test is not widely available.	Few days.
VERNIX	Easy and noninvasive collection; Sample can be easily stored until analysis.	May be contaminated with urine or milk stool; Drugs administered during labor and delivery may be detected	Last 24 weeks of gestation.
AMNIOTIC FLUID	Requires minimal sample cleanup.	Risk of possible complications is associated with collection procedure; Sampling procedure is highly invasive.	Few months.

3. Analytical Issues

3.1. Preanalytical Phase

The physicochemical characteristics of the analytes and the complexity of the sample tissue or fluid from which they are to be extracted dictate the method that can be used for sample preparation [20,21]. It takes a great deal of preanalytical processing to homogenize, digest, or otherwise prepare newborn specimens that are not liquid (such as meconium and tissue) for analysis. Further preanalytical processing (such as hydrolysis and derivatization) may be carried out to reduce analytical interferences and increase the possibility of identifying the desired analyte. These specimens' analytes are typically separated and purified using certain techniques, such as liquid–liquid extraction (LLE), solid-phase extraction (SPE), and solid-phase microextraction (SPME) [5,22].

These procedures frequently entail washing processes—i.e., an acid, base, or enzymatic hydrolysis—and lengthy incubation times [7]. The extraction of drug analytes from the intricate matrix is one of the most challenging analytical problems in regard to analyzing solid specimens. For the purposes of mass spectrometric techniques, removing lipids and proteins is crucial as they could cause ion suppression and limit the detection of drug analytes [5]. Several methods, such as liquid–liquid extraction, solid-phase extraction, and supported liquid extraction, have all been used to extract drugs from meconium or umbilical cord tissue. The recovery of the drug from the matrix and the technique's sensitivity directly impacts the window of detection that is attained, such that the significance of the extraction should not be understated. Furthermore, extraction may result in the drug analytes becoming lost. In addition, it may not be uniform across all the elements of a multianalyte panel. Furthermore, how temperature affects different matrices over time and how the long-term stability of drugs and metabolites vary may need to be better understood. Positive results need to be verified using gas chromatography/mass spectrometry because immunoassay is a relatively generic test. Additionally, opioid abuse is not always linked to opioid presence confirmation [7,8,16]. Alternative causes include passive drug exposure, consuming tainted food or drink, or taking prescription drugs that either contain the drug or are converted into it [5–8].

3.2. Screening Test

Enzyme multiplied immunoassay (EMIT), fluorescence polarization immunoassay (FPI), radioimmunoassay (RIA), or ELISA 2-6 are all frequently used for screening urine;linebreak or meconium.

When using class-based immunoassays, point-of-collection/point-of-care test cups, dipstick-type strips, or automated instrumentation, hospital laboratories routinely do urine drug screening onsite.

These tests are usually performed on automatic platforms and employ antibodies that have reactivity to ward several medications in the same class; furthermore, opioid immunoassays detect the presence of codeine, morphine, hydrocodone, and hydromorphone1,2-6. However, when compared to confirmation methods, screening assays typically have the following drawbacks: limited specificity, low sensitivity, and low reactivity in respect to specific medicines within a pharmacological class. The most commonly used screening immunoassays for opioid detection are the FPI and EMIT [30,39,40,48–52].

3.3. *Confirmation Methods*

Confirmation techniques typically use either gas chromatography (GC) or liquid chromatography (LC) to separate compounds within the matrix, followed by MS for detecting and quantifying individual drug analytes. Confirmation techniques have higher sensitivity and specificity; furthermore, they are based on a different analytical principle. Due to their well-documented capacity to generate sensitive and accurate results for the purposes of drug testing, GC-MS, liquid chromatography-tandem mass spectrometry (LC-MS/MS), and liquid chromatography time-of-flight mass spectrometry (LC-TOF-MS) are all widely used for the purposes of quantitative and/or qualitative analysis [5,21,30,47–50].

Vinner et al. investigated the gestational profile of opiate exposure. They achieved this thanks to the toxicological analysis of three different matrices: maternal and neonatal urine, as well as hair and meconium using FPI and EMIT as the screening immunoassays, and GC-MS as a confirmatory method [47]. The confirmation with GC-MS for the samples resulted in a positive for the immunoassay, which allowed us to determine different opioid metabolites, such as morphine, codeine, and 6-monoacetylmorphine [51–53]. Additionally, the analysis of meconium via GC-MS can open a wide window for the detection of fetal exposure to cocaine and opiates [45,54].

The analytical issues of the revised papers are summarized in Table 3.

Table 3. A summary of the analytical methods to detect opioids in maternal and neonatal matrices.

Biological Matrices	Authors, Year	Sample Preparation	Extraction–Separation	Analytical Methods	Opioids Identified
MECONIUM	Concheiro, 2017 [30]	///	LLE	FPIA-EMIT/GC-MS	COD-MOR-6AM-METH
	Xavier Joya, 2016 [35]	Methanol	SPE	LC-MS	COD-MOR-6AM-METH
	Lozano, 2007 [39]	///	SPE	LC-MS	6AM-MOR-COD
	Vinner, 2003 [47]	///	LLE	FPIA-EMIT/GC-MS	6AM-MOR-COD–
	Marin, 2016 [49]	Methanol	SPE	LC-MS e HPLC	COD-MOR-6AM-METH
	Kintz, 1993 [51]	///	LLE	FPIA-EMIT/GC-MS	COD-MOR-6AM
	Pichini, 2003 [54]	///	SPE	LC-MS	NBUP
UMBILICAL CORD	Xavier Joya, 2016 [35]	Formic acid	SPE	LC-MS	COD-MOR-6AM-METH
	Concheiro, 2013 [36]	Acetyl nitrile	SPE	LC-MS	COD-MOR-6AM
	Stolk, 1997 [37]	Formic acid	SPE	LC-MS	MOR-METH
NEONATAL HAIR	Marchei, 2006 [38]	///	LLE	GC-MS	6AM-MOR-COD-METH
	Lozano, 2007 [39]	///	///	FPIA-EMIT/GC-MS	6AM-MOR-COD-METH
	Ostrea, 1980 [40]	///	///	FPIA-EMIT/GC-MS	COD-MOR-6AM-METH
NEONATAL URINE	Vinner, 2003 [47]	///	LLE	FPIA-EMIT/GC-MS	6AM-MOR-COD
	Kintz, 1993 [51]	///	LLE	FPIA-EMIT/GC-MS	COD-MOR-6AM
MATERNAL HAIR	Kintz, 1993 [51]	///	LLE	ELISA	///
MATERNAL URINE	Falcon, 2010 [16]	///	///	LC-MS	COD-MOR-6AM
	Vinner, 2003 [47]	///	LLE	FPIA-EMIT/GC-MS	METH
	Kintz, 1993 [51]	///	LLE	FPIA-EMIT/GC-MS	6AM-MOR-COD
MATERNAL BLOOD	Falcon, 2010 [16]	///	///	GC-MS	COD-MOR-6AM
BREAST MILK	Falcon, 2010 [16]	///	SPE	LC-MS-MS	COD-MOR-6AM

LLE: liquid–liquid extraction; SPE: solid-phase extraction; FPIA: fluorescence polarization immunoassay; EMIT: enzyme-multiplied immunoassay; GC-MS: gas chromatography–mass spectrometry; LC-MS: liquid chromatography–mass spectrometry; HPLC: high-performance liquid chromatography; ELISA: enzyme-linked immunosorbent assay; LC-MS-MS: liquid chromatography–tandem mass spectrometry; COD: codeine; MOR: morphine; 6AM: 6 acetyl morphine; METH: methadone; and NBUP: buprenorphine.

4. Clinical Issues

Over the past 10 years, opiate use during pregnancy has drastically increased and is now considered to be a serious public health issue. Prescription opioids, illicit opioids, and opioid replacement therapy are all being used by more women. According to Walsh SL et al., they issued an increase in opioid use in pregnant women because of the widespread use of acute/chronic pain treatment during pregnancy [55].

In fact, patients may receive opioid prescriptions during pregnancy for untreated opioid-use disorder, opioid abuse, or persistent pain or addiction. In addition, as Casper et al. state, mixing benzodiazepines, alcohol, or nicotine is a practice that is fairly widespread [56]. Opioids have been utilized in maintenance therapy for heroin addicts since the 1960s, but heroin substitutes are now being administered [57].

Opioid maintenance therapy is practical for at least three reasons, according to the American College of Obstetricians and Gynecologists: it decreases the mother's risk of relapsing, reduces continued high-risk activity, and improves perinatal outcomes by preventing frequent withdrawal during pregnancy [58]. Opioid maintenance therapy regimens have traditionally relied heavily on methadone, while buprenorphine use has recently increased. Pregnant women have different methadone pharmacokinetics from the general population and these pharmacokinetics can alter dramatically over the course of the pregnancy [59]. For instance, as stated by Megan W. Stover et al., among pregnant women, the half-life of methadone, from an average of 22–24 h, is reduced to 8 h. Even though methadone is typically administered daily, split-dosing (every 12 h) can be used to account for increased clearance during pregnancy [3]. Buprenorphine is a more recent alternative to opiate maintenance therapy in pregnancy. It is a partial opioid agonist approved in 2002 for the medication-assisted treatment of opiate dependence [60].

According to Jones HE et al., Buprenorphine has been shown to be superior to methadone in several ways for the management of NAS, including a lower risk of overdose (caused by reduced intrinsic receptor efficacies), less-abrupt withdrawal, fewer drug interactions, and easier access to prescriptions [61].

The abrupt cessation of fetal exposure to substances that the mother consumed or abused while she was pregnant resulted in the formation of the NAS. The term NAS is used to describe withdrawal from substance exposure; the term neonatal opioid withdrawal syndrome (NOWS) refers to the symptoms and signs that are specifically due to opioid withdrawal. Newborns exposed to opioids in utero may develop neonatal opioid withdrawal syndrome (NOWS), lower birth weight, smaller head circumference, and a higher risk of sudden infant death syndrome [62].

NAS is a multidistrict systemic disorder. The signs of neonatal abstinence have classically been divided into four major categories: involving central nervous system, gastrointestinal system, respiratory system, and autonomic nervous system. Even though NOWS seldom results in death, it can lead to significant illness and frequently necessitates prolonged hospital stays. Depending on the kind and quantity of substance consumed, the severity of this pathology's symptoms may vary [61–63].

When compared to methadone, buprenorphine sometimes decreases in the frequency and gravity of NOWS, according to newly available research. Buprenorphine has a number of drawbacks, including high dropout rates, challenging treatment start-up, a higher risk of drug diversion, possible hepatic side effects, and lack of long-term data regarding safety during pregnancy and in young children [63].

According to the Maternal Opiate Treatment Human Experimental Research's findings, pregnant women who received buprenorphine treatment had less-severe cases of NOWS and required shorter stays in hospitals than those mothers who received methadone treatment; despite this, limited evidence is available to determine the best pharmacological agents to help with maternal opioid abstinence [64].

It is widely known that the human placenta controls how chemicals and nutrients are transferred to the fetus. Drugs, pharmaceuticals, and their metabolites can pass through the placenta and into the bloodstream of the fetus with ease. A few factors that affect this placental transfer include the specific drug, the amounts of the drug in the mother's and fetus's circulations, the way and when it is administered, the mother's and fetus's genetic makeup, and the co-administration of other medications [65]. As opioids are used more often to treat chronic benign conditions, more infants are being treated for side effects from intrauterine opioid exposure. The naturally occurring opioid morphine has been the subject of almost all prenatal exposure investigations, but since 2014, there has been a 300% increase in interactions with synthetic opioids, especially fentanyl, which is 50–100 times more powerful than morphine [66,67]. Alipio et al. found that perinatal fentanyl exposure results in neurobiological deficits that last until adolescence. The effects of this exposure include the suppression of adaptation to sensory stimuli, impairment of synaptic transmission in the S1 and ACC, suppression of cortical oscillations, abnormal dendritic morphology of cortical pyramidal neurons, and altered mRNA expression of genes that regulate synaptic transmission and dendritic morphology [67]. Due to the widespread use of synthetic opioids, especially in Western countries [68], further research should focus on determining the short- and long-term effects on newborn caused by intrauterine exposure to these substances.

Healthy infants may find the shift to extrauterine life stressful; however, the adjustment is often significantly more difficult for newborns exposed to drugs while still in the womb. Several literature studies state that opioid exposure during pregnancy also greatly raises the risk of preeclampsia, stillbirth, preterm, and sudden infant death syndrome (SIDS) [64,65,69]. As suggested by Nicole A. Bailey et al., there may be a link between prenatal opioid usage and congenital defects, such spina bifida, gastroschisis, and congenital heart disease. This assertion, however, was not supported by a recent comprehensive analysis of case-control and cohort studies on the topic [69].

The first case of a neonate who manifested opioid withdrawal signs was documented in 1875, but only in 1903 was the first case successfully treated, and it was referred to as congenital morphinism in the early 1900s and is the most frequent consequence of utero opioid exposure [70]. Congenital morphinism was termed NAS by Dr. Loretta Finnegan in the 1970s [71]. Even while other drugs—including benzodiazepines, amphetamines, cocaine, and barbiturates—can cause NAS(as revealed within the study of Krans EE et al.), babies who have been exposed to opioids are more likely to develop it [71]. While opiate maintenance therapy lessens a number of unfavorable pregnancy outcomes, it does not stop the emergence of NAS [72]. All newborns exposed to opiates in utero should be closely monitored for the development of NAS/NOWS because there is a 60–80% chance that they will develop this severe illness [64], which is a finding that is in agreement with Johnson et al.

The NAS/NOWS condition, which is intricate and extremely variable, affects the newborn when the placenta is separated from the fetus at birth. It is distinguished by gastrointestinal difficulties, autonomic nervous system dysfunction, and hyperirritability of the central nervous system [73]. Excessive impatience, bad sleep, stronger muscles, tremors, and skin excoriations caused by excessive movement, overheating, diarrhea, excessive sleepiness and sweating, stuffy nose, and sneezing are all among the most frequent symptoms. Additionally, 2–11% of newborns with NAS may experience seizures. According to the findings of Seib CA et al., newborns exposed to opiates show significant variance in the timing and presentation of symptoms [74]. The causes of this variability are unclear and probably multifaceted in nature. Examples of possible causes include differences in maternal treatment, abnormalities in placental opioid metabolism, pharmacogenomics, and neonatal comorbidities, to name a few. The signs of NOWS frequently occur between 24–48 h after delivery, 36–60 h for buprenorphine and 48–72 h for methadone, depending on the prior maternal dose (but up to 5 days because of the long half-life) [75].

As claimed by Chasnoff IJ et al., drug exposures in the past, such as from using benzodiazepines, anti-depressive medications, or smoking cigarettes, may change the development of symptoms and worsen NAS [76]. The most prevalent form of evaluation (often conducted with modifications) is the Finnegan scoring system, which can identify which newborns need pharmacologic therapy. Every 3 to 4 h, a 31-item scale from the classic Finnegan scoring system is used to evaluate the prevalence and severity of different NAS-related symptoms. Every assessment should consider the conduct that was seen throughout the preceding three to four hours. It should be noted that the Finnegan scoring system has a high intra-observer variability and is specifically intended for term newborns.

Non-pharmacologic therapy is the first line of defense in the treatment of NOWS. Usually, frequent hypercaloric meals are provided to encourage growth and reduce hunger. The care of the newborn by the mother is a crucial aspect of non-pharmacologic therapy. It is believed that non-pharmacologic care of infants with NOWS deserves more attention in the care of newborns. To develop their capacity for self-regulation, newborns and caregivers must continually alter their physiological and behavioral responses. This process is known as "co-regulation", which depends on continuing experiences of both. First, giving the dyad a secure living space and supportive environment is crucial. Rooming in and the environment for a newborn with NOWS during and after the hospitalization can provide neuroprotection for a brain that is sensitive, dysregulated, and growing quickly [77].

Furthermore, the majority of newborns with NOWS require pharmacologic treatment [78]. Opioid substances (such as morphine and methadone) are generally considered more effective than other medications in treating NOWS. However, a Cochrane review released in 2010 concluded that there was not enough proof to recommend one opioid over other sedatives (phenobarbitone or diazepam) or other supportive treatments (swaddling, relaxation baths, settling, or massage). However, the use of opiates raised the treatment efficacy compared to diazepam [79]. The most suggested first-line treatment is morphine or a diluted tincture of opium taken orally [79].

Since methadone has a longer (and more variable) half-life and needs less-frequent administration and titration, it can be used instead of morphine. It is also currently being investigated as a possible drug that could be used to treat NOWS with sublingual buprenorphine [80].

Every 3–4 h, a 31-item scale from the classic Finnegan scoring system is suggested for the evaluation of the presence and severity of various NAS-related symptoms [3]. The entire 3 to 4 h preceding the exam should be considered in each evaluation. It should be noted that the Finnegan scoring system has high intra-observer variability and is mainly designed for term newborns. The maximum Finnegan score in regard to the infant's weight, or a combination of the two, is used to determine the dosage of these drugs. Second-line medications, such as phenobarbital and clonidine, are used when symptoms are still not under proper control on the highest dose of treatment. Once symptoms have been stable for 24–48 h, the tapering of pharmacologic treatment often starts [81]. Infants and children who were exposed to opioids in utero have been reported to experience negative neurodevelopmental consequences. However, the information on long-term neurodevelopmental function is scarce [82].

As stated by Megan W. and Stover et al., NOWS occurs less frequently in preterm newborns than in term babies for a variety of reasons, including the fetal CNS's immaturity, lower cumulative drug exposure, less placental transfer, delayed hepatic and placental metabolism, and a reduced drug deposition that is due to the lower fat content. It should be noted that the absence of a corroborate scoring system created specifically for these people restricts the ability to assess NAS/NOWS in preterm infants [3]. In comparison to children born without NOWS, recent research suggests that infants with NOWS are often more prone to experience developmental delays or speech or language impairments [83]. The key points of NOWS identification are summarized in Table 4.

Table 4. A summary of the key points for the identification of NOWS.

Neonatal Opioid Withdrawal Syndrome (NOWS)	
Predictive factors	• Maternal opiate dose; • Maternal maintenance agent; • Exposure to additional substances; • Gestational age.

Table 4. *Cont.*

Neonatal Opioid Withdrawal Syndrome (NOWS)	
Timing of onset of symptoms	• For heroin: 24–48 h of life; • For buprenorphine: 36–60 h of life; • For methadone: 48–72 h of life.
Symptoms	• Hyperirritability; • Autonomic nervous system dysfunction; • Seizures; • Irritability; • Poor sleep; • Hyperthermia; • Sweating; • Sneezing.
Long-term outcomes	• Attention deficit disorders; • Disruptive behavior; • Smaller brain; • Thinner cortex; • Reduced cognitive ability.
Assessment	• 4–7 days of inpatient monitoring; • Finnegan score every 3–4 h.
Non-pharmacologic treatment	• Gentle, soothing environment; • Hypercaloric feeds; • Maternal care.
Pharmacologic treatment	• Oral morphine; • Methadone; • Phenobarbital; • Clonidine.

Bradley S. and Peterson et al. found that inborn measurements of brain anatomy, tissue architecture, and metabolites showed a direct relationship with prenatal illegal drug exposure [84]. Drug-exposed newborns, particularly those who have been exposed to heroin or methadone, had smaller head sizes overall, smaller brain volumes, and lower cognitive abilities [85]. Children who have been exposed to opioids are generally more prone to exhibit disruptive behavior, attention deficit issues, and the need for thorough psychiatric treatment.

In agreement with Honein MA et al., a longitudinal study of children exposed to opioids during pregnancy may increase our understanding of the potential teratogenic effects of opioid use, such as the confounding effects of exposure to other substances during pregnancy (such as alcohol), as well as environmental and psychosocial factors [86].

In a recent assessment of the topic of opioid use during pregnancy, healthcare professionals should routinely assess all pregnant women for drug use through history and physical examinations, as well as with proven screening tools [87]. Therefore, it is crucial that individuals who provide maternal care try to identify women who use drugs and direct them toward treatment choices.

According to the American Society of Addiction, a urine screening test to identify drug abuse should be conducted according to state regulations, which vary by state of residence, with the patient's permission, and to confirm reported or suspected drug usage [88]. Neonatal toxicology testing should start as soon as a baby is born to a mother who has used drugs previously or is suspected of doing so. All delivery staff members must be aware of drug use to help the neonate adapt to extrauterine life and provide neonatal or pediatric support.

In correspondence with the findings of Wong S. et al., the midwife may be tasked with ordering neonatal toxicological tests in the role of the intrapartum healthcare practitioner. If the collection takes place along with the first two emissions of urine, newborn pee analysis can identify recent maternal drug use [89]. As meconium toxicology tests show drug usage as early as the second trimester, the data provided a more detailed description of drug use by the pregnant mother. Umbilical blood collection is less invasive and more valuable than urine or meconium collection and is a possible third technique used for newborn toxicity testing. Finally, another form of toxicity screening involves the utilization of maternal and neonatal hair.

When a newborn toxicology test yields a positive result, healthcare professionals must take into consideration the fact that the baby had drug exposure during the pregnancy and is thus at risk for NOWS. The Finnegan neonatal abstinence scoring tool (FNAST) may be used by neonatal caregivers to thoroughly and objectively evaluate the newborn's withdrawal signs and symptoms. The scoring of the FNAST should start two hours after birth and should continue every three to four hours while the infant is receiving care. The FNAST extends for at least 48 to 72 h after withdrawal agents are stopped and includes all NOWS signs and symptoms experienced during withdrawal and management [90].

The eat, sleep, and console (ESC) approach, which was recently introduced and was first published by Grossman et al. in 2017, has introduced a different paradigm that emphasizes nonpharmacologic management of infants' symptoms and offers a framework for starting treatment based on functional impairment [91]. The clinical management of newborn opioid withdrawal syndrome is based on the ESC model (NOWS). The Finnegan scoring system and ESC system were compared in the study conducted by Kelsey Ryan et al. They found that ESC scores correlated with components of the Finnegan score system that predict the severity of NOWS; on the other hand, the ESC system did not associate with elements of the Finnegan score that do not predict the severity of NOWS. They also suggest that transitioning from the Finnegan score to the ESC system could reduce hospitalization and dependency on pharmacologic treatment for newborns affected by NOWS [92].

A neonatologist must be informed of the circumstances to adequately evaluate the child and perhaps even transfer care to a neonatal unit that is equipped to help a newborn with NOWS if the neonatal team is not currently caring for the baby. Infants and children exposed to opioids in utero have been reported to experience negative neurodevelopmental consequences. However, as most studies are small and cannot distinguish between the effects of in utero exposures, postnatal treatments, and environmental variables, there is a shortage of information addressing long-term neurodevelopmental function. Children exposed to opioids are more likely to exhibit disruptive behavior, attention deficit issues, and the requirement for a thorough psychiatric referral. Long-term follow-up is, for this reason, a relevant public health issue.

5. Medico-Legal Issues

Pregnancy-related opiate misuse carries a number of dangers, most of which are connected to the consequences of withdrawal for the mother and her fetus, or the concurrent hazards of any associated behaviors. It may be challenging for a pregnant mother to abruptly stop using opioids. Others may rely on drugs such as methadone to stop drug relapse during pregnancy [93]. A drug should be stopped if it is considered unsafe for both the mother and the fetus. In agreement with what the American Pregnancy Association states, any substance taken while pregnant must be viewed as potentially dangerous to the fetus; in addition, the risks versus the benefits of its use should be carefully weighed [94]. Furthermore, abusing these drugs puts the health of the developing child, the neonate, and the fetus at risk. As such, this represents a serious public health problem [95].

As reported by Megan T. Frey et al., many female opioid abusers engage in polysubstance misuse, frequently in an effort to treat an underlying mental health condition or alleviate withdrawal symptoms with more accessible drugs [96]. Women who use substances are more likely to self-report conditions like high poverty rates, intimate partner violence, a history of physical or sexual abuse, post-traumatic stress disorder, and mental illness [97]. Although there has been a simultaneous rise in both child welfare cases and opioid use disorders, according to Korry et al., the two developments cannot be directly connected at this time because of data limitations [98].

Local child welfare institutions state that the opioid epidemic can be blamed for the recent uptick in incidents of neglect and abuse [99]. Due to concerns about losing their children to child protection service investigations, as a study by Falletta et al. observed, some mothers were not allowed to receive treatment or were delayed, while other pregnant women avoided receiving treatment in order not to undergo drug tests [99].

According to the National Institute on Drug Abuse, addiction is a chronic condition that can be successfully managed and treated like other chronic disease processes. Social support, the quality of the patient–provider relationship, and access to therapy are all necessary to successfully treat substance-use disorders. In accordance with the ethical rule of nonmaleficence, doctors must refrain from employing humiliation or unfavorable criticism to persuade women to seek or continue receiving care. Pregnant addicts experience humiliation and criticism on top of their already high personal and societal obligations because they appear to go against the conventional moral expectation that pregnant women act in the best interest of the fetus. Criminalizing women for possessing chronic health issues while pregnant is unethical from a medical and moral standpoint and feeds societal stigmas. Regardless of existence, the right to be born healthy and protected, including throughout the intrauterine phase, must be recognized, whether interpreted as a subject or as a person, based on the many interpretations.

The implementation of integrated care systems that offer medical treatment, social services, and mental support has resulted in a great decrease in substance usage and relapse [96–99].

When faced with the suspicion that a child may suffer or risk suffering injuries, physical or mental, handicap, or pathological conditions that highlight a condition of abuse or negligence, health professionals must report the case in question. According to the Italian jurisdiction, the patient must consent before any medical procedure. If the mother does not want to agree to have blood or urine taken, these tests cannot be conducted. In the case of a minor, especially a newborn, who cannot yet act, the parents must provide consent to proceed with the medical procedures. However, suppose the doctor decides that specific investigations are required because he believes the child's life may be at risk because of negligence or drug misuse. In that case, he must contact the appropriate judicial authority. In all healthcare settings worldwide, mainly where a high rate of opioid abuse is observed during pregnancy, standard protocol and screening and clinical testing strategies should be implemented to anticipate diagnosis and point out further actions in cooperation with social services and judicial authorities to protect and guarantee adequate health and assistance for both the mother and the newborn [100].

To inform the family about the best ways to care for the infant, the mother's healthcare professional should collaborate with neonatal care specialists. The consultation of social services guarantees that the newborn's post-hospital care is adequate and suitable in accordance with the Child Abuse Prevention and Treatment Act. It is imperative to motivate women who are opioid dependent to seek out and keep up with medical care. As a result, it will be important to test not only those women who voluntarily admit to abusing opioids but also those who have medical disorders and where doctors note the risk of abuse or neonatal suffering.

A study conducted by Green et al. states that children of substance-using mothers who finish at a minimum one recovery period spend a shorter time in protective custody and are successfully reunited with their parents more frequently [101]. Although it can be challenging to obtain Child Protection Services (CPS) clients for participation in substance-misuse treatment, according to Taplin et al., half of the women who enroll in these programs are mothers of dependent children, and one-third of these have lost parental rights [102]. Knowing how other social institutions, such as the criminal justice system, can either facilitate or obstruct treatment may provide one with a more comprehensive viewpoint on the best way to include opioid abusing in the child welfare system. Supplementary studies are required to better understand how child protection services and drug misuse treatment programs interact and what effects they have on individual results.

To give clarity and direction to policymakers at the national and local levels, it is crucial to collaborate and coordinate guidelines, advocacy positions, and research projects involving prenatal substance use and NAS. This literature review highlights the necessity of a multidisciplinary approach in cases of neonatal opioid intoxication. Cooperation between different professional figures is, in fact, crucial to substantially impacting the critical public health issue confronting our vulnerable population [1,103–105]. The gynecologist has the role of following the regular course of pregnancy, identifying the risk conditions, and promoting the well-being of the fetus and mother. The pediatrician and the neonatologist must clinically identify the clinical factors suggesting an intoxication or a neonatal abstinence syndrome, thereby ensuring the newborn's health and initiating the process of protection, welfare, and judicial investigations. The role of the forensic toxicologist is essential for the purposes of detecting exposure to opioids, thereby choosing the appropriate matrix to be used and providing laboratory elements on which to base clinical, social, and forensic options [2,106,107]. A critical public health measure could consist of establishing territorial referral centers for these conditions to guarantee the presence of specialized personnel to recognize and identify neonatal opioid intoxication and NAS/NOWS. Research and development are urgently needed to improve the identification, care, and protection of high-risk neonates as the number of births impacted by maternal opiate dependency keeps growing.

6. Conclusions

Protecting newborns and mothers requires a standardized method to detect opioid use and exposure during and after pregnancy. The choice of the appropriate specimen to analyze for the purpose of detecting in utero drug exposure will depend on the availability of the specimen, as well as on specific clinical and forensic issues. Each specimen has advantages and limitations. Urine or meconium screening of the newborn typically provides essential information to clarify intrauterine and perinatal opioid exposure. Although urine screening is simple to administer, it has the drawback of only identifying recent exposures. The benefit of meconium testing is that it can screen for drug exposure going back as far as 20 weeks of gestation. Further research is required to standardize testing and to better understand the distribution of opioid derivatives in each specimen type, as well as the clinically relevant cutoff concentrations in quantitative testing results. To best care for pregnant women with opioid disorders, the fetus, and the neonate following birth, healthcare personnel must get training that promotes multidisciplinary care and cuts across barriers between specialized areas. To implement social welfare and ensure that the baby has appropriate custody when necessary, a multidisciplinary approach is required, involving the collaboration of obstetricians, pediatricians, nurses, forensic physicians and toxicologists, social workers, addiction specialists, and politicians. The healthcare system should encourage multidisciplinary activity in this field and direct suspected maternal and neonatal opioid intoxication cases to local referral centers.

Author Contributions: Conceptualization, G.D.A., C.L.S. and S.Z.; methodology, A.A., S.Z. and G.D.A.; writing—original draft preparation, C.L.S., W.P., V.M., V.T. and G.M.; writing—review and editing, A.A., S.Z. and G.D.A.; visualization, G.M. and V.T.; supervision, A.A. and S.Z. All authors have read and agreed to the published version of the manuscript.

Funding: This research received no external funding.

Institutional Review Board Statement: The study was conducted in accordance with the Declaration of Helsinki. An Institutional Ethics Committee Statement is not required for this study.

Informed Consent Statement: Not applicable.

Data Availability Statement: Data sharing is not applicable; no new data were created or analyzed.

Conflicts of Interest: The authors declare no conflict of interest.

References

1. Bhuvaneswar, C.G.; Chang, G.; Epstein, L.A.; Stern, T.A. Cocaine and opioid use during pregnancy: Prevalence and management. *Prim. Care Companion L Clin. Psychiatry* **2008**, *10*, 59–65. [CrossRef] [PubMed]
2. Guerrini, K.; Argo, A.; Borroni, C.; Catalano, D.; Dell'acqua, L.; Farè, F.; Procaccianti, P.; Roda, G.; Gambaro, V. Development and validation of a reliable method for studying the distribution pattern for opiates metabolites in brain. *J. Pharm. Biomed Anal.* **2013**, *73*, 125–130. [CrossRef] [PubMed]
3. Stover, M.W.; Davis, J.M. Opioids in pregnancy and neonatal abstinence syndrome. *Semin. Perinatol.* **2015**, *39*, 561–565. [CrossRef] [PubMed]
4. Basilicata, P.; Pieri, M.; Simonelli, A.; Capasso, E.; Casella, C.; Noto, T.; Policino, F.; Di Lorenzo, P. Diquat Poisoning: Care Management and Medico-LegalImplications. *Toxics* **2022**, *10*, 166. [CrossRef]
5. Wabuyele, S.L.; Colby, J.M.; McMillin, G.A. Detection of drug-exposed newborns. *Ther. Drug Monit.* **2018**, *40*, 166–185. [CrossRef]
6. Wang, P.; Molina, C.P.; Maldonado, J.E.; Bernard, D.W. In utero drugs of abuse exposure testing for newborn twins. *J. Clin. Pathol.* **2010**, *63*, 259–261. [CrossRef]
7. Behnke, M.; Smith, V.C. Prenatal substance abuse: Short- and long-term effects on the exposed fetus. *Pediatrics* **2013**, *131*, 1009–1024. [CrossRef] [PubMed]
8. Lozano, J.; García-Algar, O.; Vall, O.; De La Torre, R.; Scaravelli, G.; Pichini, S. Biological matrices for the evaluation of in utero exposure to drugs of abuse. *Ther. Drug Monit.* **2007**, *29*, 711–734. [CrossRef]
9. Knight, S.J.; Smith, A.D.; Wright, T.E.; Collier, A.C. Detection of opioids in umbilical cord lysates: An antibody-based rapid screening approach. *Toxicol. Mech. Methods* **2019**, *29*, 35–42. [CrossRef]
10. Jones, J.T.; Jones, M.; Jones, B.; Sulaiman, K.; Plate, C.; Lewis, D. Detection of codeine, morphine, 6-monoacetylmorphine, and meconin in human umbilical cord tissue: Method validation and evidence of in utero heroin exposure. *Ther. Drug Monit.* **2015**, *37*, 45. [CrossRef]
11. Mamillapalli, S.S.; Smith-Joyner, A.; Forbes, L.; McIntyre, K.; Poppenfuse, S.; Rushing, B.; Ravisankar, S. Screening for Opioid and Stimulant Exposure In Utero Through Targeted and Untargeted Metabolomics Analysis of Umbilical Cords. *Ther. Drug Monit.* **2020**, *42*, 787–794. [CrossRef] [PubMed]
12. Marin, S.J.; Metcalf, A.; Krasowski, M.D.; Linert, B.S.; Clark, C.J.; Strathmann, F.G.; McMillin, G.A. Detection of neonatal drug exposure using umbilical cord tissue and liquid chromatography time-of-flight mass spectrometry. *Ther. Drug Monit.* **2014**, *36*, 119–124. [CrossRef] [PubMed]
13. González-Colmenero, E.; Concheiro-Guisán, A.; Lorenzo-Martínez, M.; Concheiro, M.; Lendoiro, E.; de-Castro-Ríos, A.; Fernández-Lorenzo, J.R. Drug testing in biological samples vs. maternal surveys for the detection of substance use during whole pregnancy. *J. Addict. Dis.* **2020**, *39*, 175–182. [CrossRef] [PubMed]
14. Colby, J.M. Comparison of umbilical cord tissue and meconium for the confirmation of in utero drug exposure. *Clin. Biochem.* **2017**, *50*, 784–790. [CrossRef] [PubMed]
15. Stabler, M.; Giacobbi, P., Jr.; Chertok, I.; Long, L.; Cottrell, L.; Yossuck, P. Comparison of Biological Screening and Diagnostic Indicators to Detect In Utero Opiate and Cocaine Exposure Among Mother–Infant Dyads. *Ther. Drug Monit.* **2017**, *39*, 640–647. [CrossRef]
16. Falcon, M.; Pichini, S.; Joya, J.; Pujadas, M.; Sanchez, A.; Vall, O.; Pellegrini, M. Maternal hair testing for the assessment of fetal exposure to drug of abuse during early pregnancy: Comparison with testing in placental and fetal remains. *Forensic Sci. Int.* **2012**, *218*, 92–96. [CrossRef]
17. Argo, A.; Zerbo, S.; Buscemi, R.; Trignano, C.; Bertol, E.; Albano, G.D.; Vaiano, F. A Forensic Diagnostic Algorithm for Drug-Related Deaths: A Case Series. *Toxics* **2022**, *10*, 152. [CrossRef]
18. Barthwell, A.G.; Allgaier, J.; Egli, K. Definitive urine drug testing in office-based opioid treatment: A literature review. *Crit. Rev. Toxicol.* **2018**, *48*, 829–852. [CrossRef] [PubMed]
19. Snyder, M.L.; Fantz, C.R.; Melanson, S. Immunoassay-Based Drug Tests Are Inadequately Sensitive for Medication Compliance Monitoring in PatientsTreated for Chronic Pain. *Pain Physician* **2017**, *20*, SE1–SE9.
20. Carlier, J.; La Maida, N.; Di Trana, A.; Huestis, M.A.; Pichini, S.; Busardò, F.P. Testing unconventional matrices to monitor for prenatal exposure to heroin, cocaine, amphetamines, syntheticcathinones, and synthetic opioids. *Ther. Drug. Monit.* **2020**, *42*, 205–221. [CrossRef]
21. Gray, T.; Huestis, M. Bioanalytical procedures for monitoring in utero drug exposure. *Anal. Bioanal. Chem.* **2007**, *388*, 1455–1465. [CrossRef] [PubMed]
22. Płotka, J.; Narkowicz, S.; Polkowska, Ż.; Biziuk, M.; Namieśnik, J. Effects of addictive substances during pregnancy and infancy and their analysis in biological materials. *Rev. Environ. Contam. Toxicol.* **2014**, *227*, 55–77. [PubMed]
23. Reece-Stremtan, S.; Marinelli, K.A.; Academy of Breastfeeding Medicine. ABM clinical protocol# 21: Guidelines for breastfeeding and substance use or substance use disorder, revised 2015. *Breast Feed. Med.* **2015**, *10*, 135–141.
24. Kacinko, S.L.; Barnes, A.J.; Schwilke, E.W.; Cone, E.J.; Moolchan, E.T.; Huestis, M.A. Disposition of cocaine and its metabolites in human sweat after controlled cocaine administration. *Clin. Chem.* **2005**, *51*, 2085–2094. [CrossRef] [PubMed]
25. Schwilke, E.W.; Barnes, A.J.; Kacinko, S.L.; Cone, E.J.; Moolchan, E.T.; Huestis, M.A. Opioid disposition in human sweat after controlled oral codeine administration. *Clin. Chem.* **2006**, *52*, 1539–1545. [CrossRef]

26. Saito, T.; Wtsadik, A.; Scheidweiler, K.B.; Fortner, N.; Takeichi, S.; Huestis, M.A. Validated gas chromatographic-negative ion chemical ionization mass spectrometric method for delta(9)-tetrahydrocannabinol in sweat patches. *Clin. Chem.* **2004**, *50*, 2083–2090. [CrossRef] [PubMed]
27. Mortier, K.A.; Maudens, K.E.; Lambert, W.E.; Clauwaert, K.M.; Van Bocxlaer, J.F.; Deforce, D.L.; Van Peteghem, C.H.; De Leenheer, A.P. Simultaneous, quantitative determination of opiates, amphetamines, cocaine and benzoylecgonine in oral fluid by liquid chromatography quadrupole-time-of-flight mass spectrometry. *J. Chromatogr. B Anal. Technol. Biomed. Life Sci.* **2002**, *779*, 321–330. [CrossRef]
28. Kintz, P.; Cirimele, V.; Ludes, B. Detection of cannabis in oral fluid (saliva) and forehead wipes (sweat) from impaired drivers. *J. Anal. Toxicol.* **2000**, *24*, 557–561. [CrossRef]
29. Toennes, S.W.; Kauert, G.F.; Steinmeyer, S.; Moeller, M.R. Driving under the influence of drugs—Evaluation of analytical data of drugs in oralfluid, serum and urine, and correlation with impairment symptoms. *Forensic Sci. Int.* **2005**, *152*, 149–155. [CrossRef]
30. Concheiro, M.; Lendoiro, E.; de Castro, A.; Gónzalez-Colmenero, E.; Concheiro-Guisan, A.; Peñas-Silva, P.; Macias-Cortiña, M.; Cruz-Landeira, A.; López-Rivadulla, M. Bioanalysis for cocaine, opiates, methadone, and amphetamines exposure detection during pregnancy. *Drug Test. Anal.* **2017**, *9*, 898–904. [CrossRef]
31. Marin, S.J.; Keith, L.; Merrell, M.; McMillin, G.A. Comparison of drugs of abuse detection in meconium by EMIT II and ELISA. *J. Anal. Toxicol.* **2009**, *33*, 148–154. [CrossRef] [PubMed]
32. Gareri, J.; Klein, J.; Koren, G. Drugs of abuse testing in meconium. *Clin. Chim. Acta* **2006**, *366*, 101–111. [CrossRef] [PubMed]
33. López, P.; Bermejo, A.M.; Tabernero, M.J.; Fernández, P.; Alvarez, I. Determination of cocaine and heroin with their respective metabolites in meconium by gas chromatography-mass spectrometry. *J. Appl. Toxicol.* **2007**, *27*, 464–471. [CrossRef] [PubMed]
34. Strano-Rossi, S. Methods used to detect drug abuse in pregnancy: A brief review. *Drug Alcohol. Depend.* **1999**, *53*, 257–271. [CrossRef]
35. Joya, X.; Marchei, E.; Salat-Batlle, J.; García-Algar, O.; Calvaresi, V.; Pacifici, R.; Pichini, S. Drugs of abuse in maternal hair and paired neonatal meconium: An objective assessment of fetal exposure to gestational consumption. *Drug Test. Anal.* **2016**, *8*, 864–868. [CrossRef] [PubMed]
36. Concheiro, M.; González-Colmenero, E.; Lendoiro, E.; Concheiro-Guisán, A.; de Castro, A.; Cruz-Landeira, A.; López-Rivadulla, M. Alternative matrices for cocaine, heroin, and methadone in utero drug exposure detection. *Ther. Drug Monit.* **2013**, *35*, 502–509. [CrossRef]
37. Stolk, L.M.; Coenradie, S.M.; Smit, B.J.; van As, H.L. Analysis of methadone and its primary metabolite in meconium. *J. Anal. Toxicol.* **1997**, *21*, 154–159. [CrossRef]
38. Marchei, E.; Pellegrini, M.; Pacifici, R.; Palmi, I.; Lozano, J.; García-Algar, O.; Pichini, S. Quantification of Delta9-tetrahydrocannabinol and its major metabolites in meconium by gas chromatographic-mass spectrometric assay: Assay validation and preliminary results of the "meconium project". *Ther. Drug Monit.* **2006**, *28*, 700–706. [CrossRef]
39. Lozano, J.; García-Algar, O.; Marchei, E.; Vall, O.; Monleon, T.; Giovannandrea, R.D.; Pichini, S. Prevalence of gestational exposure to cannabis in a Mediterranean city by meconium analysis. *Acta Paediatr.* **2007**, *96*, 1734–1737. [CrossRef]
40. Ostrea, E.M., Jr.; Lynn, S.M.; Wayne, R.N.; Stryker, J.C. Tissue distribution of morphine in the newborns of addicted monkeys and humans. *Dev. Pharmacol. Ther.* **1980**, *1*, 163–170. [CrossRef]
41. De Giovanni, N.; Marchetti, D. Cocaine and its metabolites in the placenta: A systematic review of the literature. *Reprod. Toxicol.* **2012**, *33*, 1–14. [CrossRef] [PubMed]
42. Szeto, H.H. Kinetics of drug transfer to the fetus. *Clin. Obstet. Gynecol.* **1993**, *36*, 246–254. [CrossRef] [PubMed]
43. Silvestre, M.A.; Lucena, J.E.; Roxas, R., Jr.; Evangelista, E.S.; Ostrea, E.M., Jr. Effects of timing, dosage, and duration of morphine intake during pregnancy on the amount of morphine in meconiuminarat model. *Biol. Neonate* **1997**, *72*, 112–117. [CrossRef]
44. ElSohly, M.A.; Stanford, D.F.; Murphy, T.P.; Lester, B.M.; Wright, L.L.; Smeriglio, V.L.; Verter, J.; Bauer, C.R.; Shankaran, S.; Bada, H.S.; et al. Immunoassay and GC-MS procedures for the analysis of drugs of abuse in meconium. *J. Anal. Toxicol.* **1999**, *23*, 436–445. [CrossRef] [PubMed]
45. de Castro, A.; Concheiro, M.; Shakleya, D.M.; Huestis, M.A. Simultaneous quantification of methadone, cocaine, opiates, and metabolites in human placenta by liquid chromatography-mass spectrometry. *J. Anal. Toxicol.* **2009**, *33*, 243–252. [CrossRef]
46. Concheiro, M.; Jones, H.E.; Johnson, R.E.; Choo, R.; Shakleya, D.M.; Huestis, M.A. Maternal buprenorphine dose, placenta buprenorphine and metabolite concentrations and neonatal outcomes. *Ther. Drug Monit.* **2010**, *32*, 206. [CrossRef]
47. Vinner, E.; Vignau, J.; Thibault, D.; Codaccioni, X.; Brassart, C.; Humbert, L.; Lhermitte, M. Hair analysis of opiates in mothers and newborns for evaluating opiate exposure during pregnancy. *Forensic Sci. Int.* **2003**, *133*, 57–62. [CrossRef]
48. Bertol, E.; Argo, A.; Procaccianti, P.; Vaiano, F.; Di Milia, M.G.; Furlanetto, S.; Mari, F. Detection of gamma-hydroxybutyrate in hair: Validation of GC-MS and LC-MS/MS methods and application to a real case. *J. Pharm. Biomed. Anal.* **2012**, *70*, 518–522. [CrossRef]
49. Marin, S.J.; McMillin, G.A. Quantitation of Total Buprenorphine and Norbuprenorphine in Meconium by LC-MS/MS. *Methods Mol. Biol.* **2016**, *1383*, 59–68.
50. Argo, A.; Spatola, G.F.; Zerbo, S.; Sortino, C.; Lanzarone, A.; Uzzo, M.L.; Pitruzzella, A.; Farè, F.; Roda, G.; Gambaro, V.; et al. A possible biomarker for methadonerelateddeaths. *J. Forensic Leg. Med.* **2017**, *49*, 8–14. [CrossRef]
51. Kintz, P.; Mangin, P. Determination of gestational opiate, nicotine, benzodiazepine, cocaine and amphetamine exposure by hair analysis. *J. Forensic Sci. Soc.* **1993**, *33*, 139–142. [CrossRef] [PubMed]

52. Lester, B.M.; ElSohly, M.; Wright, L.L.; Smeriglio, V.L.; Verter, J.; Bauer, C.R.; Shankaran, S.; Bada, H.S.; Walls, H.H.; Huestis, M.A.; et al. The Maternal Lifestyle Study: Drug use by meconium toxicology and maternal self-report. *Pediatrics* **2001**, *107*, 309–317. [CrossRef]
53. Gray, T.R.; Choo, R.E.; Concheiro, M.; Williams, E.; Elko, A.; Jansson, L.M.; Jones, H.E.; Huestis, M.A. Prenatal methadone exposure, meconium biomarker concentrations and neonatal abstinence syndrome. *Addiction* **2010**, *105*, 2151–2159. [CrossRef] [PubMed]
54. Pichini, S.; Pacifici, R.; Pellegrini, M.; Marchei, E.; Pérez-Alarcón, E.; Puig, C.; Vall, O.; García-Algar, O. Development and validation of a liquid chromatography-mass spectrometry assay for the determination of opiates and cocaine in meconium. *J. Chromatogr. B Anal. Technol. Biomed. Life Sci.* **2003**, *794*, 281–292. [CrossRef] [PubMed]
55. Walsh, S.L.; Preston, K.L.; Stitzer, M.L.; Cone, E.J.; Bigelow, G.E. Clinical pharmacology of buprenorphine: Ceiling effects at high doses. *Clin. Pharm. Therap.* **1994**, *55*, 569–580. [CrossRef] [PubMed]
56. Casper, T.; Arbour, M.W. Identification of the pregnant woman who is using drugs: Implications for perinatal and neonatal care. *J. Midwifery Womens Health* **2013**, *58*, 697–701. [CrossRef] [PubMed]
57. Joseph, H.; Stancliff, S.; Langrod, J. Methadone maintenance treatment (MMT): A review of historical and clinical issues. *Mt. Sinai. J. Med.* **2000**, *67*, 347–364. [PubMed]
58. American College of Obstetricians and Gynecologists. Opioid abuse, dependence, and addiction in pregnancy. Committee Opinion No. 524. *Obstet. Gynecol.* **2012**, *119*, 1070–1076. [CrossRef]
59. Bell, J.R.; Butler, B.; Lawrance, A.; Batey, R.; Salmelainen, P. Comparing overdose mortality associated with methadone and buprenorphine treatment. *Drug Alcohol. Depend.* **2009**, *104*, 73–77. [CrossRef]
60. Kraft, W.K.; Dysart, K.; Greenspan, J.S.; Gibson, E.; Kaltenbach, K.; Ehrlich, M.E. Revised dose schema of sublingual buprenorphine in the treatment of the neonatal opioid abstinence syndrome. *Addiction* **2011**, *106*, 574–580. [CrossRef]
61. Jones, H.E.; Kaltenbach, K.; Heil, S.H.; Stine, S.M.; Coyle, M.G.; Arria, A.M.; O'Grady, K.E.; Selby, P.; Martin, P.R.; Fischer, G. Neonatal abstinence syndrome after methadone or buprenorphine exposure. *N. Engl. J. Med.* **2010**, *363*, 2320–2331. [CrossRef] [PubMed]
62. Velez, M.L.; Jordan, C.; Jansson, L.M. Reconceptualizing non-pharmacologic approaches to Neonatal Abstinence Syndrome (NAS) and Neonatal Opioid Withdrawal Syndrome (NOWS): A theoretical and evidence–based approach. Part II: The clinical application of nonpharmacologic care for NAS/NOWS. *Neurotoxicol. Teratol.* **2021**, *88*, 107032. [CrossRef] [PubMed]
63. Jones, H.E.; Heil, S.H.; Baewert, A.; Arria, A.M.; Kaltenbach, K.; Martin, P.R.; Coyle, M.G.; Selby, P.; Stine, S.M.; Fischer, G. Buprenorphine treatment of opioid-dependent pregnant women: A comprehensive review. *Addiction* **2012**, *107*, 5–27. [CrossRef] [PubMed]
64. Johnson, R.E.; Jones, H.E.; Fischer, G. Use of buprenorphine in pregnancy: Patient management and effects on the neonate. *Drug Alcohol. Depend.* **2003**, *70*, 87–101. [CrossRef]
65. D'Apolito, K. Neonatal opiate withdrawal: Pharmacologic management. *Newborn Infant. Nurs. Rev.* **2009**, *9*, 62–69. [CrossRef]
66. Alipio, J.B.; Haga, C.; Fox, M.E.; Arakawa, K.; Balaji, R.; Cramer, N.; Lobo, M.K.; Keller, A. Perinatal fentanyl exposure leads to long-lasting impairments in somatosensory circuit function and behavior. *J. Neurosci.* **2021**, *41*, 3400–3417. [CrossRef]
67. Nellhaus, E.M.; Murray, S.; Hansen, Z.; Loudin, S.; Davies, T.H. Novel withdrawal symptoms of a neonate prenatally exposed to a fentanyl analog. *J. Pediatr. Health Care* **2019**, *33*, 102–106. [CrossRef]
68. Spencer, M.R.; Warner, M.; Bastian, B.A.; Trinidad, J.P.; Hedegaard, H. Drug overdose deaths involving fentanyl, 2011–2016. *Natl. Vital Stat. Rep.* **2019**, *68*, 1–19.
69. Lind, J.N.; Interrante, J.D.; Ailes, E.C.; Gilboa, S.M.; Khan, S.; Frey, M.T.; Dawson, A.L.; Honein, M.A.; Dowling, N.F.; Razzaghi, H.; et al. Maternal use of opioids during pregnancy and congenital malformations: A systematic review. *Pediatrics* **2017**, *139*, e20164131. [CrossRef]
70. Bailey, N.A.; Diaz-Barbosa, M. Effect of Maternal Substance Abuse on the Fetus, Neonate, and Child. *Pediatr. Rev.* **2018**, *39*, 550–559. [CrossRef]
71. Krans, E.E.; Patrick, S.W. Opioid Use Disorder in Pregnancy: Health Policy and Practice in the Midst of an Epidemic. *Obstet. Gynecol.* **2016**, *128*, 4–10. [CrossRef]
72. Swift, R.M.; Dudley, M.; DePetrillo, P.; Camara, P.; Griffiths, W. Altered methadone pharmacokinetics in pregnancy: Implications for dosing. *J. Subst. Abuse* **1989**, *1*, 453–460. [CrossRef] [PubMed]
73. Haight, S.C.; Ko, J.Y.; Tong, V.T.; Bohm, M.K.; Callaghan, W.M. Opioid use disorder documented at delivery hospitalization—United States, 1999–2014. *Morb. Mortal. Wkly. Rep.* **2018**, *67*, 845. [CrossRef] [PubMed]
74. Seib, C.A.; Daglish, M.; Heath, R.; Booker, C.; Reid, C.; Fraser, J. Screening for alcohol and drug use in pregnancy. *Midwifery* **2012**, *28*, 760–764. [CrossRef] [PubMed]
75. Winkelman, T.N.; Villapiano, N.; Kozhimannil, K.B.; Davis, M.M.; Patrick, S.W. Incidence and costs of neonatal abstinence syndrome among infants with Medicaid: 2004–2014. *Pediatrics* **2018**, *141*, e20173520. [CrossRef] [PubMed]
76. Chasnoff, I.J.; McGourty, R.F.; Bailey, G.W.; Hutchins, E.; Lightfoot, S.O.; Pawson, L.L.; Fahey, C.; May, B.; Brodie, P.; McCulley, L.; et al. The 4P's Plus screen for substance use in pregnancy: Clinical application and outcomes. *J. Perinatol.* **2005**, *25*, 368–374. [CrossRef] [PubMed]
77. Pahl, A.; Young, L.; Buus-Frank, M.E.; Marcellus, L.; Soll, R. Non-pharmacological care for opioid withdrawal in newborns. *Cochrane Database Syst. Rev.* **2020**, *12*, CD013217. [CrossRef]

78. Seligman, N.S.; Salva, N.; Hayes, E.J.; Dysart, K.C.; Pequignot, E.C.; Baxter, J.K. Predicting length of treatment for neonatal abstinencesyn drome in methadone-exposed neonates. *Am. J. Obstet. Gynecol.* **2008**, *199*, 396-e1. [CrossRef] [PubMed]
79. Osborn, D.A.; Jeffery, H.E.; Cole, M.J. Opiate treatment for opiate withdrawal in new born infants. *Cochrane Database Syst. Rev.* **2010**, *10*. [CrossRef]
80. Wiegand, S.L.; Stringer, E.M.; Stuebe, A.M.; Jones, H.; Seashore, C.; Thorp, J. Buprenorphine and naloxone compared with methadone treatment in pregnancy. *Obstet. Gynecol.* **2015**, *125*, 363–368. [CrossRef]
81. Hudak, M.L.; Tan, R.C.; Committee on Drugs; Committee on Fetus and Newborn; Frattarelli, D.A.; Galinkin, J.L.; Green, T.P.; Neville, K.A.; Paul, I.M.; Van Den Anker, J.N.; et al. Neonatal drug withdrawal. *Pediatrics* **2012**, *129*, 540–560. [CrossRef]
82. Velez, M.L.; Jansson, L.M.; Schroeder, J.; Williams, E. Prenatal methadone exposure and neonatal neuro behavioral functioning. *Pediatr. Res.* **2009**, *66*, 704–709. [CrossRef] [PubMed]
83. Fill, M.M.A.; Miller, A.M.; Wilkinson, R.H.; Warren, M.D.; Dunn, J.R.; Schaffner, W.; Jones, T.F. Educational disabilities among children born with neonatal abstinence syndrome. *Pediatrics* **2018**, *142*, e20180562. [CrossRef] [PubMed]
84. Peterson, B.S.; Rosen, T.; Dingman, S.; Toth, Z.R.; Sawardekar, S.; Hao, X.; Liu, F.; Xu, D.; Dong, Z.; Peterson, J.B.; et al. Associations of maternal prenatal drug abuse with measures of newborn brain structure, tissue organization, and metabolite concentrations. *JAMA Pediatr.* **2020**, *174*, 831–842. [CrossRef]
85. Walhovd, K.B.; Moe, V.; Slinning, K.; Due-Tønnessen, P.; Bjørnerud, A.; Dale, A.M.; Van der Kouwe, A.; Quinn, B.T.; Kosofsky, B.; Greve, D.; et al. Volume triccerebral characteristics of children exposed to opiates and other substances in utero. *Neuro Image* **2007**, *36*, 1331–1344. [PubMed]
86. Honein, M.A.; Boyle, C.; Redfield, R.R. Public health surveillance of prenatal opioid exposure in mothers and infants. *Pediatrics* **2019**, *143*, e20183801. [CrossRef] [PubMed]
87. Terplan, M.; Minkoff, H. Neonatal abstinence syndrome and ethical approaches to the identification of pregnant women who use drugs. *Obstet. Gynecol.* **2017**, *129*, 164–167. [CrossRef] [PubMed]
88. ACOG Committee on Health Care for Underserved Women. ACOG Committee Opinion No. 524: Opioid abuse, dependence, and addiction in pregnancy. *Obstet. Gynecol.* **2012**, *119*, 1070–1076. [CrossRef]
89. Wong, S.; Ordean, A.; Kahan, M. Substance use in pregnancy. *J. Obstet. Gynaecol. Can.* **2011**, *33*, 367–384. [CrossRef]
90. Fricker, H.S.; Segal, S. Narcotic addiction, pregnancy, and the newborn. *Am. J. Dis. Child.* **1978**, *132*, 360–366. [CrossRef]
91. Hein, S.; Clouser, B.; Tamim, M.M.; Lockett, D.; Brauer, K.; Cooper, L.; Cleveland, L. Eat, sleep, console and adjunctive buprenorphine improved outcomes in neonatal opioid withdrawal syndrome. *Adv. Neonatal. Care* **2021**, *21*, 41–48. [CrossRef] [PubMed]
92. Ryan, K.; Moyer, A.; Glait, M.; Yan, K.; Dasgupta, M.; Saudek, K.; Cabacungan, E. Correlating Scores but Contrasting Outcomes for Eat Sleep Console Versus Modified Finnegan. *Hosp. Pediatr.* **2021**, *11*, 350–357. [CrossRef] [PubMed]
93. PCSAO. Available online: https://www.pcsao.org/perch/resources/downloads/opiateconfrogerwardspresentation.pdf (accessed on 15 November 2022).
94. SAMHSA. Available online: https://www.samhsa.gov/data/sites/default/files/NSDUHresults2010/NSDUHresults2010.htm (accessed on 15 November 2022).
95. National Institute on Drug Abuse. Available online: https://nida.nih.gov/publications/drugs-brains-behavior-science-addiction/preface (accessed on 15 November 2022).
96. Frey, M.T.; Meaney-Delman, D.; Bowen, V.; Yazdy, M.M.; Watkins, S.M.; Thorpe, P.G.; Honein, M.A. Surveillance for emerging threats to pregnant women and infants. *J. Womens Health* **2019**, *28*, 1031–1036. [CrossRef] [PubMed]
97. Ornoy, A.; Daka, L.; Goldzweig, G.; Gil, Y.; Mjen, L.; Levit, S.; Shufman, E.; Bar-Hamburger, R.; Greenbaum, C.W. Neurodevelopmental and psychological assessment of adolescents born to drug-addicted parents: Effects of SES and adoption. *Child Abuse Negl.* **2010**, *34*, 354–368. [CrossRef] [PubMed]
98. Youth Today. Available online: https://youthtoday.org/2016/09/is-u-s-opioid-crisis-straining-state-child-welfare-systems/ (accessed on 15 November 2022).
99. Falletta, L.; Hamilton, K.; Fischbein, R.; Aultman, J.; Kinney, B.; Kenne, D. Perceptions of child protective services among pregnant or recently pregnant, opioid-using women in substance abuse treatment. *Child. Abuse Negl.* **2018**, *79*, 125–135. [CrossRef]
100. Nigri, P.; Corsello, G.; Nigri, L.; Bali, D.; Kuli-Lito, G.; Plesca, D.; Pop, T.L.; Carrasco-Sanz, A.; Namazova-Baranova, L.; Mestrovic, J.; et al. Prevention and contrast of child abuse and neglect in the practice of European paediatricians: A multi-national pilot study. *Ital. J. Pediatr.* **2021**, *47*, 1–8. [CrossRef]
101. Green, B.L.; Rockhill, A.; Furrer, C. Does substance abuse treatment make a difference for child welfare case outcomes? A statewide longitudinal analysis. *Child. Youth Serv. Rev.* **2007**, *29*, 460–473. [CrossRef]
102. Taplin, S.; Mattick, R.P. The nature and extent of child protection involvement among heroin-using mothers in treatment: High rates of reports, removals at birth and children in care. *Drug Alcohol. Rev.* **2015**, *34*, 31–37. [CrossRef]
103. Albano, G.D.; Malta, G.; La Spina, C.; Rifiorito, A.; Provenzano, V.; Triolo, V.; Vaiano, F.; Bertol, E.; Argo, A. Toxicological Findings of Self-Poisoning Suicidal Deaths: A Systematic Review by Countries. *Toxics* **2022**, *10*, 654. [CrossRef]
104. Di Nunno, N.; Esposito, M.; Argo, A.; Salerno, M.; Sessa, F. Pharmacogenetics and Forensic Toxicology: A New Step towards a Multidisciplinary Approach. *Toxics* **2021**, *9*, 292. [CrossRef]

105. Basilicata, P.; Giugliano, P.; Vacchiano, G.; Simonelli, A.; Guadagni, R.; Silvestre, A.; Pieri, M. Forensic Toxicological and Medico-Legal Evaluation in a Case of Incongruous Drug Administration in Terminal Cancer Patients. *Toxics* **2021**, *9*, 356. [CrossRef] [PubMed]
106. Buccelli, C.; Della Casa, E.; Paternoster, M.; Niola, M.; Pieri, M. Gender differences in drugabuse in the forensictoxicologicalapproach. *Forensic Sci. Int.* **2016**, *265*, 89–95. [CrossRef] [PubMed]
107. Triolo, V.; Spanò, M.; Buscemi, R.; Gioè, S.; Malta, G.; Čaplinskiene, M.; Vaiano, F.; Bertol, E.; Zerbo, S.; Albano, G.D.; et al. EtG Quantification in Hair and Different Reference Cut-Offs in Relation to Various Pathologies: A Scoping Review. *Toxics* **2022**, *10*, 682. [CrossRef] [PubMed]

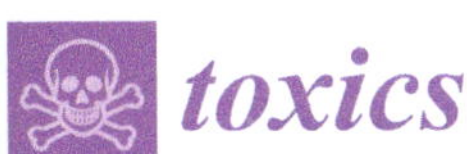 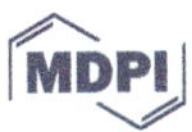

Article

Thermal (In)stability of Atropine and Scopolamine in the GC-MS Inlet

Gordana Koželj [1,*] and Helena Prosen [2]

1 Institute of Forensic Medicine, Faculty of Medicine, University of Ljubljana, Korytkova 2, SI-1000 Ljubljana, Slovenia
2 Faculty of Chemistry and Chemical Technology, University of Ljubljana, Večna pot 113, SI-1000 Ljubljana, Slovenia; helena.prosen@fkkt.uni-lj.si
* Correspondence: gordana.kozelj@mf.uni-lj.si

Abstract: The intoxication due to unintentional or intentional ingestion of plant material containing tropane alkaloids is quite frequent. GC-MS method is still widely used for the identification of these toxicologically important substances in human specimen. During general unknown analysis, high temperature of inlet, at least 270 °C, is commonly used for less volatile substances. Unfortunately, both tropanes are thermally unstable and could be overlooked due to their degradation. The temperature-related degradation of tropanes atropine and scopolamine was systematically studied in the inlet of a GC-MS instrument in the range 110–250 °C by increments of 20 °C, additionally also at 275 °C, and in different solvents. At inlet temperatures not higher than 250 °C, the degradation products were formed by elimination of water and cleavage of atropine's ester bond. At higher temperatures, elimination of formaldehyde became predominant. These phenomena were less pronounced when ethyl acetate was used instead of methanol, while *n*-hexane proved unsuitable for several reasons. At an inlet temperature of 275 °C, tropanes were barely detectable. During systematic toxicological analysis, any tropanes' degradation products should indicate the possible presence of atropine and/or scopolamine in the sample. It is not necessary to prepare thermally stable derivatives for confirmation. Instead, the inlet temperature can be decreased to 250 °C, which diminishes their degradation to a level where their detection and identification are possible. This was demonstrated in several case studies.

Keywords: atropine; scopolamine; thermal stability; GC-MS inlet; degradation

Citation: Koželj, G.; Prosen, H. Thermal (In)stability of Atropine and Scopolamine in the GC-MS Inlet. *Toxics* **2021**, *9*, 156. https://doi.org/10.3390/toxics9070156

Academic Editor: Maria Pieri

Received: 3 June 2021
Accepted: 29 June 2021
Published: 30 June 2021

1. Introduction

Gas chromatography coupled to mass spectrometry (GC-MS) is still a method widely used in toxicology for the identification of unknown substances in human specimens. In comparison to liquid chromatography coupled to mass spectrometry (LC-MS), which is nowadays the prevalent technique also in toxicological laboratories, GC-MS has the main advantage of universal ionization method (electron ionization, EI), which is negligibly influenced by sample matrix and yields reproducible spectra that can be readily used to identify the compound either by comparison with mass spectral libraries or by direct interpretation. However, the applied oven temperatures are up to 350 °C, which means that the analysis is limited to small and volatile molecules (MW < 600 Da), which is the main disadvantage of GC-MS technique and the reason it is currently less often used than LC-MS. However, GC-MS still plays a major role in screening for the responsible substance in cases of intoxication of unknown origin, which cannot be readily accomplished by more compound-specific LC-MS methods. It should also be emphasized that GC-MS equipment is much more affordable compared even to a simple LC-MS system.

Among toxicologically important substance, there are also two toxic alkaloids with a tropane skeleton, (−)-hyoscine (scopolamine, Figure 1) and (−)-hyoscyamine, which are found in plants of the family Solanaceae, e.g. *Atropa beladonna, Datura stramonium,* and *Hyoscyamus niger* [1]. The intoxication due to unintentional or intentional ingestion of plant material is quite frequent. (−)-Hyoscyamine is converted to a racemic mixture (±)-hyoscyamine (atropine, Figure 1) in the body after ingestion or during extraction from a biological sample. Frequently used methods for determination of atropine and scopolamine are gas chromatographic methods with mass-spectrometric detection [2–5]. As both alkaloids are thermally unstable, stable derivatives, such as trimethylsilyl [6–8], acetyl [5], or pentafluoropropyl [9], need to be prepared for a successful GC-MS determination. In order to avoid degradation problems, nowadays, liquid chromatography-mass spectrometry methods are used instead and are the methods of choice if quantitative analysis is required [10,11].

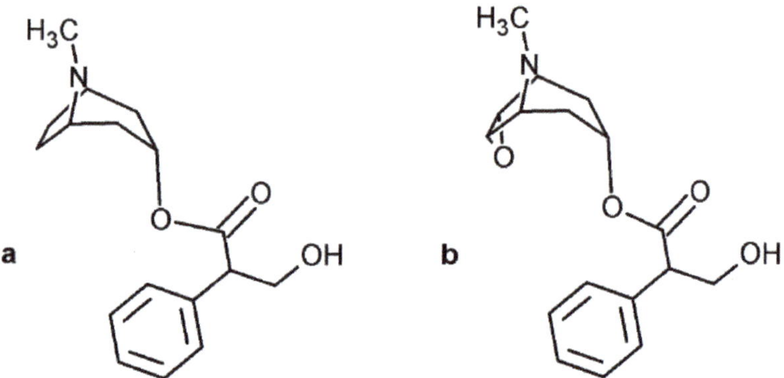

Figure 1. Chemical structure of atropine (**a**) and scopolamine (**b**).

The concentrations of both tropanes in biological samples are quite low. For atropine, therapeutic concentrations are 0.002–0.025 mg/L, toxic from 0.03 to 0.1 mg/L, and lethal around or over 0.2 mg/L. Concentrations of scopolamine in blood are almost ten times lower, in the range of 0.0001 to 0.01 mg/L [12]. Half-time of atropine in blood is 2–4 h, the majority of the dose is excreted in urine in one day, of which 13–50% as original substance and the rest as metabolites. The toxic dose can be as little as 1 mg, while the lethal dose is 50–100 mg. Scopolamine has a longer half time of 2–6 h and is excreted mostly (95%) as metabolites in urine in approximately two days. Fatal poisonings are extremely rare [12].

Due to their low concentrations in biological fluids, the risk of overlooking the presence of tropane alkaloids increases with their degradation. They could be easily missed in the general unknown GC-MS screening in cases of suspected intoxication. Thus, our intention was to study the phenomenon of their thermal degradation at different temperatures and in different solvents to establish how both compounds can be successfully recognized from their thermal degradation products. Solutions in pure solvents were used to avoid potential matrix effects besides the studied effects. The successful identification by applying the findings of our study is demonstrated in several case studies.

2. Materials and Methods

2.1. Chemicals and Reagents

Methanol Chromasolv®was purchased from Sigma-Aldrich (Steinheim, Germany), *n*-hexane and ethyl acetate from Merck (Darmstadt, Germany).

Scopolamine hydrochloride (>99%) and atropine (USP testing specifications) were purchased from Sigma-Aldrich (St. Louis, MO, USA).

2.2. GC-MS Analysis

A Hewlett Packard 6890 Plus gas chromatograph with an Agilent 7683 series injector and a 5973 mass selective detector (Hewlett Packard, Palo Alto, CA, USA) were used for qualitative analyses. The compounds were separated on an HP-5MS capillary column (5%-phenyl-methylpolysiloxane, 30 m × 0.25 mm i.d., 0.25 μm film thickness). Helium was used as a carrier gas at a constant flow of 1 mL/min. The GC inlet temperature was changed from 110 °C to 250 °C by increments of 20 °C and finally to 275 °C, which is the temperature used in our routine general unknown screening. The inlet liner was Agilent splitless single taper, deactivated liner with glass wool (Agilent, Palo Alto, CA, USA, P/N: 5062-3587). The initial oven temperature of 60 °C was held for 2 min and then ramped at 20 °C/min to 300 °C with a final hold time of 15 min. The temperature of the transfer line was 280 °C. The ion source and quadrupole temperatures were 230 °C and 150 °C, respectively. The mass selective detector was used in EI scan mode, the ionization energy was 70 eV, and the electron multiplier voltage was set 200 V above autotune value. Data were collected for a splitless injection of 1.0 μL of each tropane in methanol, ethyl acetate and *n*-hexane in the range from 50 to 550 m/z at a rate of 2.9 scans/s. The software used was MSD Chemstation D.01.02.16.

2.3. Sample Preparation

The solutions of atropine and scopolamine base were prepared in methanol, ethyl acetate and *n*-hexane with the final concentration of 40 mg/L for methanol and 200 mg/L for the other two solvents.

3. Results and Discussion

3.1. Solutions of Atropine in Scopolamine in Different Solvents

In our practice, in the case of general unknown analysis, LLE or SPE extracts of biological samples are dissolved in methanol and afterwards, screened by the GC-MS method described in the Experimental Section 2.2. Methanol, being both a proton donor and acceptor, is used as a solvent for a variety of substances that are efficiently dissolved despite their frequently quite different polarity. The sample is vaporized in the inlet and transferred to a column at a low initial temperature where condensation of solvent and sample occurs. As the temperature is increased, the methanol evaporates and the sample is preconcentrated in the residual solvent within a narrow area. Analytes are vaporized from this area at the beginning of the column at higher oven temperatures. However, a high temperature of the injector is used to vaporize less volatile substances. Because of this, the occurrence of thermal decomposition products, methylated substances, and formaldehyde adducts is possible. Several mass spectra of such compounds are included in commercial mass spectra libraries (e.g., Pfleger/Maurer/Weber, NIST) but are not necessarily marked as such, and the recognition of their origin depends on the analyst's knowledge and experience. Thermolysis is noticeable in atropine and scopolamine, as illustrated in Figure 2.

We were interested in the extent of thermal degradation at different conditions. Thus, the behavior of both substances in the solution with three solvents of different polarities was studied, with methanol being the most polar, less polar ethyl acetate, and *n*-hexane as the nonpolar one. Tropanes were also exposed to different injector temperatures. As an example, only results for methanol as solvent are presented in Figure 3, while additional results for other solvents are given in Supplementary Materials, Figure S1 and Table S1. In the temperature range from 100 to 250 °C, the thermal energy is sufficient only for low-energy reactions such as functional group elimination at the end of the chain [13]. In our case, this corresponds to elimination of water from the atropine and scopolamine molecules in the GC inlet and the cleavage of the ester bond, the latter observed only in atropine. Atropine is more degradable than scopolamine. The main structural difference lies in the cyclic ether bond, which could be the reason for increased degradability. In the temperature range from 250 to 500 °C, there is enough thermal energy to break the chemical bonds with the highest energy [13]. Consequently, also the elimination of formaldehyde becomes important for tropanes at higher inlet temperatures. Successive elution of tropanes and their degradation products from the chromatographic column, corresponding to their specific physico-chemical properties, is proof of thermal degradation taking place in the inlet of a gas chromatograph. The corresponding mass spectra are presented in Figure 4.

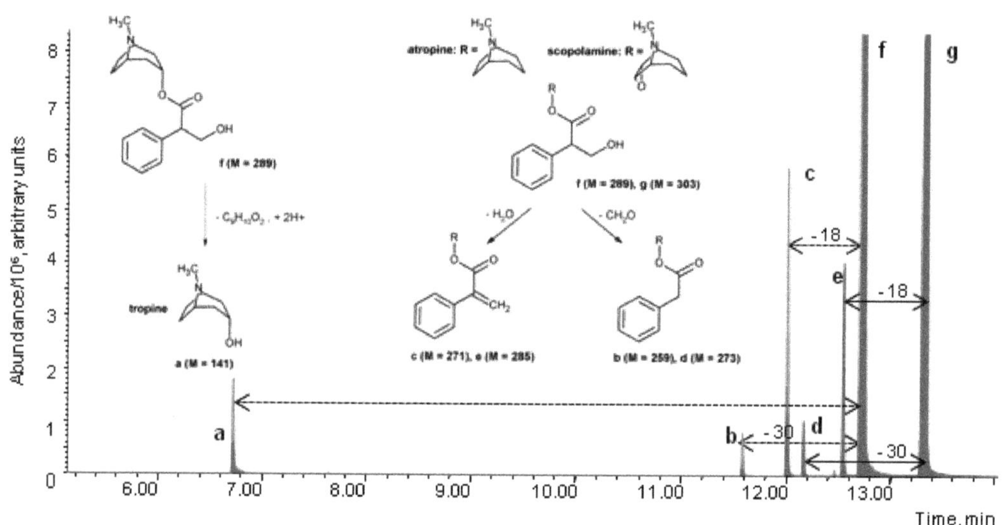

Figure 2. GC-MS chromatogram of atropine, scopolamine, and their thermolysis products with a tropane skeleton, obtained by extraction and merging of two ion currents (m/z 124–atropine related and m/z 94–scopolamine related) from TIC. The elimination of water (ΔM: −18) and formaldehyde (ΔM: −30) was observed in both tropanes while a significant cleavage of ester bond was seen only in atropine. The inlet temperature was 250 °C. Tropine (**a**), 3-phenylacetoxytropane (atropine-CH_2O) (**b**), apoatropine (atropine-H_2O) (**c**), 3-phenylacetoxyscopine (scopolamine-CH_2O) (**d**), aposcopolamine (scopolamine-H_2O) (**e**), atropine (**f**), and scopolamine (**g**).

The degradation phenomena were more pronounced in methanol. With temperatures below 250 °C, the elimination of water was predominant compared to formaldehyde elimination. Both processes were comparable but proceeded to a negligible extent in ethyl acetate again up to 250 °C. At 275 °C, atropine and scopolamine were almost completely degraded both in methanol and ethyl acetate. In the case of n-hexane as the solvent, the situation was fully unpredictable, rendering different and randomly changing ratios of peak areas, with comparable areas for atropine, scopolamine, and their degradation products and giving poor response for parent compounds. Described observations could have arisen from the properties of the applied solvents, which contributed to the degradation process. The most pronounced influence was from methanol, being both a proton acceptor and donor, and less from ethyl acetate, which is only a proton acceptor. n-Hexane is neither a proton acceptor nor proton donor. Moreover, both analytes are poorly soluble in it. Low solubility could cause their wider dispersion upon entering the GC column (at 60 °C) and lower preconcentration at the beginning of the column, leading to higher exposure to heat and consequently, a higher relative amount of thermal decomposition products, which was actually observed. To summarize: Methanol as solvent caused the highest degree of degradation both at temperatures below or above 250 °C. Ethyl acetate promoted degradation only at temperatures above 250 °C, while for n-hexane, no behavioral pattern could be established.

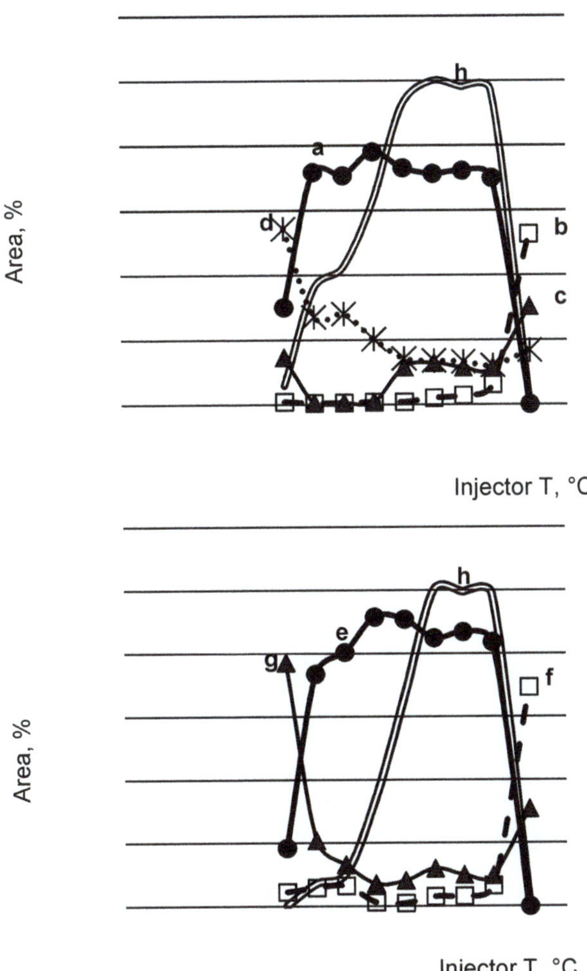

Figure 3. Influence of injector temperature on peak areas of atropine, scopolamine, and their main products of thermolysis, solvent methanol. Atropine (**a**), 3-phenylacetoxytropane (atropine-CH_2O) (**b**), apoatropine (atropine-H_2O) (**c**), tropine (**d**), scopolamine (**e**), 3-phenylacetoxyscopine (scopolamine-CH_2O) (**f**), aposcopolamine (scopolamine-H_2O) (**g**), sum of areas normalized to maximum value (**h**).

In the next step, we wanted to investigate the influence of analyte concentration on the extent of thermal degradation. We chose the following experimental conditions: The solvent was ethyl acetate and not methanol with a more pronounced influence on degradation, the inlet temperature was lowered to 250 °C to preserve the majority of parent compounds. Results for the solutions with concentration 200 and 2 mg/L (hundred-times dilution) were compared with those obtained for the same solutions at inlet temperature 275 °C (Tables 1 and 2). Atropine was significantly more degraded at the higher inlet temperature than scopolamine and additionally with dilution.

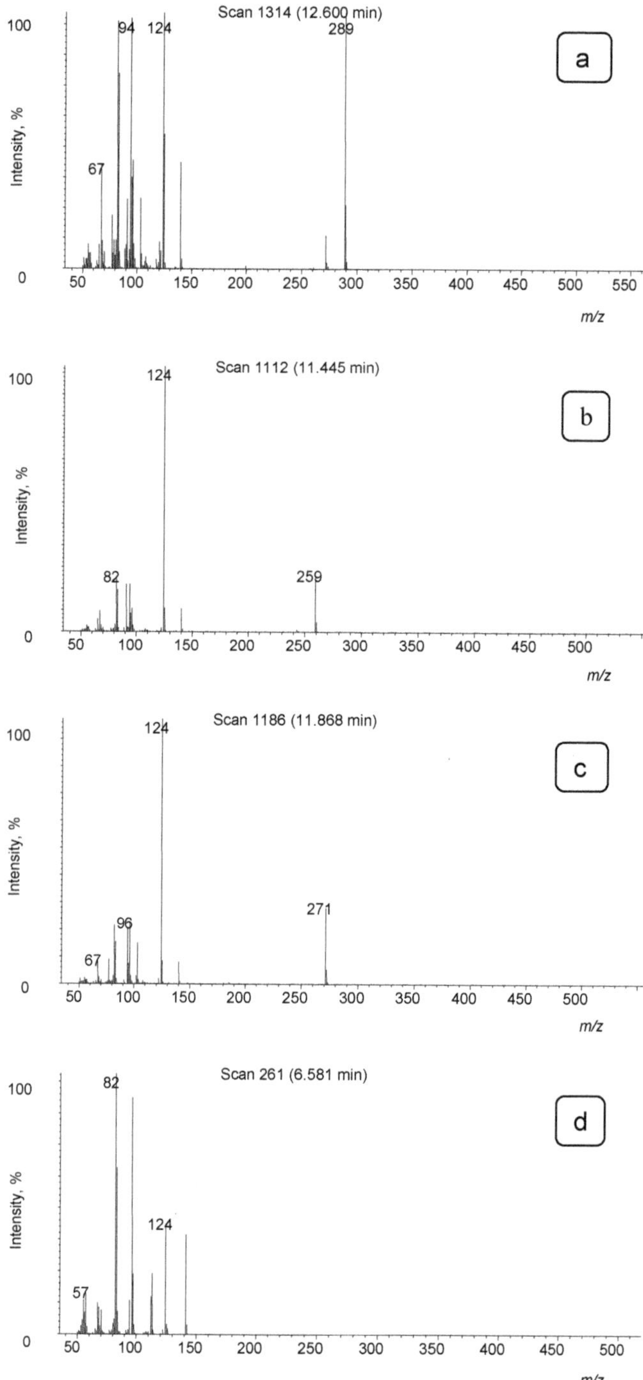

Figure 4. *Cont.*

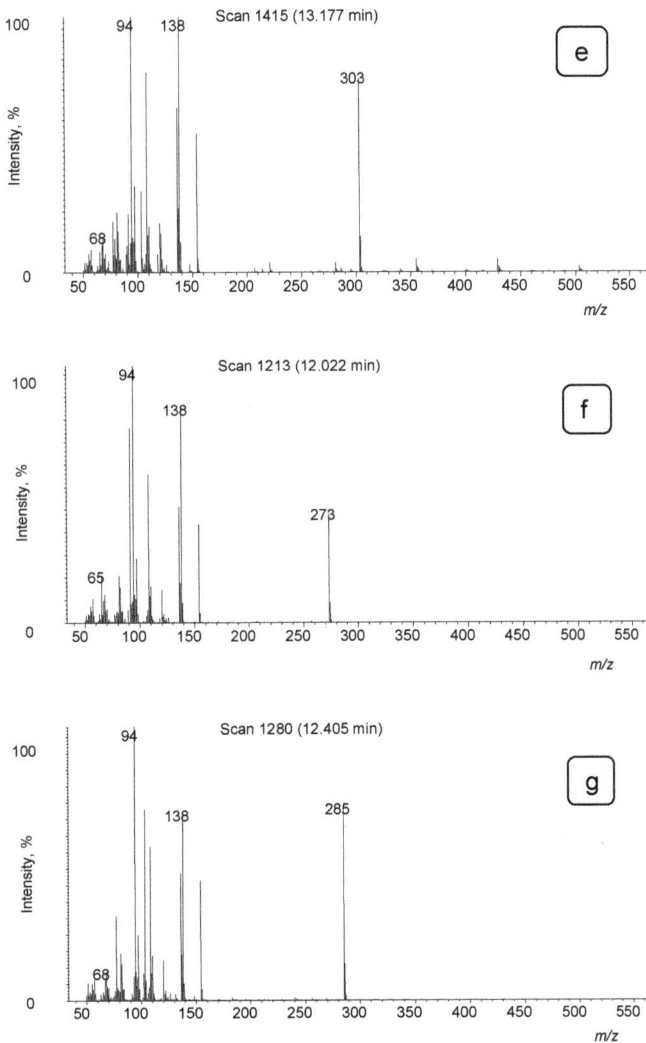

Figure 4. Mass spectra of atropine, scopolamine and their main products of thermolysis. Atropine (**a**), 3-phenylacetoxytropane (atropine-CH_2O) (**b**), apoatropine (atropine-H_2O) (**c**), tropine (**d**), scopolamine (**e**), 3-phenylacetoxyscopine (scopolamine-CH_2O) (**f**), aposcopolamine (scopolamine-H_2O) (**g**).

Table 1. Influence of inlet temperature and concentration on the ratio between atropine and its degradation products in ethyl acetate presented as percentage of a sum of areas.

Inlet *T* (°C)	Concentration (mg/L)	Atropine (%)	Atropine-H_2O (%)	Atropine-CH_2O (%)	Tropine (%)
275	200	48.1	49.6	0.5	1.8
	2	19.7	20.1	10.1	50.1
250	200	90.7	1.6	0.7	7.0
	2	91.2	2.0	2.6	4.2

Table 2. Influence of inlet temperature and concentration on the ratio between scopolamine and its degradation products in ethyl acetate presented as percentage of a sum of areas.

Inlet *T* (°C)	Concentration (mg/L)	Scopolamine (%)	Scopolamine-H_2O (%)	Scopolamine-CH_2O (%)
275	200	87.9	5.0	7.1
	2	91.2	6.0	2.8
250	200	95.9	2.6	1.5
	2	96.5	3.5	0.0

3.2. Application on Real Samples

The GC-MS method described in Experimental Section 2.2 has been used in our laboratory for more than 25 years as a general screening method in forensic, clinical, DUI, and drugs of abuse cases. From the very beginning, we have used a lower inlet temperature of 275 °C compared to usually higher reported *T* of screening procedures, for instance, 280 °C [14]. The decision was based on observed degradations of some compounds (for example, oxazepam, ß-blockers) as well as on cases with problematic or even unsuccessful primary identification. Despite the analysis of several thousands of cases per year, atropine was present in a very small number of poisonings and scopolamine even in less. Some identification problems of atropine and scopolamine will be presented in the following case studies.

- Case study 1

A young male was found irresponsive, hallucinating. After successful treatment in the hospital, he admitted taking tea prepared from thorn-apple (*Datura stramonium*), containing atropine and scopolamine. GC-MS toxicological analysis of extracted urine confirmed the presence of both alkaloids and degradation products of scopolamine, namely scopolamine-H_2O and scopolamine-CH_2O. All compounds were reliably identified with a library search algorithm. Predominant chromatographic peaks were, in this case, degradation products of scopolamine, outstanding was scopolamine-H_2O presenting 78% of a sum of areas, while for scopolamine, it was only 2%. The peak area of atropine was small compared to scopolamine. Concentrations of parent compounds were subsequently determined with a validated LC-MS/MS method [10]. The concentration of atropine in blood was 0.019 mg/L and in urine 0.30 mg/L, while concentrations of scopolamine were 0.011 and 0.95 mg/L, respectively.

- Case study 2

A young male was treated in the hospital emergency department after drinking tea. The same GC-MS method was used as above for identification of toxic compounds in extract of urine sample and extract of tea sample. Library search hits for tea extract were acetylated homatropine, atropine-H_2O, and acetylated atropine, the latter at a significantly inappropriate retention time. Based on the presence of atropine degradation products and heteroanamnestic data, typical mass fragments were extracted (m/z 84, 124, 289, 94, 138, and 303), leading to the confirmation of atropine and scopolamine as well as their degradation products formed by elimination of water and formaldehyde. Library search of mass spectra of peaks of urine extract gave only a hit for atropine-CH_2O, probably due to high background, and no other toxicologically relevant compounds were identified. With the extraction of typical mass fragments from the recorded mass spectra, the presence of atropine, atropine-H_2O and atropine-CH_2O was confirmed (estimated percentage of the sum of areas were 33%, 7%, and 60%, respectively), as well as the presence of scopolamine, scopolamine-H_2O, and scopolamine-CH_2O (estimated percentage of the sum of areas were 64%, 16%, and 20%, respectively).

- Case study 3

Buckwheat grain and flour (*Fagopyrum* sp., Polygonaceae) have an important role in the national Slovenian cuisine. Among various traditional dishes, a dish named "ajdovi žganci" is very popular (translated in English as "buckwheat spoonbread"). In September 2003, a mass food poisoning accident with the symptoms of a classic anticholinergic syndrome occurred in Slovenia. The National Institute of Public Health of Slovenia established an *ad hoc* self-reporting scheme and identified 73 cases with symptoms of tropane alkaloid toxicity. All intoxicated persons had consumed buckwheat flour food products within the last few hours. About 20 samples of disputable buckwheat products were analyzed by the presented GC-MS method after extraction of 30 g of material. All samples were dissolved in methanol and due to considerable amount of sample the presence of tropane alkaloids atropine and scopolamine was confirmed by library search. Degradation products of both compounds due to elimination of water and formaldehyde were identified after extraction of typical mass fragments from mass spectra, as well as traces of tropine. In the few delivered samples of blood and urine, tropanes or their degradation products were not identified. Further macroscopic examination of whole buckwheat grain revealed the presence of seeds of thorn-apple. At that time, temporary maximum residue levels (MRLs) of tropane alkaloids were established. To verify them, a study with volunteers was realized, and for that purpose, a validated LC-MS/MS method was developed [10,15].

- Case study 4

GC-MS analyses of blood serum samples taken from patients at the intensive care unit occasionally reveal the presence of atropine and/or atropine-H_2O in extracts as a result of medical treatment.

Although the predominant processes during thermal exposure of tropanes depend on experimental parameters, good repeatability of measurements cannot be expected, making the method inappropriate for quantitative purposes. On the other hand, the thermal degradation products can offer additional valuable information while identifying compounds in the case of a general unknown analysis. In our practice, most often, the presence of dehydrated atropine or scopolamine triggers further appropriate analyses for the confirmation of their parent compounds. Depending on other circumstances, especially if other toxicologically important substances are present, one of the following possibilities is selected for further analysis: Inlet temperature is set to 250 °C, acetylated products are additionally prepared and identified, or the LC-MS/MS method is applied.

4. Conclusions

GC-MS methods have been used for decades for identification and quantitation of countless compounds occurring in our everyday life. For quantitative purposes, these methods are validated. One of the reasons for the occurrence of non-linearity of calibration curve for target parent compound can be temperature-induced degradation in the analytical instrument. In such cases, methods are appropriately corrected so that they fulfil the expected validation demands for parent compounds, but degradation products are usually not further studied.

The greatness of GC-MS methods still lies in their screening potential. Using the accepted standard experimental parameters for acquiring mass spectra enables the transfer of their electronic version between different instruments and laboratories. That enables the use of extensive, excellent mass spectra libraries in combination with RI values for identification even without having the pure standard of the compound. Combining these collections with nowadays powerful data analysis tools enables even small laboratories, for which buying a vast array of standards is financially difficult, to successfully perform identifications. Powerful tools, on the other hand, can lead to less focused, superficial interpretation, or diminished critical evaluation and observation of analytical results. For instance, even if the degradation of a particular compound is noticed, the impact of the process on the final result is seldom evaluated. In clinical toxicology, intoxicated patients are often treated according to their symptoms and signs, thus the plasma concentration of the particular compound is usually not sought at the very first moment or not at all. However, any information about the presence of toxic compounds, metabolites, or degradation products can be of importance. On the basis of such results, other confirmation or quantitation methods can be used. The same applies to questionable or deficient results in forensic cases, DUI, and drug abuse, where there is longer affordable time to conclude the analyses.

Some of the potentially toxic compounds which are identified in extracts of biological samples by the GC-MS method are thermally unstable. Tropanes atropine and scopolamine also belong to this group. Solutions of tropanes in pure solvents were used in this study to avoid potential additional matrix effects besides the temperature and solvent effects. We have observed that the extent of their degradation depends on the inlet temperature and also on the solvent used for the dissolution of the sample extract. The major degradation products formed in the inlet and observed up to 250 °C for both tropanes occurred after water elimination and atropine's ester bond cleavage. At higher temperatures, elimination of formaldehyde became predominant and parent compounds atropine and scopolamine were barely detectable. With temperatures below 250 °C, less degradation was observed in the solvent ethyl acetate compared to methanol, while the behavior in *n*-hexane was shown to be unpredictable. Atropine is more thermally sensitive and thus more degraded than scopolamine. Thus, any estimation, that structurally very similar compounds are behaving in a similar manner, would be unjustified without actual experiments. The presence of tropanes and their degradation products should be considered during systematic toxicological analysis. If degradation products are observed, the temperature of the inlet can be lowered to 250 °C to allow for the detection and identification of parent compounds in a simpler manner compared to the time-consuming preparation of their derivatives. In the presented case studies, a comparable pattern of tropanes' degradation was recognized and used for the identification of analytes.

Supplementary Materials: The following are available online at https://www.mdpi.com/2305-6304/9/7/156/s1, Figure S1: Influence of injector temperature on peak areas of atropine, scopolamine and their main products of thermolysis in three solvents: methanol, ethyl acetate and *n*-hexane, Table S1: Relation between sums of areas of particular tropane and main degradation products in different solvents at different injector *T*.

Author Contributions: Conceptualization, G.K. and H.P.; formal analysis, G.K.; investigation, G.K.; data curation, G.K.; writing—original draft preparation, G.K.; writing—review and editing, H.P.; visualization, G.K. and H.P. All authors have read and agreed to the published version of the manuscript.

Funding: This research was funded by Slovenian Research Agency, Programme Group P1-0153.

Institutional Review Board Statement: Not applicable.

Informed Consent Statement: Not applicable.

Data Availability Statement: The data presented in this study are available on request from corresponding author.

Acknowledgments: Not applicable.

Conflicts of Interest: The authors declare no conflict of interest.

References

1. Dewick, P.M. *Medicinal Natural Products: A Biosynthetic Approach*, 3rd ed.; Wiley: Chichester, UK, 2009.
2. Dräger, B. Analysis of tropane and related alkaloids. *J. Chromatogr.* **2002**, *978*, 1–35. [CrossRef]
3. Aehle, E.; Drager, B. Tropane alkaloid analysis by chromatographic and electrophoretic techniques: An update. *J. Chromatogr. B* **2010**, *878*, 1391–1406. [CrossRef] [PubMed]
4. Beyer, J.; Drummer, O.H.; Maurer, H.H. Analysis of toxic alkaloids in body samples. *Forensic Sci. Int.* **2009**, *185*, 1–9. [CrossRef]
5. El Bazaoui, A.; Bellimam, M.A.; Soulaymani, A. Nine new tropane alkaloids from *Datura stramonium* L. identified by GC/MS. *Fitoterapia* **2011**, *82*, 193–197. [CrossRef] [PubMed]

6. Namera, A.; Yashiki, M.; Hirose, Y.; Yamaji, S.; Tani, T.; Kojima, T. Quantitative analysis of tropane alkaloids in biological materials by gas chromatography-mass spectrometry. *Forensic Sci. Int.* **2002**, *130*, 34–43. [CrossRef]
7. Oertel, R.; Richter, K.; Ebert, U.; Kirch, W. Determination of scopolamine in human serum by gas chromatography-ion trap tandem mass spectrometry. *J. Chromatogr. B* **1996**, *682*, 259–264. [CrossRef]
8. Papoutsis, I.; Nikolau, P.; Spiliopoulou, C.; Pistos, C.; Stefanidou, M.; Athanaselis, S. A simple and sensitive GC/MS method for the determination of atropine during therapy of anticholinesterase poisoning in serum samples. *Drug Test. Anal.* **2012**, *4*, 229–234. [CrossRef] [PubMed]
9. Saady, J.; Poklis, A. Determination of Atropine in Blood by Gas-Chromatography Mass-Spectrometry. *J. Anal. Toxicol.* **1989**, *13*, 296–299. [CrossRef] [PubMed]
10. Koželj, G.; Perharič, L.; Stanovnik, L.; Prosen, H. Simple validated LC-MS/MS method for the determination of atropine and scopolamine in plasma for clinical and forensic toxicological purposes. *J. Pharm. Biomed. Anal.* **2014**, *96*, 197–206. [CrossRef] [PubMed]
11. Zhang, P.T.; Li, Y.M.; Liu, G.H.; Sun, X.M.; Zhou, Y.T.; Deng, X.J.; Liao, Q.F.; Xie, Z.Y. Simultaneous determination of atropine, scopolamine, and anisodamine from *Hyoscyamus niger* L. in rat plasma by high-performance liquid chromatography with tandem mass spectrometry and its application to a pharmacokinetics study. *J. Sep. Sci.* **2014**, *37*, 2664–2674. [CrossRef] [PubMed]
12. Moffat, A.C.; Osselton, M.D.; Widdop, B. *Clarke's Analysis of Drugs and Poisons*, 3rd ed.; Pharmaceutical Press: London, UK; Chicago, IL, USA, 2004.
13. Moldoveanu, S.C. *Analytical Pyrolysis of Natural Organic Polymers*; Elsevier: Amsterdam, The Netherlands, 1998.
14. Maurer, H.H.; Pfleger, K.; Weber, A.A. *Mass Spectral Library of Drugs, Poisons, Pesticides, Pollutants: And Their Metabolites, Experimental Section*, 1st ed.; Wiley-VCH: Hoboken, NJ, USA, 2011.
15. Perharič, L.; Koželj, G.; Družina, B.; Stanovnik, L. Risk assessment of buckwheat flour contaminated by thorn-apple (*Datura stramonium* L.) alkaloids: A case study from Slovenia. *Food Addit. Contam. A* **2012**, *30*, 321–330. [CrossRef] [PubMed]

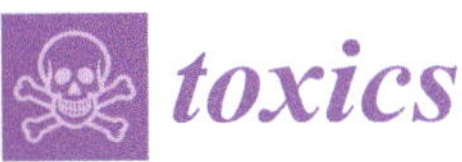

MDPI

Article

Determination of Prenatal Substance Exposure Using Meconium and Orbitrap Mass Spectrometry

Atakan Hernandez [1], Valerie Lacroze [2], Natalia Doudka [3], Jenny Becam [1], Carole Pourriere-Fabiani [1], Bruno Lacarelle [1], Caroline Solas [1,4] and Nicolas Fabresse [1,5,*]

1 Laboratory of Pharmacokinetics and Toxicology, La Timone University Hospital, 264 Rue Saint Pierre, CEDEX 5, 13385 Marseille, France; atakan.hernandez@yahoo.fr (A.H.); jenny.becam@ap-hm.fr (J.B.); carole.pourriere-fabiani@ap-hm.fr (C.P.-F.); bruno.lacarelle@ap-hm.fr (B.L.); caroline.solas@ap-hm.fr (C.S.)
2 Department of Neonatalogy, La Conception University Hospital, CEDEX 5, 13385 Marseille, France; valerie.lacroze@ap-hm.fr
3 Department of Clinical Pharmacology and Pharmacovigilance, La Timone University Hospital, 264 Rue Saint Pierre, CEDEX 5, 13385 Marseille, France; natalia.doudka@ap-hm.fr
4 Emerging Viruses Unit (UVE), IRD 190, INSERM 1207, Aix-Marseille University, CEDEX 5, 13385 Marseille, France
5 Economic and Social Sciences of Health and Medical Information Processing, INSERM, IRD, SESSTIM, Aix-Marseille University, CEDEX 5, 13385 Marseille, France
* Correspondence: nicolas.fabresse@ap-hm.fr

Abstract: The aim of this study was to develop and to validate a toxicological untargeted screening relying on LC-HRMS in meconium including the detection of the four main classes of drugs of abuse (DoA; amphetamines, cannabinoids, opioids and cocaine). The method was then applied to 29 real samples. Analyses were performed with a liquid chromatography system coupled to a benchtop Orbitrap operating in a data-dependent analysis. The sample amount was 300 mg of meconium extracted twice by solid phase extraction following two distinct procedures. Raw data were processed using the Compound Discoverer 3.2 software (Thermo). The method was evaluated and validated on 15 compounds (6-MAM, morphine, buprenorphine, norbuprenorphine, methadone, EDDP, amphetamine, MDA, MDMA, methamphetamine, cocaine, benzoylecgonine, THC, 11-OH-THC, THC-COOH). Limits of detection were between 0.5 and 5 pg/mg and limits of identification between 5 and 50 pg/mg. Mean matrix effect was between −79 and −19% (n = 6) and mean overall recovery between 18 and 73% (n = 6) at 100 pg/mg. The application allows the detection of 88 substances, including 47 pharmaceuticals and 15 pharmaceutical metabolites, cocaine and its metabolites, THC and its metabolites, and natural (morphine, codeine) and synthetic (methadone, buprenorphine, tramadol, norfentanyl) opioids. This method is now used routinely for toxicological screening in high-risk pregnancies

Keywords: meconium; mass spectrometry; toxicology; drug of abuse; orbitrap; newborn

Citation: Hernandez, A.; Lacroze, V.; Doudka, N.; Becam, J.; Pourriere-Fabiani, C.; Lacarelle, B.; Solas, C.; Fabresse, N. Determination of Prenatal Substance Exposure Using Meconium and Orbitrap Mass Spectrometry. *Toxics* **2022**, *10*, 55. https://doi.org/10.3390/toxics10020055

Academic Editors: Maria Pieri and Giovanna Tranfo

Received: 23 December 2021
Accepted: 22 January 2022
Published: 26 January 2022

1. Introduction

In 2019, according to the United Nation Office on Drug and Crime (UNODC), cannabis remains the most widely used drug, with 200 million people having used cannabis, followed by opioids (62 million people), amphetamines (27 million people) and cocaine (20 million people) [1]. In France, 45% of adults (18–64 years old) have used cannabis, 5.6% cocaine, 5.0% 3,4-methylenedioxy-N-methylamphetamine (MDMA) and 1.3% heroin [2]. Drug of abuse (DoA) exposure during pregnancy may have serious consequences on newborn health: fetal development disorders, high neonatal mortality rates and various adverse mental and physical effects [3]. These concerns justify a recognition of fetal exposure as early as possible, in order to provide treatment to the exposed neonate. Maternal interview remains the most common and economical method to detect drug exposure, however, many studies have highlighted an underreporting issue [4]. Consequently, sensitive and specific bioanalytical methods are necessary to accurately measure biomarkers of in utero exposure. Fetal drug exposure can be identified by analyzing maternal specimens during pregnancy or neonatal specimens such as hair, urine and meconium, shortly after birth.

Meconium refers to the first stool of the newborn. Meconium consists mainly of water, epithelial cells, lanugo, bile acids and salts, cholesterol and sterol precursors, blood group of substances, mucopolysaccharides, sugars, lipids, proteins and other compounds from swallowed amniotic fluid [5]. It accumulates during the last three months of pregnancy, thus allowing exploration of the exposure of the newborn during the last trimester of pregnancy.

Meconium is accepted as a gold standard matrix for in utero drug exposure. It allows for a wide detection window and a non-invasive sample collection from a soiled diaper. However, it is susceptible to contamination by urine, there is a possible detection of drugs given to the newborn after birth and painkiller drugs used by the mother during labor, the specimen volume is limited and extensive extraction procedures are required for sample preparation [6]. Several studies dedicated to meconium analysis have been published [7–20]. Most of the methods have focused on the analysis of specific drug groups such as amphetamines, opioids, cannabinoids, cocaine, alcohol biomarkers, benzodiazepines or antidepressants [7–16]. Typically, each drug group is extracted and analyzed separately in meconium; this may cause problems due to the limited amount of sample, and the time-consuming procedures required for multiple drugs analysis. Very few methods devoted to large screening of meconium have been published. The first broad-spectrum drug screening of meconium was developed by Ristimaa et al. in 2010 [17]. This method relies on liquid chromatography coupled to high resolution mass spectrometry (LC-HRMS) and an in-house database containing 869 molecular drugs. More recently (2021), López-Rabuñal et al. proposed another large screening devoted to new psychoactive substances (NPS) [21]. This method allows the simultaneous determination of 137 NPS in meconium by LC-HRMS. These two methods are efficient and innovative; however, they are targeted. To our knowledge, there is no untargeted LC-HRMS method devoted to toxicological screening in meconium, and none allowing the simultaneous detection of the four main classes of DoA (amphetamines, cannabinoids, opioids and cocaine) in the current literature.

The aim of this study was to develop and to validate a toxicological untargeted screening relying on high resolution mass spectrometry (Orbitrap) in meconium, including the detection of the four main classes of DoA. The method was then applied to real samples.

2. Materials and Methods

2.1. Chemicals and Reagents

Water purity was 18.2 mΩ/cm (Millipore, Molsheim, France). Methanol was supplied by Biosolve (Dieuze, France). Formic acid and orthophosphoric acid were ordered to Carlo Erba (Val de Reuil, France). Acetonitrile and sodium dihydrogen phosphate (NaH_2PO_4) were supplied by Fisher Scientific (Illkirch, France). Sodium hydrogen phosphate (Na_2HPO_4) was ordered from Merck (Darmstadt, Germany). β-glucuronidase was purchased by MP Biomedicals (Illkirch, France). LGC standards (Molsheim, France) supplied vials for 11-hydroxy-Δ^9-tetrahydrocannabinol (11-OH-THC), 11-nor-9-carboxy-Δ^9-tetrahydrocannabinol-D3 (THC-COOH-D3), Δ^9-tetrahydrocannabinol-D3 (THC-D3), methamphetamine, cocaine, 3,4-methylenedioxyamphetamine (MDA), 3,4-methylenedioxymetamphetamine (MDMA), MDMA-D5, morphine-D3, buprenorphine, methadone, 6-monoacetylmorphine (6-MAM), 6-MAM-D3. Vials of 11-OH-THC, THC-COOH, THC, methampethamine-D5, amphetamine, amphetamine-D5, cocaine, cocaine-D3, MDA-D5, benzoylecgonine, benzoylecgonine-D3, morphine, buprenorphine-D4 and methadone-D3 were supplied by Euromedex (Souffelweyersheim, France).

2.2. Solutions Preparation

Phosphate buffer pH = 5 was made with 1.70 g Na2HPO4 and 12.14 g NaH2PO4 in 1000 mL of distilled water. The pH was adjusted with orthophosphoric acid. The elution phase was prepared with 90 mL acetonitrile and 10 mL methanol. A stock solution at 10 μg/mL was prepared in methanol by mixing all the standards with appropriates volumes. The internal standard solution was a mixture of all the deuterated compounds at 5 μg/mL in methanol.

2.3. Sample Preparation

Meconium samples are stored at −80 °C before analysis. Two solid phase extractions (SPE) are carried out from the sample: (1) a first extraction devoted to DoA non cannabinoids, and (2) a second one devoted to cannabinoids. The sample amount is 300 mg of meconium (±10 mg) and 900 μL of phosphate buffer pH = 5 were added. The mixture is vortexed for 20 s following by 10 min in an ultrasonic bath. The mixture is then hydrolyzed with 100 μL of β-glucuronidase at 48 °C for 1 h. A first centrifugation is done, 10 min at rpm. (1) The supernatant is transferred into an Oasis HLB Prime column (Waters, Milford, CT, USA), which were not previously conditioned. The column is rinsed with 2 mL of water and dried for 10 min under vacuum. The molecules are then eluted with 1 mL of an acetonitrile/methanol mixture (90/10; *v/v*). (2) Residual meconium is reconstituted with 600 μL of buffer pH = 5 and 300 μL of acetonitrile with 1% formic acid, the sample is vortexed for 20 s and then centrifuged for 10 min at rpm. The supernatant is transferred into a novel Oasis HLB Prime column without pretreatment. After introducing the sample, the column is rinsed by adding 2 mL of methanol/water (25/75; *v/v*) and dried for 10 min under vacuum. The molecules are then eluted with 1 mL of an acetonitrile/methanol (90/10; *v/v*). The eluates are collected before being evaporated to dryness under nitrogen flow at +48 °C. The dry residue is reconstituted with 100 μL of mobile phase A (2 mM ammonium formate in water and 0.1% formic acid)/methanol (70/30; *v/v*). Five μL is injected into the chromatographic system. A schematic description of the procedure is presented in Figure 1.

2.4. Instruments

2.4.1. Liquid Chromatography

Liquid chromatography was performed on a Vanquish UHPLC system (Thermo, Les Ulis, France). The compounds were separated on a Luna Omega Polar C18 column (2.1 mm × 100 mm; 1.6 μm, Phenomenex, Le Pecq, France) with an oven temperature set at 50 °C. The flow rate was fixed at 0.4 mL/min. The mobile phase A was a mixture of 2 mM ammonium formate in water and 0.1% formic acid; mobile phase B was methanol. The chromatographic gradient was as follows: 100% A for 1 min, linear gradient to 55% A in 5 min, linear gradient to 50% A in 1 min held for 1 min, follow by a linear gradient to 0% A in 4 min held for 1 min. The column re-equilibration was performed by a linear gradient to 100% A in 0.1 min held for 2 min.

2.4.2. Mass Spectrometry

Ionization was performed with a heated electrospray ionization (HESI) source operating in positive mode. Nitrogen was employed as sheath gas (60 UA) and auxiliary gas (10 UA). Vaporization temperature was set at 320 °C. Capillary voltage was set at 3.5 kV and S-lens at 70 eV. The ions were then analyzed by high-resolution mass spectrometry (Orbitrap Exploris 120, Thermo, Les Ulis, France) in data-dependent mode. The full scan analysis was realized over a window ranging from 125 to 650 m/z with a resolution of 60,000 FWHM. The MS2 analysis was performed with a parent ion isolation window of 1 m/z, a dynamic exclusion of 6 s and a resolution of 16,000 FWHM. Mass spectrometer was calibrated once a week with a MRFA solution (L-methionyl-arginyl-phenylalanyl-alanine acetate) 1 μg mL^{-1}, caffeine 2 μg mL^{-1} and Ultramark® 1621 0.001% over a mass range of 50–2000 m/z.

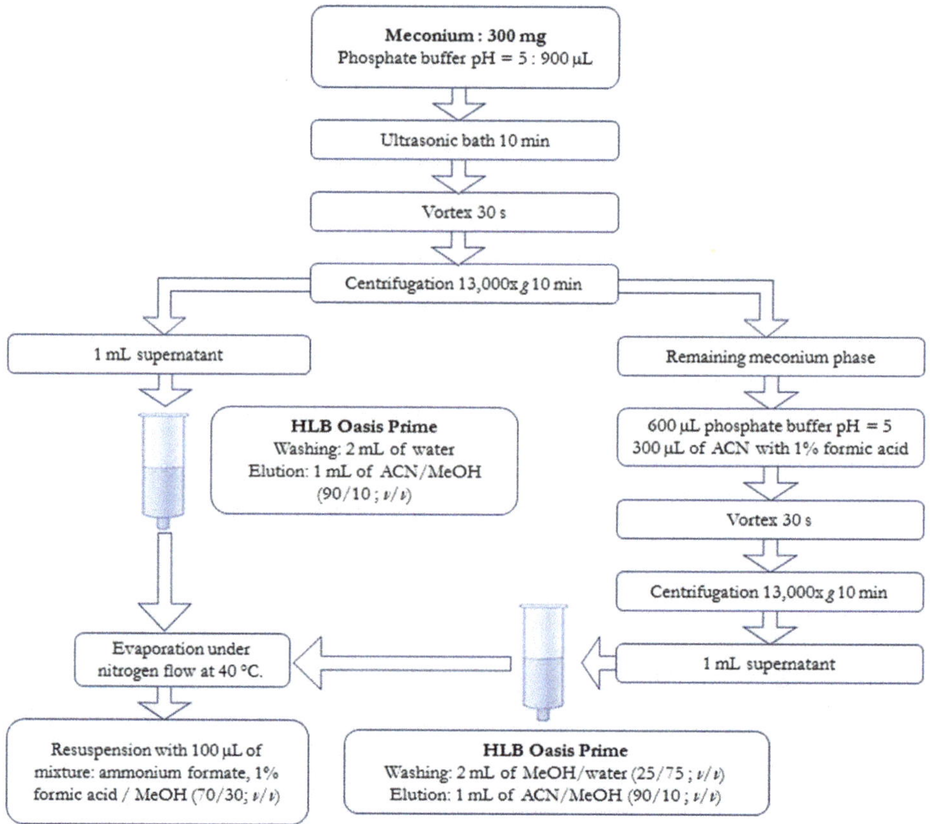

Figure 1. Schematic representation of the extraction procedure.

2.5. Data Reprocessing

Data were processed using the Compound Discoverer 3.2 (Thermo, Les Ulis, France) software following a specific workflow. All ions presenting a signal over 3 times the background noise and a peak intensity over 500,000 were taken into account to create the extracted ion chromatogram (EIC). MS and MS2 spectra were then used to identify ions. Three processes were used for compound identification:

(1) MassList: this process includes an in-house library containing 150 molecules. Identification is carried out using exact mass, isotopic profile and retention time.
(2) MzCloud: mzCloud™ is an online library containing 19,521 molecules with MS and MS2 spectra [22]. The mzCloud™ database contains 17 compound classes, screening was performed including all classes. Identification was performed using the HighChem HighRes algorithm.
(3) NIST: the NIST is a downloaded library constituted by the National Institute of Standards and Technology, recently a spectra database compatible with LC-HRMS technology has been released. This library contained 26,000 molecules with MS and MS2 spectra. The identification is performed using the NIST identification algorithm.

These three processes include monoisotopic mass and isotopic pattern for compound identification with a tolerance of 5 ppm.

2.6. Method Validation

The method was validated for 15 molecules: 6-MAM, morphine, buprenorphine, norbuprenorphine, methadone, EDDP, methamphetamine, amphetamine, MDA, MDMA, cocaine, benzoylecgonine, THC, 11-OH-THC and THC-COOH. SWGTOX guidelines were followed for the validation procedure [23]. The following criteria were considered for a qualitative method validation: specificity, limit of detection, limit of identification, matrix effect, extraction yield and cross-contamination (carry over).

2.6.1. Specificity

Specificity was assessed by analyzing five drug-free meconium samples from healthy newborns. Currently, no commercial proficiency test is available for meconium toxicological screening.

2.6.2. Matrix Effect and Extraction Yield

Three procedures (A, B and C) were performed on six different blank meconium samples at two concentrations (100 pg/mg and 500 pg/mg) in order to evaluate extraction yield and matrix effect (ME): (A) Analytes and the IS were spiked in the mobile phase and directly injected; (B) Analytes and the IS were spiked afterwards in extracted blank matrix samples and injected; and (C) Analytes and IS were spiked in meconium samples, the complete extraction procedure was carried through, and the samples were injected into the system. The mean chromatographic peaks obtained using the three procedures were compared. The ratios C/B, B/A and C/A determined the extraction yield, the matrix effect and the process efficiency, respectively, and were calculated for each analyte.

2.6.3. Limit of Detection and Identification

Sensitivity was evaluated by injecting 3 different meconium matrices spiked with a mixture of the 15 substances at different concentrations (0.05 pg/mg, 0.1 pg/mg, 0.5 pg/mg, 1 pg/mg, 5 pg/mg, 10 pg/mg, 50 pg/mg, and 100 pg/mg). Limit of identification (LOI) was defined by the lowest concentration of analyte that could be correctly identified by the processing software. Limit of detection (LOD) was defined as the lower concentration exhibiting a signal at least three-fold the background noise.

2.6.4. Cross-Contamination

Cross-contamination was assessed by injecting a blank sample immediately after a blank sample spiked at 500 pg/mg (50 pg/mg for 6-MAM, buprenorphine, norbuprenorphine, THC, THC-COOH and 11-OH-THC). For a quantitative method, the signal generated must be lower than 20% of the limit of quantification for the analytes and 5% for the internal standards. In the development of this qualitative method, we consider that no signal should be generated on the blank sample.

2.6.5. Application

The method was applied to real samples addressed to the Pharmacokinetics and Toxicology Laboratory of Marseille. Meconium samples were collected between 0 and 3 days after birth, and sent to the laboratory at ambient temperature. Samples were then stored at −80 °C till analysis. Stability after 3 freeze/thaw cycles was evaluated in previous studies. No relevant degradation was observed for 6-MAM, morphine, cocaine, benzoylecgonine, buprenorphine, norbuprenorphine, THC, THC-COOH and 11-OH-THC (<10%), for amphetamine, metamphetamine, MDA, MDMA (<15%) and for methadone and EDDP (<20%) [7,24–30].

3. Results and Discussion

3.1. Method Development and Validation

The aim of this study was to develop a new analytical method devoted to meconium toxicological screening relying on Orbitrap mass spectrometry. Meconium remains the gold standard matrix to evaluate in utero exposure to xenobiotics, however two major limits reduce its use. The matrix is very pasty and sticky, requiring a complex analytical pre-treatment and the sample amount is sometimes limited, allowing a single analysis. In the method presented here, a small amount of sample was necessary, 300 mg, which is acceptable in comparison to previous publications using between 200 and 2000 mg [7–18]. Several extraction procedures have been applied to meconium toxicological analysis including liquid–liquid extraction [9], salting out assisted liquid–liquid extraction [14] and solid-phase extraction (SPE) [11–13,15–18]. SPE is widely employed to prepare and clean up complex matrices in the field of forensic analysis and is the most widely used method for the preparation of meconium. SPE was therefore chosen in this method development. The chromatographic run was completed in 12 min and initial conditions were restored in 2 min. No interferences were observed for the 15 compounds included in the method evaluation after the analysis of 5 blank meconium samples.

Mean matrix effects and extraction recoveries results are presented in Table 1. An ion suppression was observed for all compounds between −79 and −19% at 100 pg/mg and −89% and −16% at 500 pg/mg. These modifications of ionization were well corrected with internal standards, providing ME between −15 and +15% with the exception of 6-MAM at 100 pg/mg (+28%). Coefficients of variation were under 15%, highlighting a good precision, although this method is not devoted to quantitation. Cannabinoids (THC, 11-OH-THC and THC-COOH) presented the most important ion suppression (between −89 and −49%). Prego-Meleiro et al. noticed a similar matrix effect in meconium (between −71 and −26%) [16]. However, this does not affect the sensitivity with a limit of detection for cannabinoids at 5 pg/mg and a limit of identification at 10 pg/mg (with the exception of THC-COOH, not identified). Extraction recoveries were over 50% for most compounds except norbuprenorphine at 500 pg/mg (47%) and cannabinoids (between 18 and 45%). Ristimaa et al. obtained a lower extraction recovery (16%) for THC-COOH after liquid–liquid extraction [17]. Prego-Meleiro et al. observed a higher extraction yield, between 50 and 68%, however their sample pretreatment relying on a SPE was specifically devoted to the detection and quantification of cannabinoids and their metabolites in meconium [16].

Limits of detection and identification are presented in Table 2. The LOD are in good agreement with previously published methods. LOD obtained for 6-MAM, EDDP, metamphetamine, amphetamine, MDMA, cocaine and THC are slightly higher than those reported in the literature. This could be attributed to the mass spectrometer acquisition mode. The detection is carried out from the spectrum acquired in fullscan mode, which is more affected by the background noise than data acquired following a LC-MS/MS acquisition (MRM) used in the majority of the methods indicated in Table 2. A comparison of LOD and meconium concentrations measured in real samples is also provided in Table 2. The developed method is sensitive enough to detect all compounds. The only compound exhibiting a LOD overlapping meconium concentrations is THC: LOD = 5 pg/mg and concentrations measured in real samples = 4.2–7.7 pg/mg. However, THC is always detected in association with at least one metabolite, and exhibits concentration lower than THC-COOH in meconium samples [16]. Therefore, this limit is easily compensated for by the detection of THC-COOH. To our knowledge, limits of identification have never been evaluated before in meconium for these compounds with high resolution mass spectrometry and an untargeted approach (no inclusion list). All molecules have been successfully identified at low concentrations (<50 pg/mg) with the exception of THC-COOH. Interestingly, LOI were lower enough to identify most compounds at the concentrations found in real samples. The only class requiring a targeted approach remains cannabinoids. Regarding carry-over, blank samples injected after meconium samples spiked at 500 pg/mg did not present any traces for the 15 validated molecules.

Table 1. Matrix effect and coefficient of variation observed for the 15 compounds at 100 pg/mg and 500 pg/mg (compounds marked with an asterisk (*) were evaluated at 10 pg/mg and 50 pg/mg).

	100 pg/mg (n = 6)					500 pg/mg (n = 6)				
Compounds	Raw (%)	Matrix Effect Normalized with Internal Standard (%)	CV (%)	Extraction Yield (%)	Process Efficiency (%)	Raw (%)	Matrix Effect Normalized with Internal Standard (%)	CV (%)	Extraction Yield (%)	Process Efficiency (%)
6-MAM *	−29	+28	10.8	52	37	−29	+15	14.9	53	38
Morphine	−42	+4	9.6	61	35	−31	+11	10.7	55	38
Buprenorphine *	−25	−3	5.3	66	50	−27	+11	10.5	61	45
Norbuprenorphine *	−31	−4	9.1	62	43	−39	+4	11.7	47	29
Methadone	−19	0	10.2	70	57	−18	+13	11.6	61	50
EDDP	−22	−3	5.8	71	55	−19	+11	11.2	72	58
Amphetamine	−35	−1	12	73	47	−22	+23	12.2	61	48
MDA	−29	−1	9.6	61	43	−16	+15	12.2	68	57
MDMA	−31	−3	6.7	60	41	−25	+16	9.3	62	47
Methamphetamine	−31	−5	7.4	69	48	−23	+13	9.7	65	50
Cocaine	−25	−5	6.1	61	46	−21	+11	12.7	64	51
Benzoylecgonine	−25	−2	7.6	62	47	−26	+10	10.9	63	47
THC *	−79	−2	8.2	24	5	−89	−12	14.9	19	2
11-OH-THC *	−49	+5	10.1	45	23	−65	+6	8.3	31	11
THC-COOH *	−69	+14	11.6	18	6	−72	+10	14.4	18	5

Table 2. Limit of detection (LOD) and limit of identification (LOI) observed for the 15 compounds, LOD retrieved in previous studies and concentrations.

Compounds	LOD (pg/mg)	LOI (pg/mg)	LOD Found in the Literature (pg/mg)	Concentrations Found in the Literature (pg/mg)	References
6-MAM	5	5	0.3–1.5	5–142 (n = 3)	[7,17,28]
Morphine	0.5	10	1.2–6	397 (n = 1)	[7,17,28]
Buprenorphine	0.5	5	5–10	23.9–240.5 (n = 9)	[17,31,32]
Norbuprenorphine	5	10	5–10	323.9–1880.2 (n = 10)	[17,31,32]
Methadone	0.1	5	0.25–10	85–21,980 (n = 48)	[17,28,33]
EDDP	0.5	5	0.25–25	4431–101,021 (n = 48)	[28,33]
Methamphetamine	1	50	0.2–10	18–13,325 (n = 16)	[14,17,27]
Amphetamine	5	5	0.5–10	41–2220 (n = 15)	[14,17,27]
MDA	5	5	2–4	No data	[14,17]
MDMA	5	10	0.3–4	No data	[14,17]
Cocaine	1	50	0.5–0.9	72–903 (n = 3)	[7,28]
Benzoylecgonine	0.5	5	1–1.2	134–847 (n = 3)	[7,28]
THC	5	10	1	4.2–7.7 (n = 4)	[16]
11-OH-THC	5	10	1	11.9 (n = 1)	[16]
THC-COOH	5	NI	1–20	24.1–288.8 (n = 4)	[16,17]

3.2. Application

The results of meconium analyses (n = 29 samples) are presented in Table S1. The application allowed the identification of different biomarkers in meconium samples. All molecules included in the validation were detected with the exception of amphetamines (amphetamine, metamphetamine, MDMA and MDA) and 6-MAM. However, these molecules were included in the method validation, and presented LOD lower than the concentrations observed in the literature. These molecules were therefore probably absent from the samples analyzed. THC-COOH (not identified during LOI evaluation) was successfully identified in 3 samples; the THC-COOH LOI probably corresponds to a high concentration, higher than those evaluated in the method validation. EIC of the molecules identified in samples 4 and 14 are presented in Figure 2.

The untargeted screening allowed the detection of 88 different substances, each substance being detected in 1 to 22 samples. They include 47 pharmaceuticals and 15 pharmaceutical metabolites (antalgic, antibiotics, anticonvulsants, antidepressants, antiemetic, anti-histaminics, antihypertensives, antipyretic, antiretrovirals, benzodiazepines, beta-2-agonist, beta-blocker, H2 blocker, local anesthetics, antifungal, neuroleptics, opiates, proton pump inhibitor, and stimulant). Most of these molecules are classically prescribed to pregnant woman for nausea, gastroesophageal reflux, peripartum anesthesia, infection prevention during cesarean section and eclampsia treatment.

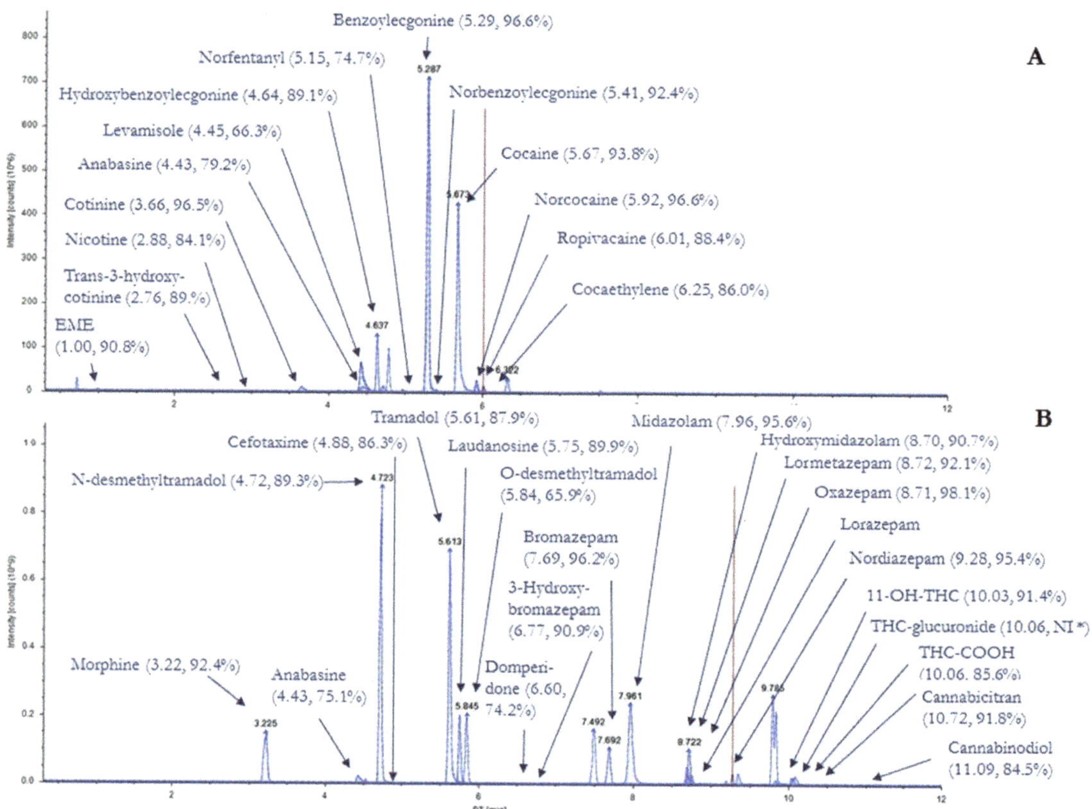

Figure 2. Presentation of the extracted ion chromatograms (EIC) for the substances identified in sample n° 4 (**A**) and sample n° 14 (**B**) (retention time, similarity score with the MzCloud™ spectral library). * THC-glucuronide was not identified with MzCloud™ and NIST library (NI), but solely with the house made library.

Cocaine and its metabolites were successfully identified (benzoylecgonine (n = 5), cocaethylene (n = 1), cocaine (n = 4), ecgonine methyl ester (n = 2), hydroxybenzoylecgonine (n = 1), norbenzoylecgonine (n = 2), norcocaine (n = 1)). These substances are commonly identified in meconium [7,28,34]. The identification of cocaethylene in one sample is of particular importance since this metabolite allows the identification of fetal alcohol exposure in addition to cocaine. Levamisole, a cocaine adulterant, was detected in one sample. To our knowledge, levamisole is identified for the first time in meconium. Cannabinoids were identified in 10 samples (11-OH-THC (n = 5), cannabicitran (n = 1), cannabidiol (n = 1), cannabinol (n = 8), THC (n = 4), THC-COOH (n = 7), THC-COOH-glucuronide (n = 7)). This class is of particular importance since this is the main DoA used in France and especially in the Marseille region [2,35]. Natural opioids (codeine (n = 2), norcodeine (n = 1), morphine (n = 5), morphine-3-glucuronide (n = 1), normorphine (n = 1)), synthetic opioids (tramadol (n = 3), N-desmethyltramadol (n = 2), O-desmethyltramadol (n = 1), norfentanyl (n = 16)) and opioid substitution treatments (methadone (n = 2), EDDP (n = 2), buprenorphine (n = 1), norbuprenorphine (n = 1)) were well detected. Interestingly, solely norfentanyl (n = 16) was identified and fentanyl was not detected even following a manual identification. Conversely, López-Rabuñal et al. identified fentanyl in four meconium samples without norfentanyl (included in the screening) [21]. Ristimaa et al. detected fentanyl in 2 out of 209 meconium samples, however they do not indicate if norfentanyl was screened for [17]. Fentanyl is known to cross the placenta barrier and has been detected in umbilical cord plasma [36]. Therefore, this compound should be detected in meconium samples. This discrepancy could be explained by a lack of sensitivity, as fentanyl LOD and LOI were not evaluated here. Additionally, several biomarkers of tobacco exposure were identified (anabasine (n = 22), nicotine (n = 3), cotinine (n = 20), cotinine-N-oxide (n = 3), trans-3-hydroxycotinine (n = 4)).

Most of the analytical methods described in the literature for the determination of DoA in meconium are based on LC-MS/MS [10–16,18]. All these methods are targeted, therefore limiting the number of compounds analyzed. LC-HRMS allows the inclusion of hundreds of compounds in the database without compromising on sensitivity. In addition, retrieval of new compounds in the acquisition data is easy because the formula database is updatable with literature data for current substances, such as designer drugs. These results highlight the interest of this untargeted analytical method in the context of high-risk pregnancies. The application to samples collected in the framework of the care of newborns has made it possible to highlight most of the molecules of interest. This made it possible to document in a precise and almost exhaustive manner the exposure of newborns in utero, to adapt medical monitoring and care at birth and in particular to adjust treatment in the event of a withdrawal syndrome. The main limitation of this method is the absence of biomarker of exposure to alcohol. The qualitative aspect of the developed method may be a second limitation; however, interpretation of quantitative results is difficult due to contamination of meconium with urine [37–39]. A further limitation of this procedure is the cumbersome analytical preparation prior the analysis (two SPE). However, meconium is a tricky matrix which requires an extensive analytical pre-treatment.

4. Conclusions

This study enabled the development of a sensitive untargeted method devoted to meconium analysis, using low amount of meconium. To our knowledge, this is the first untargeted method allowing the simultaneous detection of the four categories of DoA (opioids, amphetamines, cannabinoids, cocaine). The application to real samples demonstrates the efficacy of this protocol in identifying DoA and pharmaceuticals. This method is now used routinely for toxicological screening in high-risk pregnancies. This procedure, by revealing the presence of drugs and metabolites beyond the ordinary scope of abused drugs, will significantly help pediatricians and will make it possible to quickly adapt the care of newborns.

Supplementary Materials: The following are available online at https://www.mdpi.com/article/10.3390/toxics10020055/s1, Table S1: Substances identified in meconium samples.

Author Contributions: Conceptualization, N.F.; methodology, J.B.; formal analysis, A.H., C.P.-F. and N.D.; investigation, V.L.; writing—original draft preparation, N.F.; writing—review and editing, B.L. and C.S.; supervision, B.L., C.S. and N.F. All authors have read and agreed to the published version of the manuscript.

Funding: This research received no external funding.

Institutional Review Board Statement: The study was conducted according to the guidelines of the Declaration of Helsinki, and approved by the Institutional Review Board of the AP-HM (PADS21-331, 21 December 2021).

Informed Consent Statement: Patient consent was waived because the analyzes described in this study were performed as part of normal medical care and not as part of a research protocol.

Data Availability Statement: Not applicable.

Conflicts of Interest: The authors declare no conflict of interest.

References

1. United Nations Office on Drug and Crime World Drug Report 2021. Available online: https://www.unodc.org/unodc/en/data-and-analysis/wdr2021.html (accessed on 13 October 2021).
2. Observatoire Français des Drogues et des Toxicomanies. Available online: https://www.ofdt.fr/publications/collections/periodiques/drogues-chiffres-cles/drogues-chiffres-cles-8eme-edition-2019 (accessed on 13 October 2021).
3. Ostrea, E.M.; Brady, M.; Gause, S.; Raymundo, A.L.; Stevens, M. Drug screening of newborns by meconium analysis: A large-scale, prospective, epidemiologic study. *Pediatrics* **1992**, *89*, 107–113. [CrossRef] [PubMed]
4. Gray, T.R.; Choo, R.E.; Concheiro, M.; Williams, E.; Elko, A.; Jansson, L.M.; Jones, H.E.; Huestis, M.A. Prenatal methadone exposure, meconium biomarker concentrations and neonatal abstinence syndrome. *Addict. Abingdon Engl.* **2010**, *105*, 2151–2159. [CrossRef] [PubMed]
5. Moore, C.; Negrusz, A.; Lewis, D. Determination of drugs of abuse in meconium. *J. Chromatogr. B Biomed. Sci. Appl.* **1998**, *713*, 137–146. [CrossRef]
6. Tamama, K. Advances in drugs of abuse testing. *Clin. Chim. Acta* **2021**, *514*, 40–47. [CrossRef] [PubMed]
7. Pichini, S.; Pacifici, R.; Pellegrini, M.; Marchei, E.; Pérez-Alarcón, E.; Puig, C.; Vall, O.; García-Algar, O. Development and validation of a liquid chromatography-mass spectrometry assay for the determination of opiates and cocaine in meconium. *J. Chromatogr. B Anal. Technol. Biomed. Life Sci.* **2003**, *794*, 281–292. [CrossRef]
8. Bearer, C.F.; Santiago, L.M.; O'Riordan, M.A.; Buck, K.; Lee, S.C.; Singer, L.T. Fatty acid ethyl esters: Quantitative biomarkers for maternal alcohol consumption. *J. Pediatr.* **2005**, *146*, 824–830. [CrossRef] [PubMed]
9. Sampériz, S.; Millet, V.; Arditti, J.; Lacroze, V.; Masset, D.; Bourdon, H.; Jouglard, J.; Unal, D. Value of toxicological research in newborn infants of addicted mothers by the study of several samples (urine, meconium, hair). *Arch. Pediatr. Organe Off. Soc. Francaise Pediatr.* **1996**, *3*, 440–444. [CrossRef]
10. Colby, J.M.; Adams, B.C.; Morad, A.; Presley, L.D.; Patrick, S.W. Umbilical cord tissue and meconium may not be equivalent for confirming in utero substance exposure. *J. Pediatr.* **2019**, *205*, 277–280. [CrossRef]
11. Joya, X.; Marchei, E.; Salat-Batlle, J.; García-Algar, O.; Calvaresi, V.; Pacifici, R.; Pichini, S. Drugs of abuse in maternal hair and paired neonatal meconium: An objective assessment of foetal exposure to gestational consumption. *Drug Test. Anal.* **2016**, *8*, 864–868. [CrossRef]
12. Meyer-Monath, M.; Chatellier, C.; Rouget, F.; Morel, I.; Lestremau, F. Development of a multi-residue method in a fetal matrix: Analysis of meconium. *Anal. Bioanal. Chem.* **2014**, *406*, 7785–7797. [CrossRef]
13. López-Rabuñal, A.; Lendoiro, E.; Concheiro, M.; López-Rivadulla, M.; Cruz, A.; de-Castro-Ríos, A. LC–MS-MS method for the determination of antidepressants and benzodiazepines in meconium. *J. Anal. Toxicol.* **2020**, *44*, 580–588. [CrossRef] [PubMed]
14. Nemeškalová, A.; Bursová, M.; Sýkora, D.; Kuchař, M.; Čabala, R.; Hložek, T. Salting out assisted liquid-liquid extraction for liquid chromatography tandem-mass spectrometry determination of amphetamine-like stimulants in meconium. *J. Pharm. Biomed. Anal.* **2019**, *172*, 42–49. [CrossRef] [PubMed]
15. Abernethy, C.; McCall, K.E.; Cooper, G.; Favretto, D.; Vaiano, F.; Bertol, E.; Mactier, H. Determining the pattern and prevalence of alcohol consumption in pregnancy by measuring biomarkers in meconium. *Arch. Dis. Child. Fetal Neonatal* **2018**, *103*, F216–F220. [CrossRef] [PubMed]
16. Prego-Meleiro, P.; Lendoiro, E.; Concheiro, M.; Cruz, A.; López-Rivadulla, M.; de Castro, A. Development and validation of a liquid chromatography tandem mass spectrometry method for the determination of cannabinoids and phase I and II metabolites in meconium. *J. Chromatogr. A* **2017**, *1497*, 118–126. [CrossRef]
17. Ristimaa, J.; Gergov, M.; Pelander, A.; Halmesmäki, E.; Ojanperä, I. Broad-Spectrum drug screening of meconium by liquid chromatography with tandem mass spectrometry and time-of-flight mass spectrometry. *Anal. Bioanal. Chem.* **2010**, *398*, 925–935. [CrossRef] [PubMed]
18. Malaca, S.; Marchei, E.; Barceló Martín, B.; Minutillo, A.; Pichini, S. Novel fast ultra-performance liquid chromatography-tandem mass spectrometry (UHPLC-MS/MS) and extraction of Ethylglucuronide in meconium samples. *Drug Test. Anal.* **2019**, *11*, 1471–1475. [CrossRef] [PubMed]
19. Coles, R.; Kushnir, M.M.; Nelson, G.J.; McMillin, G.A.; Urry, F.M. Simultaneous determination of codeine, morphine, hydrocodone, hydromorphone, oxycodone, and 6-Acetylmorphine in Urine, Serum, Plasma, whole blood, and meconium by LC-MS-MS. *J. Anal. Toxicol.* **2007**, *31*, 1–14. [CrossRef]
20. De Carvalho Mantovani, C.; Silva, J.P.E.; Forster, G.; de Almeida, R.M.; de Albuquerque Diniz, E.M.; Yonamine, M. Simultaneous Accelerated Solvent Extraction and Hydrolysis of 11-nor-Δ9-Tetrahydrocannabinol-9-Carboxylic Acid Glucuronide in Meconium Samples for Gas Chromatography-Mass Spectrometry Analysis. *J. Chromatogr. B Anal. Technol. Biomed. Life Sci.* **2018**, *1074–1075*, 1–7. [CrossRef]
21. López-Rabuñal, Á.; Di Corcia, D.; Amante, E.; Massano, M.; Cruz-Landeira, A.; de-Castro-Ríos, A.; Salomone, A. Simultaneous determination of 137 drugs of abuse, new psychoactive substances, and novel synthetic opioids in meconium by UHPLC-QTOF. *Anal. Bioanal. Chem.* **2021**, *413*, 5493–5507. [CrossRef]
22. MzCloud Database. Available online: https://www.mzcloud.org/home (accessed on 13 October 2021).
23. Scientific Working Group for Forensic Toxicology. Scientific working Group for Forensic Toxicology (SWGTOX) standard practices for method validation in forensic toxicology. *J. Anal. Toxicol.* **2013**, *37*, 452–474. [CrossRef]

24. Kacinko, S.L.; Shakleya, D.M.; Huestis, M.A. Validation and application of a method for the determination of buprenorphine, norbuprenorphine, and their glucuronide conjugates in human meconium. *Anal. Chem.* **2008**, *80*, 246–252. [CrossRef] [PubMed]
25. Marchei, E.; Pellegrini, M.; Pacifici, R.; Palmi, I.; Lozano, J.; García-Algar, O.; Pichini, S. Quantification of Delta9-Tetrahydrocannabinol and its major metabolites in meconium by gas chromatographic-mass spectrometric assay: Assay validation and preliminary results of the "meconium project". *Ther. Drug Monit.* **2006**, *28*, 700–706. [CrossRef] [PubMed]
26. Pichini, S.; Pacifici, R.; Pellegrini, M.; Marchei, E.; Lozano, J.; Murillo, J.; Vall, O.; García-Algar, Ó. Development and validation of a high-performance liquid chromatography−mass spectrometry assay for determination of amphetamine, methamphetamine, and methylenedioxy derivatives in meconium. *Anal. Chem.* **2004**, *76*, 2124–2132. [CrossRef] [PubMed]
27. Gunn, J.A.; Sweeney, B.; Dahn, T.; Bell, S.; Newhouse, R.; Terrell, A.R. Simultaneous Quantification of amphetamine and methamphetamine in meconium using ISOLUTE HM-N-Supported liquid extraction columns and GC-MS. *J. Anal. Toxicol.* **2008**, *32*, 485–490. [CrossRef]
28. De Castro, A.; Concheiro, M.; Shakleya, D.M.; Huestis, M.A. Simultaneous quantification of methadone, cocaine, opiates, and metabolites in human placenta by liquid Chromatography–Mass spectrometry. *J. Anal. Toxicol.* **2009**, *33*, 243–252. [CrossRef]
29. Concheiro, M.; Gutierrez, F.M.; Ocampo, A.; Lendoiro, E.; González-Colmenero, E.; Concheiro-Guisán, A.; Peñas-Silva, P.; Macías-Cortiña, M.; Cruz-Landeira, A.; López-Rivadulla, M.; et al. Assessment of biological matrices for the detection of in utero cannabis exposure. *Drug Test. Anal.* **2021**, *13*, 1371–1382. [CrossRef]
30. Kelly, T.; Gray, T.R.; Huestis, M.A. Development and validation of a liquid chromatography-atmospheric pressure chemical ionization-tandem mass spectrometry method for simultaneous analysis of ten amphetamine-, methamphetamine- and 3,4-methylenedioxymethamphetamine-related (MDMA) analytes in human meconium. *J. Chromatogr. B Anal. Technol. Biomed. Life Sci.* **2008**, *867*, 194–204.
31. Marin, S.J.; McMillin, G.A. Quantitation of total buprenorphine and norbuprenorphine in meconium by LC-MS/MS. *Methods Mol. Biol. Clifton NJ* **2016**, *1383*, 59–68. [CrossRef]
32. Kacinko, S.L.; Jones, H.E.; Johnson, R.E.; Choo, R.E.; Huestis, M.A. Correlations of Maternal buprenorphine dose, buprenorphine, and metabolite concentrations in meconium with neonatal outcomes. *Clin. Pharmacol. Ther.* **2008**, *84*, 604–612. [CrossRef]
33. Di Trana, A.; La Maida, N.; Tittarelli, R.; Huestis, M.A.; Pichini, S.; Busardò, F.P.; Carlier, J. Monitoring prenatal exposure to buprenorphine and methadone. *Ther. Drug Monit.* **2020**, *42*, 181–193. [CrossRef]
34. D'Avila, F.B.; Limberger, R.P.; Fröehlich, P.E. Cocaine and crack cocaine abuse by pregnant or lactating mothers and analysis of its biomarkers in meconium and breast milk by LC–MS—A review. *Clin. Biochem.* **2016**, *49*, 1096–1103. [CrossRef] [PubMed]
35. Observatoire Français des Drogues et des Toxicomanies. Available online: https://www.ofdt.fr/publications/collections/rapports/portraits-de-territoire/addictions-en-provence-alpes-cote-dazur-consommations-de-substances-psychoactives-et-offre-medicosociale/ (accessed on 13 October 2021).
36. Fleet, J.-A.; Belan, I.; Gordon, A.L.; Cyna, A.M. Fentanyl concentration in maternal and umbilical cord plasma following intranasal or subcutaneous administration in labour. *Int. J. Obstet. Anesth.* **2020**, *42*, 34–38. [CrossRef] [PubMed]
37. Gareri, J.; Klein, J.; Koren, G. Drugs of abuse testing in meconium. *Clin. Chim. Acta Int. J. Clin. Chem.* **2006**, *366*, 101–111. [CrossRef] [PubMed]
38. Gray, T.; Huestis, M. Bioanalytical procedures for monitoring in utero drug exposure. *Anal. Bioanal. Chem.* **2007**, *388*, 1455–1465. [CrossRef] [PubMed]
39. Lombardero, N.; Casanova, O.; Behnke, M.; Eyler, F.D.; Bertholf, R.L. Measurement of Cocaine and metabolites in urine, meconium, and diapers by gas chromatography/mass spectrometry. *Ann. Clin. Lab. Sci.* **1993**, *23*, 385–394. [PubMed]

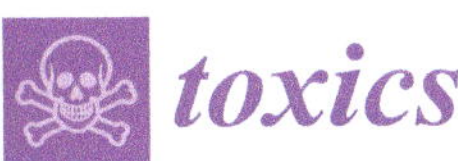 toxics

MDPI

Article

Diquat Poisoning: Care Management and Medico-Legal Implications

Pascale Basilicata [1], Maria Pieri [1], Angela Simonelli [1,*], Emanuele Capasso [1], Claudia Casella [1], Tina Noto [2], Fabio Policino [1] and Pierpaolo Di Lorenzo [1]

[1] Department of Advanced Biomedical Science-Legal Medicine Section, University of Naples "Federico II", 80138 Naples, Italy; pascale.basilicata@unina.it (P.B.); maria.pieri@unina.it (M.P.); emanuele.capasso@unina.it (E.C.); claudia.casella@unina.it (C.C.); fabio.policino@unina.it (F.P.); pierpaolo.dilorenzo@unina.it (P.D.L.)

[2] Department of Forensic and Forensic Medicine, University of Murcia, 30100 Murcia, Spain; tina.noto@um.es

* Correspondence: angela.simonelli@unina.it; Tel.: +39-0817463474; Fax: +39-0817464726

Abstract: Acute chemical intoxication represents one of the major causes of Emergency Room admittance, and possible errors in diagnosis are extremely frequent, especially when patients present generic and non-specific symptoms. Diquat, a bipyridyl class of herbicides, exerts high intrinsic toxicity as a consequence of free oxygen radicals, leading to cellular death and organ dysfunctions. Following ingestion, with the major source of absorption for suicidal purposes, the chemical induces local irritating effects; systemic symptoms appear later, while specific symptoms can occur in the following 48 h. A smoker and hypertensive 50-year-old man arrives at the E.R., reporting that an episode of herbicide inhalation occurred few hours earlier. Physical examination evidenced alkalosis with hypoxemia, leucocytosis, mild hyperglycaemia and moderate increase in creatine kinase and myoglobin. Despite blood creatine kinase and myoglobin values that were higher than normal, he was prescribed with hydration and anti-pain therapy. During the night, the man left the hospital; he returned the next morning at 8:45 a.m., with cardiorespiratory arrest, medium fixed non-reactive mydriasis, diffused cyanosis of the skin and of the mucous membranes, as well as imperceptible pulse and peripheral pressure. Despite resuscitation attempts, the patient died at 9:30 a.m.; the body was immediately transferred to the morgue. Autopsy and toxicological analyses were carried out nine days later, evidencing paraquat ingestion for suicidal purposes. GC/MS analyses to verify the presence of diquat were performed on body fluids and gastric and colon contents; all specimens resulted positive, thus confirming the cause of death as herbicide ingestion (blood diquat concentration of 1.2 mg/L; more than twice the minimum to observe a systemic poisoning). The procedure followed for patient management resulted to be not in line with the provisions of both guidelines and good clinical practices. Staff did not perform clinical-diagnostical monitoring of the patient's condition or ask for more specific analyses (i.e., serum creatine phosphokinase monitoring). This misconduct led to a decrease in the patient's chances to survive.

Keywords: diquat; suicidal ingestion; patient management; professional liabilities

Citation: Basilicata, P.; Pieri, M.; Simonelli, A.; Capasso, E.; Casella, C.; Noto, T.; Policino, F.; Di Lorenzo, P. Diquat Poisoning: Care Management and Medico-Legal Implications. *Toxics* **2022**, *10*, 166. https://doi.org/10.3390/toxics10040166

Academic Editor: David R. Wallace

Received: 4 March 2022
Accepted: 29 March 2022
Published: 30 March 2022

Publisher's Note: MDPI stays neutral with regard to jurisdictional claims in published maps and institutional affiliations.

1. Introduction

Exposure to chemicals represents a major source of accidents and hospitalizations; applications for compensation may derive from incorrect patient management [1,2]. The XII edition of the MadMed survey report on errors related to medical malpractice in Italy between 2004 and 2019 showed that Orthopaedics and Traumatology Operative Units together with Emergency Rooms (E.R.; the principal unit involved in the management of patients showing chemical poisoning) present the highest frequency of adverse events (20.1% and 14.2%, respectively), followed by General Surgery Departments, showing 13.2% of adverse events [3]. In the E.R., errors can derive from incorrect diagnosis (59.9%) and therapies (25.2%), both resulting in severe consequences in terms of permanent disability or death; estimated costs related to each error amounts to about 92.547 euros [3].

Acute intoxication derives from a dynamic process characterized by a rapid negative evolution with possible lethal consequences, even when symptoms are initially mild; exposure to xenobiotics represents a major source of acute intoxication, and severity is generally dose-related [4]. Symptoms deriving from poisoning vary according to the chemical/physical characteristics of the xenobiotic involved. Absorption route, exposure time, interpersonal variability, and the subject's general health condition also play a critical role in determining the specific effects registered in each patient. The times of evolution may differ, as the manifestations of toxicity can be delayed by the exposure time. Clinical manifestations are strictly related to chemical and physical properties of the substance and can be used to determine the duration of the exposure and the absorption routes. These include stomatitis, enteritis, or perforations of the gastrointestinal tract mucous membrane as a consequence of caustic/corrosive substance ingestion; halitosis, in the case of alcohol or hydrocarbon ingestion; erythema, pain, or blisters after dermal absorption (frequent in the case of accidents); lesions in the cornea, sclera, and lens, with eye pain, redness, and loss of vision associated with liquid spills. Anatomical localization of lesions can differ in accordance with solubility (inhalation of toxic water-soluble substances, i.e., chlorine or ammonia, can cause symptoms in the upper airways; otherwise, lesions may occur at the lower airway region or involve non-cardiogenic pulmonary oedema).

Diquat (6,7-dihydrodipyrido[1,2-a:2′,1′-c]pyrazine-5,8-diium dibromide) is a non-selective contact herbicide characterized by a high toxic capacity, commercialized as a paraquat substitute [5]. Treatment of poisoning due to this herbicide requires extensive experience. Clinical manifestations associated with diquat poisoning imply gastroenteritis and acute renal failure, but in severe cases it can lead to respiratory failure, cardiovascular collapse, arrhythmias, seizures, coma with cerebral haemorrhage, and heart attack [6]. Inhalation of the aerosol is generally associated with mild symptoms, rarely resulting in fatal outcomes [7,8]. Ingestion of high diquat doses for suicidal purposes, the most common cause of poisoning, may result in the subject's death during the next one or two days, as reported for a man who ingested about 160 mL of enriched diquat (20 g per 100 mL) [9]. Diquat intoxication can lead to severe toxic effects on the central nervous system, with manifestations including nervousness, irritability, restlessness, aggression, disorientation, senseless reasoning, inability to recognize family or friends, and reduced reflexes. Neurological effects can progress to coma, accompanied by tonic-clonic seizures, and culminate in the patient's death [5,10]. Moreover, diquat ingestion produces corrosive manifestations on digestive tract tissues, with the appearance of burnings in the mouth, throat, chest, and abdomen; intense nausea and vomiting and diarrhoea can appeal up to two days after exposure to low doses, and blood may appear in vomit and stool.

Once absorbed, diquat is excreted through the kidney, the target organ and a useful intoxication index for clinicians [5,6]. Proteinuria, haematuria, and pyuria can progress to renal failure and uraemia. Toxic effects can include liver, pancreatic, heart, and muscle damage; jaundice and liver lesions may arise as evidenced by an increase in alkaline phosphatase, transaminase, and LDH values. If the patient survives several hours or days, cardiocirculatory failure due to dehydration may occur, as well as hypotension and tachycardia, with shock progressing to death. The picture can evolve towards cardiorespiratory problems, including toxic cardiomyopathy, or a secondary infection, such as bronchopneumonia [11].

Case Report

A smoker and hypertensive 50-year-old man came to the E.R. at 9:00 p.m., reporting an episode of accidental inhalation of herbicide happening few hours earlier. The toxic substance and duration of exposure time were not specified.

Physical and laboratory examination: 170/100 SBP, 97% SaO_2; alkalosis with hypoxemia (ABG test: 7.55 pH, pCO_2 23 mmHg, pO_2 69 mmHg), leucocytosis (WBC 14.07 × 10^3/μL—v.n.

4.5–10), mild hyperglycaemia (glucose 123 mg/dL—v.n. 60–110) and moderate increase in creatine kinase (307 UL/L—v.n. ≤ 170) and myoglobin (145.6 ng/dL—25–72). Renal (urea 35 mg/dL—v.n. 15–50; creatinine 0.62 mg/dL—v.n. 0.6–1.3) and hepatic (AST 26 UI/L—v.n. < 40; ALT 30 UI/L—v.n. < 40; GGT 23 UI/L—v.n. 10–71) function parameters were normal. A chest contrast-enhanced CT (ECCT) evidenced blurred and diffuse centrilobular opacities of both upper lobes; an angio-ECCT scan of the abdomen and pelvis excluded internal organ lesions. The patient was hospitalized in the Short Stay Observation Unit at 11:00 p.m., because he suffered from burning in the lower limbs. Physicians prescribed hydration and pain relief therapy (paracetamol in 500 mL saline solution). Vital signs (blood pressure, heart rate, respiratory rate, body temperature, diuresis) were not monitored, nor was the onset of a more specific symptomatology. The next day physicians decided on discharge, but at 8:30 a.m. the man was not in his room. At 8:45 a.m. he arrived at the E.R. in critical condition, presenting cardiorespiratory arrest with medium fixed non-reactive mydriasis, diffuse cyanosis of the skin and mucous membranes, as well as imperceptible pulse and peripheral pressure.

Despite the attempts to resuscitate him, the patient died at 9:30 a.m., and the body was immediately transferred to the morgue. Both autopsy and toxicological analyses were performed nine days later, to clarify the exact cause of death (with particular attention to possible poisoning due to herbicide) as well as to verify eventual professional liabilities.

The identification of the toxic substance was made possible by toxicological examination of the liquids and the biological remains obtained during the autopsy.

There was no evidence that the patient took an additional dose of herbicide when he left the hospital; no further intake by family members was reported.

2. Material and Methods

Certified standard solutions of chemicals used for confirmatory analysis in gas chromatography/mass spectrometry (GC/MS) were from Cerilliant-Merck (Milan, Italy), *N,O*-bis(trimethylsilyl)trifluoroacetamide (BSTFA) derivatizing agent from Acros (Morris Plains, NJ, USA), and HPLC grade solvents from Carlo Erba (Milan, Italy). Solid phase extraction was made using Strata-C18.

Immunochemical screening tests were carried out on a Randox Evidence Investigator (Randox Toxicology, Country Antrim, UK), using DoA I + WB SQ and DoA II WB whole blood tests for AMP/MAMP/MDMA, barbiturates, benzodiazepines, buprenorphine, cannabinoids, cocaine, methadone, opiates, phencyclidine, tricyclic antidepressants, fentanyl, ketamine, LSD, methaqualone, oxycodone, and propoxyphene.

GC/MS analyses were performed using a DSQ single quadrupole mass spectrometer directly linked to a AS3000 gas chromatograph equipped with a *split-splitless* autosampler, all from ThermoFisher (San José, CA, USA). Gas chromatographic separations were made with a Rxi®-5MS (30 m × 0.25 mm × 0.25 µm) capillary column (Restek, Bellefonte, PA, USA). Data were processed using the Xcalibur software (version 2.0.7) from ThermoFisher.

Head-space gas chromatographic/mass spectrometric (HS-GC/MS) analyses were performed on an HP6890 series gas chromatographer provided with a HP7694E autosampler and a 5973 single quadrupole mass spectrometer (Hewlett-Packard, Palo Alto, CA, USA); chromatographic separation was accomplished by a CP PorabondQ capillary column (Varian, Crawley, UK), and data were analyzed using the MSD Chemstation software (D.02.0.275 version) from Agilent Technologies (Santa Clara, CA, USA).

2.1. Toxicological Analysis

Biological fluids (peripheral blood, urine, and bile) and gastric and colon contents (g.c. and c.c., respectively) were used for complete toxicological analyses. Screening tests were initially carried out on 100 µL aliquot of peripheral blood and processed according to immunoassay system specifications.

Specific conformation analyses were performed on all biological matrices by GC/MS, after proper purification through solid phase extraction and eventual derivatization [12–14].

For GC-MS analyses, all samples were acquired both in *full scan* and selected ion monitoring mode (GC/MS-SIM). Specific GC/MS analyses to verify the presence of diquat were done on body fluids, g.c., and c.c. At this stage, 1.5 mL aliquots of each biological sample were treated with 10 mg $NaBH_4$ at 60 °C for 10 min to allow diquat reduction. Samples were subsequently purified by solid phase extraction. Cartridges were conditioned with 2 mL methanol and 2 mL phosphate buffer (pH 8); after sample loading, cartridges were washed with 2 mL bidistilled water, then dried for 5 min before elution with 2 mL methanol. Eluted samples were dried under nitrogen stream and then redissolved in 200 µL methanol for GC/MS *full scan* and SIM analyses.

The possible presence of ethyl alcohol or any other volatile chemical was also verified by analysing aliquot peripheral blood using HS-GC/MS.

2.2. *Diquat Quantification*

2.2.1. Sample Preparation and Purification

A four-point standard addition protocol was used to quantify diquat (DQ) in blood, bile, urine, and gastric and colon contents using paraquat (PQ) as an internal standard (i.s.).

For each biological sample, four aliquots (1 mL for blood and urine; 0.5 mL for bile, gastric and colon contents) were analyzed. The specimens were added with 50 µL of a 20 ng/µL paraquat solution.

Standard addition samples were prepared as follows: "zero" point, biological matrix was spiked with i.s.; A–C samples, biological matrix was spiked with 50 µL of diquat solutions at concentrations of 80, 40, and 20 ng/µL, respectively, and corresponding to urine diquat concentrations of 4, 2, and 1 µg/mL in blood and urine and 8, 4, and 2 µg/mL in bile, gastric and colon contents, respectively.

Conversion of quaternary ammonium compounds, such as DQ and PQ, in thermally stable and volatile substances is essential for gas chromatographic analysis. The reaction is successfully carried out with sodium borohydride and applied to the gas chromatographic/mass spectrometric analysis of blood, urine, bile, and gastric and colon contents samples. Samples were treated with 10 mg of sodium borohydride ($NaBH_4$) to reduce diquat into a more volatile compound. The reaction was conducted for 10 min at 60 °C. SPE extraction was performed with Strata-C18 E (200 mg/3 mL), involving drop-to-drop elution at 5 mmHg and the following extraction procedure: conditioning: 2 mL methanol and 2 mL phosphate buffer (pH 8); sample loading; washing: 2 mL bidistilled water; elution: 2 mL methanol. The eluted fraction, dried under nitrogen stream, was reconstituted in 100 µL methanol and 1 µL was injected into the GC/MS system, then analyzed according to de Almeida et al. [15].

2.2.2. GC/MS Analysis and Quantification

The GC oven temperature was kept at 150 °C for 1 min; then, the temperature was increased up to 300 °C at 20 °C/min. Helium (purity: 99.5%) was used as carrier gas at 1 mL/min, with a constant flow mode. The MS detector (source temperature, 240 °C) operated in the selected ion monitoring (SIM) mode; acquired ions: *m/z* 108, 135, and 190 for diquat; *m/z* 134, 148, and 192 for paraquat.

The ratio of peak areas between diquat and paraquat was worked out and considered as the detector response. According to the standard addition approach [16], quantification was based on detector responses recorded for "zero point" and A–C spiked samples versus spiked analyte amount. A straight line was drawn, and the value of the x intercept represented the amount of the analyte in the unknown sample.

3. Results

3.1. *Autopsy*

The autopsy evidenced the following: congestion of meningeal vessels; oedema and congestion of both lungs; left ventricular hypertrophy with widespread congestion and sclerosis of both valves and coronaries; inflammation of small intestine and stomach, both presenting a greenish liquid with a very intense smell (see Figure 1); congestion of spleen and kidneys.

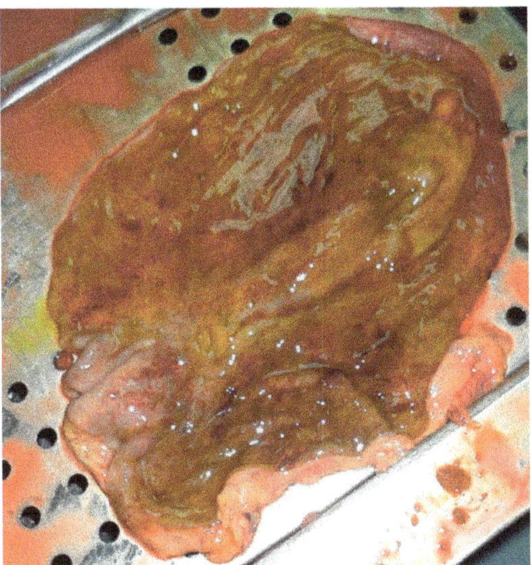

Figure 1. Internal stomach walls with areas of inflammation.

3.2. Histological Analyses

Histological exams showed a degenerative myocardiopathy and segmental vascular insufficiency, associated with myocardial micronecrosis foci. Lungs presented diffuse alveolar damage, with chronic interstitial pulmonary disease. Kidney showed necrotic degenerative changes of the tubules and glomeruli with interstitial nephritis (see Figure 2). The presence of the greenish liquid was confirmed in the stomach and in the small intestine, with both presenting mucosal inflammation and gastric necrotic areas (see Figure 3). Finally, there was mild fatty liver disease.

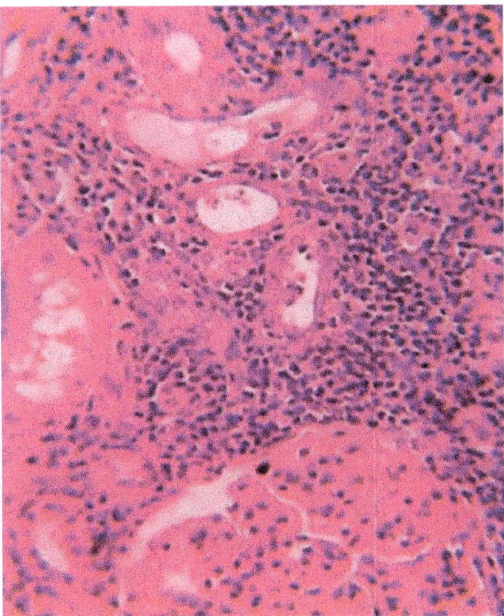

Figure 2. Tubular degeneration and necrosis of the kidney.

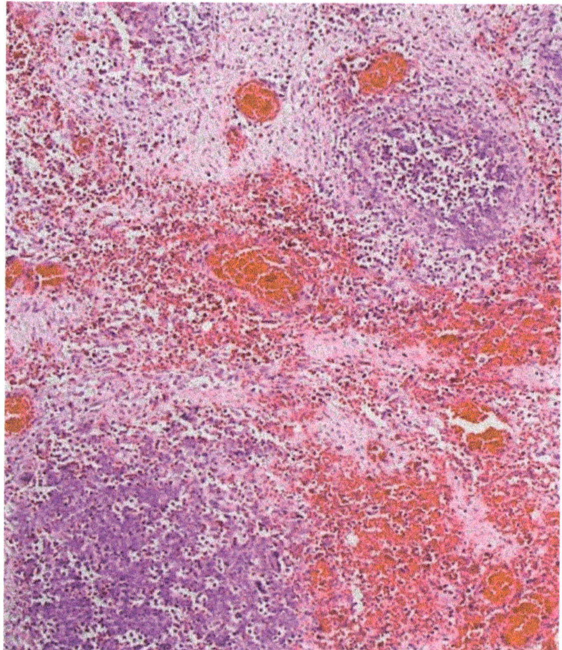

Figure 3. Mucosal inflammation and necrotic areas of the stomach.

3.3. *Toxicological Analyses*

The standard addition approach is suitably used as a quantification procedure when a blank matrix is not available. In the case presented here, the need to analyze autoptic samples such as gastric and colon contents was the main reason to choose this quantification procedure. Three aliquots of biological samples were added with three known diquat amounts, while the third was not spiked and was analyzed as a "zero" sample.

GC/MS-SIM analyses confirmed positivity to diquat in blood, urine, bile, and gastric and colon contents at the concentrations reported in Table 1.

Table 1. Diquat concentrations evidenced by GC/MS analyses performed on post-mortem blood, urine, bile, and gastric and colon contents.

Matrix	Diquat (mg/L)
blood	1.2
bile	106.3
urine	0.03
gastric content	83.1
colon content	6.3

3.4. *Practitioners' Work Analysis*

The patient's treatment procedure did not follow established guidelines or good clinical practices. Staff did not perform any clinical-diagnostical monitoring of the patient's conditions, and this led to the lack of clarity about his clinical status. When the patient arrived at the E.R., his blood creatine kinase and myoglobin values were higher than normal, thus requiring careful clinical monitoring, further exams (i.e., echocardiogram), and more specialized evaluations in order to exclude possible lethal evolution linked to the evidenced muscular damage and to establish the possible consequences and origin of the evidenced abnormal parameters. The decision to simply prescribe a pain relief therapy without starting a close monitoring of the patient's conditions cannot be endorsed. According to the guidelines, blood pressure, heart rate, respiratory rate, body temperature, and diuresis had to be strictly monitored, also to evidence the eventual onset of a more specific symptomatology.

4. Discussion

Diquat is a dipyridyl compound commonly used as a herbicide and structurally related to the commonly used paraquat. Diquat toxicity is a consequence of free oxygen radicals able to react with the cell membrane via lipid peroxidation; the final effect is cellular death and organ disfunction [17,18]. Reports on intoxication are usually related to suicidal ingestion, since its inhalation is not related to systemic toxicity (symptoms are normally reversible, with positive outcomes) [8,19]. After ingestion, specific symptoms can occur up to 48 h [5]. Due to its limited use, reports on diquat intoxication are few compared to those on paraquat. Tanen et al. reported 13 cases referred to diquat ingestion, with 9 of the 13 characterized by fatal outcomes [20]. Mortality rate was about 70%, with deaths related to gastrointestinal complications, pneumonia, paramedian pontine infarction, and renal failure [20]. In reviewing the literature on toxicity after diquat poisoning, Magalhães et al. [18] summarized the data since 1968, when the first man died from accidental oral absorption "of undiluted 20% formulation". The authors schematized 57 cases, detailing the therapy administered and related effects: 30 of the 57 poisonings evolved into fatal outcomes, and death occurred from 5.5 h up to 1 month later [18]. As schematized by Magalhães et al., several analytical procedures are available for diquat analyses, involving different extraction/purification methods as well as detectors (colorimetric tests, UV-absorption, or mass spectrometric analysis). It must be stressed that obtaining an irrefutable result is mandatory in forensic toxicology, and consequently forensic determinations are almost entirely based on mass spectrometry.

Poisoning following diquat ingestion requires a timely and rapid diagnosis, since only supportive care therapies (often non-resolutive) are available.

Dipyridyl compounds present a wide distribution volume. Intestinal absorption is low, but organ and tissue uptake can reach lethal amounts within 6 to 18 h. Once distributed from blood to tissues, the toxicant is scarcely removed [21]. Usually, the absorbed dose plays a key role in determining the severity of intoxication or even death. The International Programme on Chemical Safety reports a lethal diquat dose of 6–12 g [22], with such amount fixed in 10 mL by the producers of a commercially available solution [23]. According to Schultz et al. [24], blood diquat concentrations in the range of (0.1–0.4) mg/L are associated with toxic effects; concentrations in the range (0.4–4.5) mg/L can result in coma/fatal outcomes. Literature data report fatal outcomes with less than 6 g of diquat; plasma concentrations of 0.5 mg/L within the first 24 h after ingestion are associated with systemic poisoning [25]. In the case presented here, toxicological analyses evidenced a blood diquat concentration of 1.2 mg/L, more than twice the minimum needed to observe a systemic poisoning. Moreover, given the diquat half-life and the estimated time between death and autopsy (in Italy, judicial autopsy cannot be performed before 24 h), it is more than reasonable to deduce that ante-mortem levels were even higher, and in line with the ingestion of a lethal dose. On his arrival at the E.R., the man declared a herbicide inhalation, without specifying which one, and complained of pain in his legs and feet; physicians performed general checks (blood analyses; ECG; chest, abdomen, and pelvis CT-angio with contrast agent). The clinical picture was normal, except for some values, which were attributed to a general nonspecific inflammation and a respiratory alkalosis, probably due to hypoxia or pulmonary hyperventilation. This hypothesis was in line with the patient's declarations. Physicians transferred the man in the Short-Stay Observation and gave him antipyretic/analgesic (paracetamol) therapy and hydration.

Yu et al. [26] studied three cases of acute diquat poisoning with resulting encephalopathy. The data highlighted renal failure, neurological disorders, and respiratory failure following ingestion of 50–100 mL of a 20 g/100 mL diquat formulation; blood diquat concentrations were determined in two out of three cases, as 0.43 µg/mL and 0.93 µg/mL. One of the patients died after 18 days of hospitalization due to cardiac arrest. The second patient still presented dystasia and trouble walking three months after the adverse event; the last one had nearly total symptom relief after 57 days.

Hanston et al. [27] published results obtained in a case of suicide by ingestion of about 300 mL of 20% diquat solution (corresponding to about 60 g). The man arrived at the E.R. 4 h after the poisoning, presenting neurological disorders and progressive anuria (after 14 h, he became anuric). Gastric lavage and treatment with active charcoal were performed. The serum diquat concentration was 64 µg/mL. His hemodynamic status worsened within 22 h from diquat ingestion, and he died from refractory cardiocirculatory collapse 26 h after the poisoning. At autopsy, the brain presented abnormalities probably due to status epilepticus, although not specific for diquat poisoning; abundant necrotic lesions characterized renal tubules, and fibrin deposits were present in the glomeruli; the pancreas had signs of necrosis; lung and myocardium showed interstitial oedema [27]. Post-mortem toxicological analyses performed on organs evidenced higher diquat concentrations in the kidney (4.5 µg/g tissue), followed by lung (3.4 µg/g tissue), liver (2.3 µg/g tissue), brain (1.6 µg/g tissue), and heart (1.1 µg/g tissue) [27].

After a correct diagnosis of diquat ingestion, a prompt gastrointestinal decontamination can reduce/prevent the absorption [4,10]. Adsorbent agents such as bentonite (7.5% suspension) and Fuller earth (15% suspension) are useful, and if not available, active carbon can be of help up to one hour after the ingestion (beyond that time, use of active carbon requires special care to avoid bleeding, perforations, or injuries due to additional trauma on already traumatized tissues) [11,18]. No literature studies support the efficacy of active carbon-based treatments to avoid death. Five out of seven cases for which gastrolus was immediately performed resulted in a fatal outcome within 1–7 days; the other two patients ingested low diquat amounts (5 mL), and in one case, such an amount was fatal after seven days [10,28–32].

Post-mortem toxicological analyses performed in the case discussed here evidenced positivity in all specimens (83.1 mg/L in gastric content, 6.3 mg/L in colon content, 106.3 mg/L in bile, and 0.03 mg/L in urine). Gastric and colon content positivities, with concentrations higher than urinary results, attested to the analyte accumulation in gastrointestinal fluids. According to data from Crabtree et al. [33] showing such a mechanism develops rapidly within 24 h from absorption, it is reasonable to assume that the patient ingested diquat long before 8 p.m. of the first day of E.R. admittance. As in other diquat intoxication reports [10,20,34], the patient presented non-specific symptoms; was vigilant, without any discomfort; and his lips, tongue, and gums were not burned. Moreover, there was no airway oedema, and chest X-ray evidenced no infiltration. Very often in literature reports, family members or the patient themselves declares the ingestion of the pesticide upon arrival at the hospital, thus facilitating a correct diagnosis. Despite this, a fatal outcome occurred in 70% of the cases. In the case presented here, the patient declared a herbicide inhalation, without specifying the exact compounds or commercial formulation. Data from the gastric contents confuted this, since ingestion was the most reasonable absorption method.

Healthcare professionals are required to comply with the rules of conduct and good practices defined in specific guidelines. In Italy, such recommendations are mandatory when guidelines are validated by the Ministry of Health [35]. Among others, physicians are asked to correctly draw up and archive health records for a prescribed time [36]. They must take the necessary precautions to avoid the onset of complications for the patients [37] and inform them about the health treatment and its foreseeable consequences [38,39].

The most frequent source of errors in the E.R. is related to the definition of the colour code assigned during the triage and the diagnosis process. Regardless of the possible exposure to chemicals, decisional flow-charts are available to help to choose the triage code, also indicating the most appropriate analyses (laboratory and instrumental) and the most pertinent therapy [40]. According to the Italian guidelines for Short-Stay Observation [41], hospitalization is appropriate with altered state of consciousness, persistent altered vital functions, and foreseeable late toxicity. When the results of laboratory tests are within normal parameters and symptoms subside in 4–6 h, most patients can be discharged. If a voluntary chemical ingestion is reasonable, a psychiatric evaluation could be necessary. A correct treatment of intoxications in adults must include clinical and laboratory investigations as well as a diagnostic analysis of the patient in order to define the exact chemical absorbed and establish a general and specific therapy [41].

Acute intoxication can derive from accidental ingestion, injection, inhalation, or body exposure (through skin, eyes, and mucous membranes), mostly occurring for children and older people (as consequence of an altered mental status or visual disturbances) or because of the precise suicidal intent of the subject. The collection of anamneses can be of great utility to define both the chemicals involved and the absorption route. Clinical examination must highlight any alterations in vital functions, through clinical monitoring of breathing (airway patency, ventilation), circulation (PA, cardiac arrhythmias), and central nervous system (convulsions, coma).

Serum creatine phosphokinase (SCK), whose concentration reflects the extent of acute muscle necrosis, is considered a predictive index, as it can be used to assess the severity of poisoning [42–45]. Damage to muscle tissues is reported for dipyridyls intoxications [46]. Monitoring creatine phosphokinase is useful to predict the patient's prognosis, since an increase in serum values can act as an alarm signal to start an intensive monitoring. Instrumental investigations (electrocardiogram, x-ray of the chest and abdomen, esophagogastroduodenoscopy) can provide additional information that is useful for diagnostic and therapeutic purposes.

Once ingested, treatment of diquat poisoning includes skin and eye decontamination (with copious amounts of water in the case of skin contact) and gastrointestinal decontamination with adsorbents (with bentonite, Fuller's earth, or activated carbon). The effectiveness of gastric lavage in diquat poisoning has not been proven; it should not be performed later than one hour after ingestion, to avoid the risk of bleeding, perforation, or injury due to additional trauma to already traumatized tissues. Pain derived from the deep erosion of the mucous membranes of the digestive tract may require the use of morphine; mouthwashes, cold liquids, ice cream, or anaesthetic can help relieve pain in the mouth and throat. It is essential to maintain adequate diuresis by fluid infusion (physiological solution, ringer acetate, 5% glucose). Such therapy is extremely advantageous in the early stages of intoxication to correct dehydration and accelerate the elimination of the toxin. A careful monitoring of fluid balance allows prevention of fluid overload if renal failure develops. If kidney failure occurs, the intravenous infusion of liquids must be stopped, and haemodialysis is recommended, although it is not effective in purifying blood and tissues from the diquat. Oxygen should be administered only when the patient develops severe hypoxemia; high concentrations of oxygen in the lungs may increase the extent of damage induced by diquat [11]. In severe poisoning, treatment must be guaranteed in the intensive care unit (IUC), to allow appropriate monitoring of vital functions and for invasive medical procedures.

If diquat has spread to the tissues, procedures and treatment to remove the toxin from the blood are insufficient.

In the clinical case presented, the behaviour of Intensive Brief Observation (OBI) department doctors was considered incorrect due to the omission of clinical and laboratory monitoring. Such improper conduct prevented the assessment of the foreseeable worsening of the clinical conditions. The incorrect conduct resulted in a loss of the patient's chance in terms of survival. Death was not avoidable with certainty, as diquat is very toxic, and the decontaminating treatment has limited efficacy (the patient also suffered from cardiovascular comorbidities).

The misconduct of the physicians was judged to be the cause of damages in a civil action, while it was deemed to have no consequences in penal trial. This difference relates to the different criteria of conviction for professional liability in civil and criminal law:

in the civil court, the causal relationship is recognized if the misconduct has a greater probability than other possible causes to produce damages to the psycho-physical integrity of the person, whereas in criminal proceedings, the causal link must be demonstrated "beyond any reasonable doubt" (degree of probability close to certainty). Moreover, in the civil judgement, loss of survival chance and/or worsening of life quality are considered among possible personal injuries [47].

5. Conclusions

The clinical management of the subject poisoned with diquat (and, more generally, of a person who is intoxicated by any chemical) is quite complex and requires great experience. In addition to a correct initial diagnostic framework, it also requires careful clinical and laboratory monitoring; in fact, acute intoxication is a dynamic process that can quickly worsen and lead to lethal complications, although onset symptoms may be blurred.

After diquat poisoning, SCK is a valid biological parameter to evaluate the severity of the intoxication, and its monitoring can give prognostic indications.

Author Contributions: P.B.: formal analysis, conceptualization; M.P.: conceptualization, writing—review and editing; A.S.: formal analysis; E.C.: medico-legal considerations; C.C.: medico-legal considerations; T.N.: medico-legal considerations; F.P.: medico-legal considerations; P.D.L.: conceptualization, writing—review and editing. All authors have read and agreed to the published version of the manuscript.

Funding: This research received no external funding.

Institutional Review Board Statement: Research was carried out following the rules of the Declaration of Helsinki of 1975. Approval from the local institutional review board was not necessary since all analyses were performed in accordance with Prosecutor Office requests.

Informed Consent Statement: Patient consent was waived since all analyzes had been authorized by the Prosecutor Office.

Data Availability Statement: Not applicable.

Conflicts of Interest: The authors declare no conflict of interest.

References

1. Descamps, A.M.K.; Vandijck, D.M.; Buylaert, W.A.; Mostin, M.A.; Paepe, P.D. Characteristics and costs in adults with acute poisoning admitted to the emergency department of a university hospital in Belgium. *PLoS ONE* **2019**, *14*, e0223479. [CrossRef] [PubMed]
2. Mehrpour, O.; Akbari, A.; Jahani, F.; Amirabadizadeh, A.; Allahyari, E.; Mansouri, B.; Ng, P.C. Epidemiological and clinical profiles of acute poisoning in patients admitted to the intensive care unit in eastern Iran (2010 to 2017). *BMC Emerg. Med.* **2018**, *18*, 30. [CrossRef] [PubMed]
3. Report MedMal. Study on Medical Malpractice Risk in Private and Public Healthcare Systems. XII Edition. 2021. Available online: https://www.simlaweb.it/wp-content/uploads/2021/07/12%C2%B0-Report-Med-Mal.pdf (accessed on 17 February 2022).
4. O'Malley, G.F.; O'Malley, R. General Principles of Poisoning. MSD Manual for the Professional. 2020. Available online: https://www.msdmanuals.com/professional/injuries-poisoning/poisoning/general-principles-of-poisoning (accessed on 25 January 2022).
5. Jones, G.M.; Vale, J.A. Mechanisms of toxicity, clinical features, and management of diquat poisoning: A review. *J. Toxicol. Clin. Toxicol.* **2000**, *38*, 123–128. [CrossRef] [PubMed]
6. Jović-Stosić, J.; Babić, G.; Todorović, V. Fatal diquat intoxication. *Vojnosanit. Pregl.* **2009**, *66*, 477–481. [CrossRef] [PubMed]
7. Coge, J.C. Toxicity of paraquat and diquat aerosols generated by a size-selective cyclone: Effect of particle size distribution. *Br. J. Ind. Med.* **1968**, *25*, 304–314.
8. Wood, T.E.; Edgar, H.; Salcedo, J. Recovery from inhalation of diquat aerosol. *Chest* **1976**, *70*, 774–775. [CrossRef]
9. Huang, Y.; Zhang, R.; Meng, M.; Chen, D.; Deng, Y. High-dose diquat poisoning: A case report. *J. Int. Med. Res.* **2021**, *49*, 03000605211026117. [CrossRef]
10. McCarthy, L.G.; Speth, C.P. Diquat intoxication. *Ann. Emerg. Med.* **1983**, *12*, 394–396. [CrossRef]
11. Lanza, V.; Ruskin, R.J. Intossicazioni da Paraquat e Diquat. *Educ. Synop. Anesthesiol. Crit. Care Med.* **2003**, *8*, 5. Available online: http://www.anestit.org/esiait/052003_01.htm (accessed on 17 February 2022).

12. Basilicata, P.; Pieri, M.; Simonelli, A.; Faillace, D.; Niola, M.; Graziano, V. Application of a chemiluminescence immunoassay system and GC/MS for toxicological investigations on skeletonized human remains. *Forensic Sci. Int.* **2019**, *300*, 120–124. [CrossRef]
13. Basilicata, P.; Pieri, M.; Settembre, V.; Galdiero, A.; Della Casa, E.; Acampora, A.; Miraglia, N. Screening of several drugs of abuse in Italian workplace drug testing: Performances comparison of an on-site screening tests and a Fluorescence Polarization ImmunoAssay-based device. *Anal. Chem.* **2011**, *83*, 8566–8574. [CrossRef] [PubMed]
14. Basilicata, P.; Giugliano, P.; Vacchiano, G.; Simonelli, A.; Guadagni, R.; Silvestre, A.; Pieri, M. Forensic toxicological and medico-legal evaluation in a case of incongruous drug-administration in terminal cancer patients. *Toxics* **2021**, *9*, 356. [CrossRef] [PubMed]
15. De Almeida, R.M.; Yonamine, M. Gas chromatographic-mass spectrometric method for the determination of the herbicides paraquat and diquat in plasma and urine samples. *J. Chromatogr. B Anal. Technol. Biomed. Life Sci.* **2007**, *853*, 260–264. [CrossRef]
16. Basilicata, P.; Miraglia, N.; Pieri, M.; Acampora, A.; Soleo, L.; Sannolo, N. Application of the standard addition approach for the quantification of urinary benzene. *J. Chromatogr. B Anal. Technol. Biomed. Life Sci.* **2005**, *818*, 293–299. [CrossRef] [PubMed]
17. Niesink, J.M.; de Vries, J.; Hollinger, M.A. *Toxicology: Principles and Applications*; CRC Press: Boca Raton, FL, USA, 1996.
18. Magalhães, N.; Carvalho, F.; Dinis-Oliveira, R.J. Human and experimental toxicology of diquat poisoning: Toxicokinetics, mechanisms of toxicity, clinical features, and treatment. *Hum. Exp. Toxicol.* **2018**, *37*, 1131–1160. [CrossRef]
19. Weirich, J. Intoxication with diquat ("reglone"). *Dtsch. Gesundh.* **1969**, *24*, 1986–1988.
20. Tanen, D.A.; Curry, S.C.; Laney, R.F. Renal failure and corrosive airway and gastrointestinal injury after ingestion of diluted diquat solution. *Ann. Emerg. Med.* **1999**, *34 Pt 1*, 542–545. [CrossRef]
21. United States Environmental Protection Agency. Chapter 12: Paraquat and Diquat. In *Recognition and Management of Pesticide Poisonings*, 6th ed.; United States Environmental Protection Agency: Washington, DC, USA, 2013.
22. IPCS. *Diquat: Health and Safety Guide*; No. 52; World Health Organization: Geneva, Switzerland, 1991.
23. Reglone Ion. Safety Data Sheet. Syngenta. Version 2.0. 29 September 2021. Available online: https://assets.syngenta.ca/pdf/ca/msds/Reglone_ION_31058_en_SDS.pdf (accessed on 17 February 2022).
24. Schulz, M.; Schmoldt, A.; Andresen-Streichert, H.; Iwersen-Bergmann, S. Revisited: Therapeutic and toxic blood concentrations of more than 1100 drugs and other xenobiotics. *Crit. Care* **2020**, *24*, 195–198. [CrossRef]
25. Tormey, W.P.; Moore, T. Poisonings and clinical toxicology: A template for Ireland. *Ir. J. Med. Sci.* **2013**, *182*, 17–23. [CrossRef]
26. Yu, G.; Jian, T.; Cui, S.; Shi, L.; Kan, B.; Jian, X. Acute diquat poisoning resulting in toxic encephalopathy: A report of three cases. *Clin. Toxicol.* **2022**, *4*, 647–650. [CrossRef]
27. Hantson, P.; Wallemacq, P.; Mahieu, P. A case of fatal diquat poisoning: Toxicokinetic data and autopsy findings. *Clin. Toxicol.* **2000**, *38*, 149–152. [CrossRef] [PubMed]
28. Oreopoulos, D.G.; McEvoy, J. Diquat poisoning. *Postgrad. Med. J.* **1969**, *45*, 635–637. [CrossRef] [PubMed]
29. Schönborn, H.; Schuster, H.P.; Kössling, F.K. Clinical and morphologic findings in an acute oral intoxication with Diquat (Reglone). *Arch. Toxikol.* **1971**, *27*, 204–216. [CrossRef] [PubMed]
30. Fél, P.; Zala, I.; Szüle, E.; Varga, L. Diquat-dibromide (Reglone) poisoning treated with hemodialysis. *Orv. Hetil.* **1976**, *117*,1773–1774. [PubMed]
31. Vanholder, R.; Colardyn, F.; De Reuck, J.; Praet, M.; Lameire, N.; Ringoir, S. Diquat intoxication: Report of two cases and review of the literature. *Am. J. Med.* **1981**, *70*, 1267–1271. [CrossRef]
32. Okonek, S. Paraquat and diquat poisoning. Toxicologic findings and new therapeutic possibilities. *Med. Welt* **1976**, *27*, 1401–1405.
33. Crabtree, H.C.; Lock, E.A.; Rose, M.S. Effects of diquat on the gastrointestinal tract of rats. *Toxicol. Appl. Pharmacol.* **1977**, *41*, 585–595. [CrossRef]
34. Ruha, A.M.; Wallace, K.; Tanen, D.A.; Patel, P. Dilute diquat death. *Am. J. Emerg. Med.* **2001**, *9*, 527–528. [CrossRef]
35. Buccelli, C.; Abignente, I.; Niola, M.; Paternoster, M.; Graziano, V.; Di Lorenzo, P. Relevance of guidelines in determining medical liability. The novelties introduced by Balduzzi law, related problems, attempts at solutions. *Riv. Ital. Med. Leg. Dirit. Campo Sanit.* **2016**, *2*, 663–681.
36. Di Lorenzo, P.; Niola, M.; Buccelli, C.; Re, D.; Cortese, A.; Pantaleo, G.; Amato, M. Professional responsibility in dentistry: Analysis of an interdepartmental case study. *Dent. Cadmos* **2015**, *83*, 324–340. [CrossRef]
37. Polistena, A.; Di Lorenzo, P.; Sanguinetti, A.; Buccelli, C.; Conzo, G.; Conti, A.; Niola, M.; Avenia, N. Medicolegal implications of surgical errors and complications in neck surgery: A review based on the Italian current legislation. *Open Med.* **2016**, *11*, 298–306. [CrossRef] [PubMed]
38. Di Lorenzo, P.; Casella, C.; Capasso, E.; Conti, A.; Fedeli, P.; Policino, F.; Niola, M. The central importance of information in cosmetic surgery and treatments. *Open Med.* **2018**, *13*, 153–157. [CrossRef] [PubMed]
39. Niola, M.; Di Lorenzo, P.; Capasso, E.; Dalessandri, D.; Conti, A. Information and consent in dentistry. *J. Clin. Diagn. Res.* **2018**, *12*, ZE05–ZE07. [CrossRef]
40. Pesci, C.; Magnani, A.; Semprini, C.; Garattoni, D.; Sciamanna, M.; Perin, T.; Galletti, M. Emergenza tossicologica in Pronto Soccorso: Organizzazione logistica, sistematizzazione delle risorse e algoritmo gestionale. *Emerg. Care J.* **2010**, *6*, 35–36.
41. Italian Ministry of Health. Guidelines for Short-Stay Observation. 2019. Available online: https://www.salute.gov.it/imgs/C_17_notizie_3849_listaFile_itemName_0_file.pdf (accessed on 17 February 2022).

42. Gao, Y.; Liu, L.; Li, T.; Yuan, D.; Wang, Y.; Xu, Z.; Hou, L.; Zhang, Y.; Duan, G.; Sun, C.; et al. A novel simple risk model to predict the prognosis of patients with paraquat poisoning. *Sci. Rep.* **2021**, *11*, 237. [CrossRef]
43. Lokesh, N.K.; Shivakumar, K.M.; Anikethan, G.V. Serum creatine phosphokinase as predictor of intermediate syndrome in organophosphorus poisoning. *Int. J. Contemp. Med. Res.* **2018**, *5*, F1–F4.
44. Subathra, C.; Balasubramaniyan, S.; Balaji, I.; Haynes Raja, K. Creatine Phosphokinase: A Prognostic Marker in Organophosphorus Compound Poisoning. *J. Med. Sci. Clin. Res.* **2018**, *6*, 936–941.
45. Sen, R.; Nayak, J.; Khadanga, S. Study of serum cholinesterase, CPK and LDH as prognostic biomarkers in Organophosphorus Poisoning. *Int. J. Med. Res. Rev.* **2014**, *2*, 185–189. [CrossRef]
46. Tabata, N.; Morita, M.; Mimasaka, S.; Funayama, M.; Hagiwara, T.; Abe, M. Paraquat myopathy: Report on two suicide cases. *Forensic Sci. Int.* **1999**, *100*, 117–126. [CrossRef]
47. Di Lorenzo, P.; Paternoster, M.; Nugnes, M.; Pantaleo, G.; Graziano, V.; Niola, M. Professional dental and oral surgery liability in Italy: A comparative analysis of the insurance products offered to health workers. *Open Med.* **2016**, *11*, 256–263. [CrossRef]

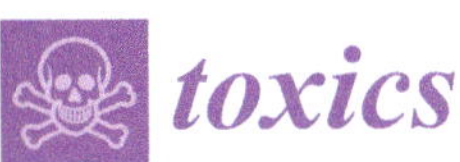

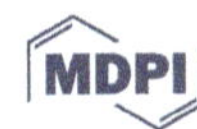

Article

Suicide by Pesticide (Phorate) Ingestion: Case Report and Review of Literature

Angela Simonelli [1], Anna Carfora [2], Pascale Basilicata [1,*], Bruno Liguori [3], Pasquale Mascolo [3], Fabio Policino [1], Massimo Niola [1] and Carlo Pietro Campobasso [2]

[1] Department of Advanced Biomedical Science, Legal Medicine Section, University of Naples "Federico II", Via S. Pansini, 5, 80138 Napoli, Italy; angela.simonelli@unina.it (A.S.); fabio.policino@unina.it (F.P.); masniola@unina.it (M.N.)
[2] Forensic Toxicology Unit, Department of Experimental Medicine, University of Campania "L. Vanvitelli", Via L. Armanni, 5, 80138 Napoli, Italy; anna.carfora@unicampania.it (A.C.); carlopietro.campobasso@unicampania.it (C.P.C.)
[3] Department of Experimental Medicine, Institute of Legal Medicine, University of Campania "L. Vanvitelli", Via L. Armanni, 5, 80138 Napoli, Italy; bruno.liguori@gmail.com (B.L.); studiomedicolegalemascolo@gmail.com (P.M.)
* Correspondence: pbasilic@unina.it; Tel.: +39-081-746-3474; Fax: +39-081-746-4727

Abstract: It has been estimated that approximately one in seven of all global suicides is due to pesticide self-poisoning, mostly in rural areas of developing countries. Organophosphorus (OP) compounds are a group of pesticides exerting their toxicological effects through non-reversible inhibition of the enzyme acetylcholinesterase (AChE). Among these compounds, phorate (thimet) is one of the most dangerous compounds, the use of which is restricted in many countries. A case of intentional suicide after phorate ingestion in a 24-year-old Bengali male is described. This is the second case of suicidal ingestion of phorate reported in the forensic literature, and the first presenting complete toxicological findings.

Keywords: phorate; suicidal ingestion; pesticides

Citation: Simonelli, A.; Carfora, A.; Basilicata, P.; Liguori, B.; Mascolo, P.; Policino, F.; Niola, M.; Campobasso, C.P. Suicide by Pesticide (Phorate) Ingestion: Case Report and Review of Literature. *Toxics* **2022**, *10*, 205. https://doi.org/10.3390/toxics10050205

Academic Editor: Luc P. Belzunces

Received: 4 March 2022
Accepted: 11 April 2022
Published: 21 April 2022

1. Introduction

Based on the Food and Agriculture Organization of the United Nations definition [1], pesticides can be broadly described as chemical products used for the control of unwanted animals, plants and microbes. Pesticides are often classified according to the pest organism, to which they are designed (rodenticides, insecticides, weedicides, fungicides, acaricide, et cetera), however, the most useful classification is based on their chemical composition: organochlorines; organophosphorus; carbamates; and pyrethrin and pyrethroids [2,3]. Organophosphate pesticides are the most common pesticides used in agriculture, however, they can have a negative impact on both the environment and human health [4,5]. Several ecological and health concerns have been raised on the recurrent usage of organophosphate pesticides. Epidemiological studies of pesticide poisoning indicate three main categories of circumstances, under which poisoning occurs: occupational accidents after occupational exposures; domestic accidents; and suicide due to intentional ingestion [6–9]. A literature review of mortality studies related to suicide by organophosphate pesticides has suggested that the wide availability of highly toxic pesticides may have a causal relationship to suicide [9].

According to the World Health Organization hanging, pesticide self-poisoning and use of fire arms are globally the most common methods of suicide [10]. A systematic review of world data for 2010–2014 estimated that around one in seven of global suicides were due to pesticide self-poisoning (approximately 110,000 deaths each year) [11]. Mostly these deaths occur among people living in rural areas of low-income and middle-income countries, especially in South Asia, South East Asia and China [11,12].

Organophosphorus compounds (OP) are widely used as insecticides or acaricide and exert their toxicological effects through non-reversible inhibition of the acetylcholinesterase enzyme (AChE). Inhibition of AChE results in accumulation of acetylcholine (ACh) at autonomic postganglionic and central synapses and at neuromuscular junctions [13,14]. As a consequence, ACh binds to and over-stimulates muscarinic and nicotinic receptors. AChE inhibition is irreversible, therefore new synthesis of the enzyme in the liver is necessary to restore enzymatic activity [15].

Phorate is an OP compound available as a liquid or in granules. According to the WHO Recommended Classification of Pesticides by Hazard [10] it is classified as 'extremely hazardous' (class Ia-see Table 1), with an oral LD50 8.0 mg/kg mice, and 1.1–3.2 mg/kg to rats [15,16]. Although phorate is an extremely hazardous poison, only a few cases of fatal poisoning by phorate (both intentional and accidental) are reported in the literature [17–19]. This could be partially due to its limited use, since it is not approved for use in the EU [20]. The Environmental Protection Agency has authorized restrictions on its use in the US since 1990 [21]; in China, phorate and the metabolites of phorate sulfone are forbidden in food stuffs [16].

Table 1. World Health Organization classification for pesticides toxicity.

WHO Class		**LD50 for the Rat (mg/kg Body Weight)**	
		Oral	Dermal
Ia	Extremely hazardous	<5	<50
Ib	Highly hazardous	5–50	50–200
II	Moderately hazardous	50–2000	200–2000
III	Slightly hazardous	Over 2000	Over 2000
U	Unlikely to present acute hazard	5000 or higher	

The present paper reports a case of suicide by phorate ingestion in a rural area of Southern Italy. To the best of our knowledge this is the second paper reporting toxicological data after suicidal phorate ingestion in Italy. Toxicological data and autopsy findings are discussed with respect to the literature data and recommendations for safety pesticides management.

2. Case Report

A 24-year-old Bengali male was found dead in a rural area of Southern Italy. The body was found on the ground in a supine position. Post-mortem changes were consistent with an early post-mortem interval of approximately 3–6 h, with no signs of putrefaction. At external examination, a marked miosis (pinpoint pupils) was observed along with a white foam coming out of the mouth and nostrils and semen leakage. Body weight was 56 kg and height 152 cm. At autopsy, performed according to a Prosecutor Office request, no evidence of traumatic injuries or relevant diseases were observed, except for an overdistension of the lungs with an overlap of their anterior edges over the midline.

Stomach contents were represented by 300 mL of an oily, sharp-smelling liquid containing pieces of a partially digested yellow citrus fruit. Hemorrhagic erosions of the gastric mucosa were observed along with diffuse visceral congestion; blood appeared fluid and dark red in color. According to the international recommendations on sample collection [22,23], 10 mL peripheral blood was taken from the right femoral vein. Urine, bile, and stomach contents were also sampled for toxicological analysis.

3. Materials and Methods

The certified standard solutions of drugs of abuse used for confirmation analysis in gas chromatography/mass spectrometry (GC/MS) were from Cerilliant-Merck (Milan,

Italy), *N,O*-bis(trimethylsilyl)trifluoroacetamide (BSTFA) derivatizing agent from Acros (Morris Plains, NJ, USA), and HPLC grade-solvents from Carlo Erba (Milan, Italy).

Enzyme Linked ImmunoSorbent Assay (ELISA) screening tests were performed on a Dynex-DSX system from Technogenetics (Chantilly, VA, USA), using forensic blood kits from Abbott for AMP/MAMP/MDMA, barbiturates, benzodiazepines, buprenorphine, cannabinoids, cocaine, fentanyl, ketamine, methadone, opiates, oxycodone, tricyclic antidepressants, zolpidem. The immunoassay system is based on a heterogeneous assay with a fixed and constant antibody coating on the plate. All the antibodies are poly-clonal, except for amphetamine and methadone, which are mono-clonal ones. The enzyme conjugate contains a fixed titer of an enzyme (horseradish peroxidase) labelled drug. The immunoassay exploits a competitive binding between the antibody and the antigen.

GC/MS analyses were performed using a DSQII single quadrupole mass spectrometer directly linked to a FocusGC gas chromatograph equipped with a *full scan* AS3000 autosampler, all from ThermoFisher (San José, CA, USA). Gas chromatographic separations were performed with a DB-5ms Ultra Inert (30 m × 0.25 mm × 0.25 μm) (J and W Scientific, Folsom, CA, USA). Data were processed using the Xcalibur software (version 2.0.7) from ThermoFisher.

Head-space gas chromatographic/mass spectrometric (HS-GC/MS) analyses were performed on an HP6890 series gas chromatographer provided with a HP7694E autosampler and a 5973 single quadrupole mass spectrometer (Hewlett-Packard, Palo Alto, CA, USA); chromatographic separation was accomplished by a CP PorabondQ capillary column (Varian, Palo Alto, CA, USA), and data analyzed using the MSD Chemstation, with software (D.02.0.275 version) from Agilent Technologies.

Toxicological Analysis

Biological fluids were used for complete toxicological analyses. ELISA screening tests were initially performed on a blood sample, after dilution (1:10, v:v) of a proper aliquot with bidistilled water, according to the manufacturer's specifications.

Generic analyses were performed on blood, urine, bile and gastric contents, after purification through solid phase extraction (SPE) using BondElut Certified cartridges (Agilent Santa Clara, CA, US) with and without acidic hydrolysis [24–26]. Generic analysis with acidic hydrolysis. Sample preparation: 1 mL matrix diluted with 2 mL bidistilled water and added with 200 μL 37% HCl. Acidic hydrolysis: samples were kept at 120 °C for 20 min, then cooled at room temperature and added with 800 μL TRIS buffer and 200 μL 10 M KOH saturated with $KHCO_3$ (samples' pH 8–9). Samples were centrifuged at 4000 rpm for 40 min then purified. SPE purification procedure, involving a drop-to-drop elution at 5 mmHg, was performed as follows: conditioning, 1 mL methanol, 2 mL 0.1 M phosphate buffer (pH 6); sample loading; washing: 6 mL bidistilled water, 3 mL 0.1 N HCl; 9 mL methanol; cartridges were dried for 5 min, then clean test tubes loaded; elution: 2 × (3 mL dichloromethane/methanol = 80/20, 2% ammonia, v:v). Eluted fractions, dried under nitrogen stream, were derivatized by adding 50 μL BSTFA at 75 °C for 20 min; samples were cooled at room temperature and analyzed in GC/MS. Generic analysis without acidic hydrolysis. Sample preparation: 1 mL matrix diluted with 2 mL bidistilled water. Each sample was centrifuged at 4000 rpm for 40 min then purified. SPE purification procedure was performed as follows: conditioning, 1 mL ethyl acetate, 1 mL methanol, 1 mL bidistilled water, 1 mL 0.1 M phosphate buffer (pH 6); sample loading; washing: 3 mL bidistilled water, 3 mL 0.1 M phosphate buffer 3% acetonitrile; 3 hexane; cartridges were dried for 5 min, then clean test tubes loaded; elution: 2 × (3 mL ethylacetate, 2% ammonia, v:v). Eluted fractions, dried under a nitrogen stream, were derivatized by adding 50 μL BSTFA at 75 °C for 20 min; samples were cooled at room temperature and analyzed in GC/MS.

Toxicological analyses aimed to verify the presence of pesticides involved a liquid/liquid purification through TOXI-A and TOXI-B cartridges (Agilent, Santa Clara, CA, USA); solutions recovered by TOXI tubes were dried under nitrogen stream and redissolved in 50 μL acetonitrile prior to GC/MS analyses. Analyses were performed on fluids and gastric content; no hydrolysis nor derivatization were performed. Qualitative GC-MS *full scan* analyses were performed on all samples; selected ion monitoring mode (GC/MS-SIM) was used for quantifications of active principles, eventually evidenced by *full scan*. The eventual presence of ethyl alcohol or any other volatile chemicals in the blood sample were also verified by HS-GC/MS.

A five-point calibration curve in the range (0.016–0.250) mg/L was used for phorate quantification, using ethion as internal standard. GC/MS-SIM analyses were based on the following transitions: phorate, *m/z* (260, 231, 121); ethion, *m/z* (231, 153, 125); in both cases the first ion was selected as quantifier.

4. Results and Discussion

ELISA analyses were negative with respect to considered analytes. Generic analyses performed on samples purified by SPE with and without acidic hydrolysis were negative as well. No volatile compounds were evidenced in the blood sample by HS-GC/MS.

GC/MS *full scan* analyses on samples purified by TOXI-A and TOXI-B cartridges evidenced a positivity towards phorate. Quantification in blood, urine, bile and stomach contents involved GC/MS-SIM analyses of sample aliquots spiked with ethion (used as internal standard) and purified by TOXI-A. Specificity towards phorate identification was verified through the analysis of drug-free blood and urine samples spiked with the internal standard only and processed according to the previously described method. Results evidenced the absence of any signal corresponding to the analyte of interest. Limit Of Detection (LOD) and Lower Limit Of Quantification (LLOQ) were determined as concentrations corresponding to a signal-to-noise ratio of 3/1 and 5/1, respectively: LOD, 8.5 ng/mL; LLOQ, 14.1 ng/mL. Recovery and accuracy of the applied method were calculated for drug-free blood and urine spiked with phorate standard solution to obtain concentrations of 0.150, 0.075 and 0.037 mg/L (each sample was prepared in triplicate). After purification and GC/MS-SIM analysis, a mean recovery and an accuracy of 87% and 95% were obtained, respectively. Quantification involved the use of a calibration curve. Since to the best of our knowledge a toxic interval for human absorption was not available (in terms of expected blood concentrations), the calibration curve concentrations' range was optimized to balance between the need of optimal ions' intensities and to avoid the analysis of unnecessary excessively concentrated solutions—resulting in the need of frequent instrumental cleaning. Quantitative results are reported in Table 2 (bile and gastric content analyses were repeated after proper sample dilution with bidistilled water, in order to obtain concentration within the calibration curve range).

Table 2. Quantitative results of phorate in analyzed biological samples.

Samples	Phorate (mg/L)
Blood	0.18
Urine	0.01
Bile	1.12
Stomach contents	11.52

In samples purified by TOXI-A, GC/MS *full scan* analysis was able to detect the presence of phorate main metabolites like phorate sulphone and phorate sulphoxide. Both metabolites are reported to be more toxic than phorate [27]. The majority of toxicokinetic studies reported in the literature were based on laboratory animals, while data on humans are extremely limited [28].

Although a specific oral toxic or lethal dose for phorate in humans has not been established [29], the blood concentration of phorate found in this case study was very similar to the lethal concentration reported by Thompson et al. [30], and here considered as "reference" for assessing lethal phorate levels in humans. In describing the case of fatal ingestion of phorate-containing insecticide in a 17-year-old restaurant assistant, the authors reported a post-mortem blood insecticide concentration of 0.25 mg/L. In our case phorate blood concentration was close to the "lethal" concentration published by Thompson et al. [30]. The case discussed by Thompson et al. is one of the very few cases published in the literature where quantitative results of toxicological analyses are reported. Khatiwada et al. [18], for instance, published a case of accidental intoxication after ingestion of phorate granules with a fatal outcome in one of the two victims, however, results of toxicological analyses are not reported. Peter et al. [31] reported a non-fatal case of a 28-year-old woman who swallowed 50 mL of phorate. She survived after five days in a deep coma, during which findings largely consistent with brain death were observed.

In our case study high phorate concentration was also determined in the stomach content (11.52 mg/L). Considering the entire volume of matrix present at autoptic examination, an ingestion of at least 3.4 mg of phorate can be estimated. In a recent study, Montana and colleagues [19] published the case of a suicide following phorate ingestion by a 70-year-old farmer, who had been exposed for several years to phorate at low doses and died after ingestion of a granular pesticide powder mixed with water. Reported toxicological datum refers to gastric content only and phorate levels of 3.29 mg/L were determined. In our case, the main histological findings were represented by brain and pulmonary oedema associated to alveolar hemorrhages consistent with an acute fatal event. Similar histological findings have been also observed by Montana et al. [19], consistent with the acute toxicological effects of OP poisoning on the nervous and respiratory systems along with additional signs of chronic obstructive pulmonary disease, such as scattered bronchopneumonia outbreaks and peribronchiolar lymphocytes infiltrations and alterations of kidney due to chronic exposure to OP.

In our case toxicological findings, along with those derived from the autopsy, were consistent with an acute intoxication due to phorate intentional ingestion. Among others, the pungent smell typical of pesticides coming from the stomach contents, signs of overstimulation of the parasympathetic nervous system (miosis, white foam that comes out of the mouth and nostrils, ejaculation of the semen), were found along with the exclusion of traumatic lesions or relevant underlying diseases as possible causes of death. Miosis has been found to be one of the most prevalent signs in insecticide poisoning in a range between 44–83% of cases [32,33]. Miosis and tightness in the chest may occur as the result of the severity of local anti-AChE effects [13]. Such autopsy findings are consistent with the lethal effects of OP insecticide poisoning. These compounds can produce a variety of toxicological effects on the nervous (central and peripheral) system, as well as cardiovascular and pulmonary systems such as: ventricular arrhythmias and tachyarrhythmias belonging to the 'torsades de pointes' types, which may progress to ventricular fibrillation and/or asystole; twitching of muscles followed by convulsions and paralysis with respiratory failure associated to nasal and bronchial hypersecretion (rhinorrhea and bronchorrhea) as a result of bronchoconstriction, cyanosis and respiratory depression [13]. In the case presented here both circumstantial and toxicological findings were in agreement and provided evidence to confirm the diagnosis of OP poisoning.

With respect to the particular absorption route, OP pesticides can efficiently enter the organisms by all routes, including inhalation, ingestion, and dermal absorption [14]. The latter two routes of absorption concern mostly agricultural workers, accidentally exposed either during pesticide application to crops or due to incorrect or careless storage. Symptoms may occur within five minutes of massive ingestion and almost always within twelve hours [13]. Work-related poisoning can be ruled out in the case discussed here due to the high concentration present in the gastric contents and signs evidenced during the autopsy, which were consistent with an ingestion of the toxicant.

In cases of acute OP poisoning, antidotal treatment with the combined use of atropine sulfate and pyridine-2-aldoxine methochloride (2-PAM) is recommended. Atropine sulfate acts by blocking the muscarinic Ach receptors (mAChRs) [15]. In case of ingestion, gastric lavage can be considered especially in the first hours after poisoning occurs, although its value is unproven [34], also in consideration of the potential harm it can cause if the patient, at risk of seizures or rapid loss of consciousness, has not been intubated [35]. Ventilation must be maintained in patients with acute OP poisoning; eventually patients must be intubated and sustained by mechanical ventilation [13]. Finally, careful attention must be given to fluid and electrolyte balance along with heart rate and blood pressure monitoring by ECG. Unfortunately, there are conflicting recommendations on the general management of poisoned patients and the lack of evidence for the treatment of acute OP poisoning has been raised [36–38].

5. Conclusions

Pesticide self-poisoning is very common in rural areas of developing countries. Unfortunately, few details are available about phorate toxicity on humans. Further studies dealing with toxicokinetic and toxicodynamic of OP compounds are still needed. According to the autopsy findings, the effects of OP poisoning can determine a rapid death due to brain and respiratory alterations through non-reversible inhibition of the enzyme AChE.

Author Contributions: A.S.: formal analysis and conceptualization; A.C.: toxicological considerations; P.B.: writing/review and editing; B.L.: writing; P.M.: autopsy; F.P.: medico-legal considerations; M.N.: conceptualization; review; C.P.C.: writing/conceptualization and review. All authors have read and agreed to the published version of the manuscript.

Funding: This research received no external funding.

Institutional Review Board Statement: Research was carried out following the rules of the Declaration of Helsinki of 1975. Approval from local institutional review board was not necessary since all analyses were performed in accordance with Prosecutor Office requests.

Informed Consent Statement: Patient consent was waived since all analyses were authorized by the Prosecutor Office.

Data Availability Statement: Not applicable.

Conflicts of Interest: The authors declare no conflict of interest.

References

1. Food and Agriculture Organization of the United Nations. *International Code of Conduct on the Distribution and Use of Pesticides;* FAO, Information Division: Rome, Italy, 2005; ISBN 92-5-105411-8.
2. Drum, C. *Soil Chemistry of Pesticides;* PPG Industries, Inc.: Pittsburgh, PA, USA, 1980.
3. Buchel, K.H. *Chemistry of Pesticides;* John Wiley & Sons, Inc.: Hoboken, NJ, USA, 1980.
4. Dar, M.A.; Baba, Z.A.; Kaushi, G. A review on phorate persistence, toxicity and remediation by bacterial communities. *Pedosphere* **2022**, *32*, 171–183. [CrossRef]
5. Kim, K.H.; Kabir, E.; Jahan, S.A. Exposure to pesticides and the associated human health effects. *Sci. Total Environ.* **2017**, *1*, 525–535. [CrossRef] [PubMed]
6. Torchio, P.; Lepore, A.R.; Corrao, G.; Comba, P.; Settimi, L.; Belli, S.; Magnani, C.; di Orio, F. Mortality study on a cohort of Italian licensed pesticide users. *Sci. Total Environ.* **1994**, *149*, 183–191. [CrossRef]
7. Parron, T.; Hernandez, A.F.; Villanueva, E. Increased risk of suicide with exposure to pesticides in an intensive agricultural area. A 12-year retrospective study. *Forensic Sci. Int.* **1996**, *79*, 53–63. [CrossRef]
8. Stallones, L. Suicide and potential occupational exposure to pesticides, Colorado, 1990–1999. *J. Agromed.* **2006**, *11*, 107–112. [CrossRef]
9. London, L.; Flisher, A.J.; Wesseling, C.; Mergler, D.; Kromhout, H. Suicide and exposure to organophosphate insecticides: Cause or effect? *Am. J. Ind. Med.* **2005**, *47*, 308–321. [CrossRef]
10. World Health Organization. *The WHO Recommended Classification of Pesticides by Hazard and Guidelines to Classification;* World Health Organization: Geneva, Switzerland, 2009.
11. Mew, E.; Padmanathan, P.; Konradsen, F.; Eddleston, M.; Chang, S.; Phillips, M.; Gunnell, D. The global burden of fatal self-poisoning with pesticides 2006-15: Systematic review. *J. Affect. Disord.* **2017**, *219*, 93–104. [CrossRef]
12. Gunnell, D.; Knipe, D.; Chang, S.; Pearson, M.; Konradsen., F.; Lee, W.; Eddleston, M. Prevention of suicide with regulations aimed at restricting access to highly hazardous pesticides: A systematic review of the international evidence. *Lancet Glob. Health.* **2017**, *5*, e1026–e1037. [CrossRef]
13. Vale, A.; Lotti, M. *Handbook of Clinical Neurology*, 3rd ed.; Elsevier B.V.: Amsterdam, The Netherlands, 2015; Volume 131.

14. Colovic, M.; Krstic, D.; Lazarevic-Pasti, T.; Bondzic, A.; Vasic, V. Acetylcholinesterase inhibitors: Pharmacology and toxicology. *Curr. Neuropharmacol.* **2013**, *11*, 315–335. [CrossRef]
15. Gupta, R.C.; Sachana, M.; Mukherjee, I.M.; Doss, R.B.; Malik, J.K.; Milatovic, D. Organophosphates and Carbamates. In *Veterinary Toxicology-Basic and Clinical Principles*, 3rd ed.; Academic Press: Cambridge, MA, USA, 2018; pp. 495–508.
16. Guo, H.; Ye, J.; Liu, Y.; Lin, L.; Yang, C.; Li, Q. Determination of phorate and its metabolite phorate sulfone residues in the egg by high performance liquid chromatography-tandem mass spectrometry. In Proceedings of the Second International Conference on Materials Chemistry and Environmental Protection (MEEP 2018), Sanya, China, 23–25 November 2018; pp. 63–68, ISBN 978-989-758-360-5.
17. Young, R.J.; Jung, F.P.; Ayer, H.E. Phorate intoxication at an insecticide formulating plant. *Am. Ind. Hyg. Assoc. J.* **1979**, *40*, 1013–1016. [CrossRef]
18. Khatiwada, S.; Tripathi, M.; Pokharel, K.; Acharya, R.; Subedi, A. Ambiguous phorate granules for sesame seeds linked to accidental organophosphate fatal poisoning. *J. Nepal Med. Assoc.* **2012**, *52*, 171–175. [CrossRef]
19. Montana, A.; Rapisarda, V.; Esposito, M.; Amico, F.; Cocimano, G.; Di Nunno, N.; Ledda, C.; Salerno, M. A rare case of suicide by ingestion of phorate: A case report and a review of the literature. *Healthcare* **2021**, *9*, 131. [CrossRef] [PubMed]
20. Pohanish, R.P. *Sittig's Handbook of Pesticides and Agricultural Chemicals*, 2nd ed.; William Andrew: Norwich, NY, USA, 2015; pp. 657–661.
21. Devine, G.J.; Furlong, M.J. Insecticide use: Contexts and ecological consequences. *Agric. Human Values* **2007**, *24*, 281–306. [CrossRef]
22. The International Association of Forensic Toxicologists-Committee of Systematic Toxicological Analysis Recommendations on Sample Collection. (TIAFT-Bulletin XXIX-Number 1). 1999. Available online: http://www.tiaft.org/data/uploads/documents/tiaft-sta-recommendations-on-sample-collection.pdf (accessed on 10 April 2022).
23. Society of Forensic Toxicologists (SOFT) and American Academy of Forensic Sciences (AAFS) Forensic Laboratory Guidelines. 2006. Available online: http://www.the-ltg.org/data/uploads/guidelines/soft-guidelines_2006.pdf (accessed on 10 April 2022).
24. Basilicata, P.; Pieri, M.; Simonelli, A.; Faillace, D.; Niola, M.; Graziano, V. Application of a chemiluminescence immunoassay system and GC/MS for toxicological investigations on skeletonized human remains. *Forensic Sci. Int.* **2019**, *300*, 120–124. [CrossRef]
25. Basilicata, P.; Pieri, M.; Settembre, V.; Galdiero, A.; Della Casa, E.; Acampora, A.; Miraglia, N. Screening of several drugs of abuse in Italian workplace drug testing: Performances comparison of an on-site screening tests and a Fluorescence Polarization ImmunoAssay-based device. *Anal. Chem.* **2011**, *83*, 8566–8574. [CrossRef]
26. Carfora, A.; Campobasso, C.P.; Cassandro, P.; La Sala, F.; Maiellaro, A.; Perna, A.; Petrella, R.; Borriello, R. Fatal inhalation of volcanic gases in three tourists of a geothermal area. *Forensic Sci Int.* **2019**, *297*, e1–e7. [CrossRef]
27. Hogdson, E.; Rose, R.L.; Ruy, D.-Y.; Falls, G.; Blake, B.L.; Levi, P.E. Pesticide-metabolizing enzymes. *Toxicol. Lett.* **1995**, *82*, 73–81.
28. Henderson, M.C.; Krueger, S.K.; Siddens, L.K.; Stevens, J.F.; Williams, D.E. S-Oxygenation of the thioether organophosphate insecticides phorateand disulfoton by human lung flavin-containing monooxygenase 2. *Biochem. Pharmacol.* **2004**, *68*, 959–967. [CrossRef]
29. Schulz, M.; Schmoldt, A.; Andresen-Streichert, H.; Iwersen-Bergmann, S. Revisited: Therapeutic and toxic blood concentrations of more than 1,100 drugs and other xenobiotics. *Crit. Care* **2020**, *24*, 195–198. [CrossRef]
30. Thompson, J.; Casey, P.; Vale, J. Deaths from pesticide poisoning in England and Wales 1990–1991. *Hum. Exp. Toxicol.* **1995**, *14*, 437–445. [CrossRef]
31. Peter, J.V.; Prabhakar, A.T.; Pichamuthu, K. In-laws, insecticide-and a mimic of brain death. *Lancet* **2008**, *371*, 622. [CrossRef]
32. Hirshberg, A.; Lerman, Y. Clinical Problems in Organophosphorus Insecticide Poisoning: The Use of a Computerized Information System. *Fundam. Appl. Toxicol.* **1984**, *4*, S209–S214. [CrossRef]
33. Lee, P.; Tai, D.Y.H. Clinical features of patients with acute organophosphate poisoning requiring intensive care. *Intensive Care Med.* **2001**, *27*, 694–699. [CrossRef] [PubMed]
34. Li, Y.; Tse, M.L.; Gawarammana, I.; Buckley, N.; Eddleston, M. Systematic review of controlled clinical trials of gastric lavage in acute organophosphorus pesticide poisoning. *Clin Toxicol.* **2009**, *47*, 179–192. [CrossRef]
35. American Academy of Clinical Toxicology and European Association of Poisons Centres and Clinical Toxicologists. Position statement: Gastric lavage. *J. Toxicol. Clin. Toxicol.* **1997**, *35*, 711–719. [CrossRef]
36. Eddleston, M.; Buckley, N.A.; Checketts, H.; Senarathna, L.; Mohamed, F.; Rezvi Sheriff, M.H.; Dawson, A. Speed of initial atropinisation in significant organophosphorus pesticide poisoning-a systematic comparison of recommended regimens. *J. Toxicol. Clin. Toxicol.* **2004**, *42*, 865–875. [CrossRef]
37. Eddleston, M.; Phillips, M.R. Self poisoning with pesticides. *BMJ* **2004**, *328*, 42–44. [CrossRef]
38. Srinivas Rao, C.; Venkateswarlu, V.; Surender, T.; Eddleston, M.; Buckley, N. Pesticide poisoning in south India: Opportunities for prevention and improved medical management. *Trop. Med. Int. Health* **2005**, *10*, 581–588. [CrossRef]

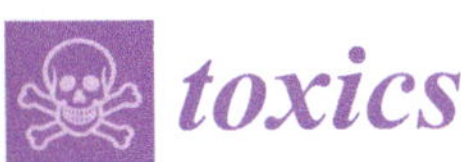

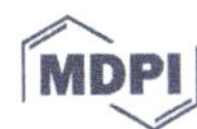

Article

Carbamazepine Overdose after Psychiatric Conditions: A Case Study for Postmortem Analysis in Human Bone

Lucia Fernández-López [1,2], Rosanna Mancini [3], Maria-Concetta Rotolo [3], Javier Navarro-Zaragoza [1,2,*], Juan-Pedro Hernández del Rincón [4] and Maria Falcón [2,4]

1 Department of Pharmacology, Faculty of Medicine, University of Murcia, 30120 Murcia, Spain; lucia.fernandez2@um.es
2 Instituto Murciano de Investigación Biosanitaria IMIB-Arrixaca, 30120 Murcia, Spain; falcon@um.es
3 National Centre on Drug Addiction and Doping, Istituto Superior di Sanitá, 00161 Rome, Italy; rosanna.mancini@iss.it (R.M.); mariaconcetta.rotolo@iss.it (M.-C.R.)
4 Forensic and Legal Medicine, Faculty of Medicine, University of Murcia, 30120 Murcia, Spain; jphrincon@um.es
* Correspondence: jnavarrozaragoza@um.es; Tel.: +34-868889286

Abstract: Carbamazepine is the main option used as a preventive medication to treat bipolar disorder when there is no response to lithium. Carbamazepine toxicity is defined as serum levels greater than 12 μg/mL, with severe toxicity occurring over 40 μg/mL, reduced to 30 μg/mL when combined with pharmacological treatment, i.e., benzodiazepines or antidepressants. For these reasons, it is necessary to find a validated tool to determine carbamazepine levels in an autopsy to rule out suicide or to know if the death was a consequence of an adverse drug reaction (ADR), especially when only bones can be accessed. We have validated a tool to detect and quantify drug concentration in bone. Our results showed a peak for carbamazepine at minute 12 and a mass fragment of 193 *m/z*. This case study is the first time in the literature that carbamazepine has been detected and quantified in bone. These results demonstrate that carbamazepine can be detected in bone tissue from forensic cases, but almost more importantly, that the method proposed is valid, reliable, and trustworthy.

Keywords: carbamazepine; bipolar; bone tissue; blood; matrix; concentration

Citation: Fernández-López, L.; Mancini, R.; Rotolo, M.-C.; Navarro-Zaragoza, J.; Hernández del Rincón, J.-P.; Falcón, M. Carbamazepine Overdose after Psychiatric Conditions: A Case Study for Postmortem Analysis in Human Bone. *Toxics* **2022**, *10*, 322. https://doi.org/10.3390/toxics10060322

Academic Editor: Maria Pieri

Received: 17 May 2022
Accepted: 11 June 2022
Published: 13 June 2022

1. Introduction

Carbamazepine is a dibenzazepine, a drug indicated for use as an antiepileptic drug, but it is also useful to treat other disorders that generate pain, such as trigeminal neuralgia and neuropathic pain and psychiatric conditions including depression and bipolar disorder [1]. Moreover, carbamazepine is the main option used as a preventive medication to treat bipolar disorder when there is no response to lithium [2]. Indeed, it has more effectiveness in avoiding manic episodes than other drugs, with 50% efficacy, and is even more powerful than lithium in preventing relapses [3]. One of the reasons why carbamazepine is not the first choice to treat bipolar disorder is the high rate of toxicity that this drug produces. According to the US Poison Control Center, there are nearly 2000 cases each in the US [4]. Carbamazepine produces a metabolite named oxcarbazepine that has similar effects but fewer adverse drug reactions (ADR) [5]. The recommended plasmatic concentration levels are approximately 4–12 μg/mL with a daily dose of 400 to 1200 mg; meanwhile, carbamazepine toxicity is defined as serum levels greater than 12 μg/mL, with severe toxicity occurring over 40 μg/mL (Table 1) [6,7].

Additionally, patients with combined pharmacological treatment, i.e., benzodiazepines or antidepressants, can generate severe toxicity over 30 μg/mL, affecting the heart and other organs. Furthermore, combination with alcohol can heighten these toxic effects and lead to overdose and, finally, death [6,8] when the use of activated charcoal is not enough [9].

Table 1. Carbamazepine indications, pharmacokinetics, and reference blood levels.

Indication	Pharmacokinetic	Blood Levels
Main indication: epilepsy Other indications: trigeminal neuralgia neuropathic pain psychiatric conditions (depression, bipolar disorder, manic episodes)	Distribution: 70–80% protein binding Reaches breast milk and crosses placental barrier. Metabolism: hepatic Elimination: 70% renal, 30% hepatic $t_{1/2}$ 36 h	Terapeutic: 4–12 µg/mL Toxic: >12 µg/mL Severe toxicity: 40 µg/mL (in combination with antidepressants or alcohol: 30 µg/mL)

These data, together with the fact that psychiatric patients sometimes have suicidal intentions, show that carbamazepine might be observed and quantified in problematic patients [10]. Nevertheless, when a patient known to be treated with carbamazepine dies, it is necessary to determine the drug levels during the autopsy in order to discard suicide or ADR as a potential cause of death. An autopsy includes post-mortem toxicological analysis to confirm if any drug or toxic has been involved in the death of the person [11]. The matrices usually analyzed are blood, urine, vitreous humor, or pericardial fluid, when available. Some scenes are complicated, and it can be difficult to come to a conclusion about the cause of the death when the body has been buried or hidden for a long time and the matrices are affected [12–14]. Sometimes, in post-mortem analysis, blood and urine are not available, so other specimens are submitted, i.e., stomach contents, bile, vitreous humor, liver and other tissues, muscle, or bone marrow [15,16]. In these cases, it can be hard to test and interpret data as these matrices are not frequently analyzed, and therefore there is a lack of literature and published results to compare with [17,18]. The problem becomes larger when the body is fully discomposed, and only bones remain. Toxicological analysis in bones can be performed, although the correlation to blood concentration to complete the post-mortem toxicology is not accessible for carbamazepine, oxcarbazepine, and other similar drugs that have never been quantified in bone. This deficit of data makes it necessary to validate a precise and highly specific method that correlates drug concentration levels in bone to drug concentration levels in blood. The aim of this research was to analyze different post-mortem human rib samples to establish a correlation between carbamazepine levels from bones to blood.

2. Materials and Methods

2.1. Chemicals and Reagents

We used two internal standards (IS) for carbamazepine and sertraline (Salars, Como, Italy). N,O-Bis(trimethylsilyl)trifluoroacetamide (BSTFA) with trimethylchlorosilane (TFMC) (Sigma-Aldrich, Milano, Italy) is a reagent commonly used in identification and quantification. BSTFA + TMCS has been used as a derivatizing reagent for GC-MS determination of both drugs.

2.2. Preparation of Standard Solutions

The standard solutions were prepared according to the following steps. The internal standard solution (100 ng/mL) and the stock solution for the drug studied (1 mg/mL) were stored at 20 °C in methanol. Subsequently, the stock solution was diluted with methanol for the calibration curves and quality control spots. Standards were prepared each day at LOQ values, 5, 50, 100, 250, and 500 ng/mg of the rib by spiking a pre-checked naïve pool with different volumes of methanol. A total of 3 quality control (QC) samples were obtained: 400 ng/mg (high control, QCH), 150 ng/mg (medium control, QCM), and 10 ng/mg (low control, OCL).

2.3. Samples

Samples in this research were collected at the Legal Medicine Institute of Murcia, Spain. All the samples were taken from the ribs; specifically, they are the fifth and the sixth ribs' central parts. This bone was selected because of its vascularity, and it is easily accessed. The length of the bone was 5 cm for all the specimens. Three rib samples from subjects whose blood was free of carbamazepine were collected in order to contrast the data. The institutional Ethical Committee of the University of Murcia approved the study.

2.4. Preparation of the Samples and Extraction Procedure

Soft tissues were removed from the surface using a scalpel, and bone samples were chopped into approximately 1 cm fragments using a scalpel and scissors. Samples were dried at 50 °C in an oven overnight and pulverized using a ball mill (Millmix 20, Biogen, Madrid, Spain). The resulting bone powder was restored at −80 °C until the analysis was performed. The analysis of carbamazepine in human bone was carried out according to a validated method [19] with the following steps. A total of 300 mg of bone powder with 1 mg/mL IS solution and 2 mL of methanol were vortexed and incubated for 1 h under ultrasounds. Then, samples were centrifuged, and the supernatants were recovered and evaporated. Phosphate buffered saline (PBS; 0.1 M, pH 6) was added, and samples were subjected to a solid-phase extraction using CleanScreen PKG50 extraction columns (3 cc, 200 mg, United Chemical Technologies, Bristol, PA, USA). Columns were preconditioned with methanol and PBS and samples were loaded. The columns were then washed with deionized water and 0.1 M hydrochloric acid, dried under vacuum, and washed again with methanol. Substances were eluted using 2 mL of dichloromethane:isopropanol:ammonia (78:20:2, $v/v/v$), and then they were evaporated. Samples were reconstituted with 100 µL of ethyl acetate, vortexed, and pipetted into GC injector vials.

2.5. Gas Chromatography–Mass Spectrometry (GC-MS) Analysis

We used a 6890 Series Plus gas chromatograph equipped with an Agilent 7683 autosampler and coupled to a 5973N mass selective detector (Agilent Technologies, Palo Alto, CA, USA) together with a fused silica capillary column (ZB-SemiVolatiles, 30 m, 0.25 mm i.d., 0.25 µm film) from Phenomenex (Torrance, CA, USA). First, 1 µL of the sample was inserted into the injection port held at 260 °C in splitless mode. We maintained the oven temperature at 100 °C for 2 min increasing 30 °C per minute until reaching 190 °C. This temperature was held for 20 min. After this period, we increased 40 °C per minute again. The final selected temperature was 290 °C, which was held for 10 min.

The electron-impact (EI) mass spectra were recorded in total ion monitoring mode (scan range 40–550 m/z) to determine retention times and characteristic mass fragments of the compounds. Afterward, the instrument was operated in selected-ion-monitoring (SIM) mode. The qualifying ions monitored in SIM mode are displayed in Table 2; the underlined ions were collected and quantified. The ion ratio acceptance criterion was a deviation of ≤20% of the average ion ratios of all the calibrators.

Table 2. Retention times and characteristic ions of analyzed substances by GC-MS.

Substance	RT (min)	Characteristic Mass Fragments (m/z)
Carbamazepine	12.9	<u>193</u>–165–139
Sertraline (IS)	26.8	159–262–<u>274</u>–304

2.6. Validation Procedure

Selectivity, carryover, matrix effect, linearity, limits of detection (LOD) and quantification (LOQ), precision, accuracy, recovery, and stability were the parameters calculated in accordance with the criteria described in previous research [20–23]. Five different daily replicates of the three QC samples were used to calculate validation parameters along three successive working days.

We studied possible interferences by endogenous substances and between carbamazepine and the IS, but also possible carryovers at the drug retention times. Calibration curves were performed in triplicate to analyze linearity. Moreover, peak area ratios between the compound and the IS were quantified. Along with these data, five replicates of blank samples were measured, obtaining a standard deviation (S.D.) of the mean noise level at the retention time window of the compound, which was used for the determination of LOD (3S.D.) and LOQ (10S.D.) of the method. Following this, we analyzed the accuracy and precision of the method at the three QC concentrations, expressed as standard deviation and error (%) of the measured values. Other values such as recovery, matrix effects, and process efficiency were calculated [24]. Finally, we analyzed 3 cycles on QC samples to obtain the mid-term stability of the analytes and their capacity to avoid thaw in bone after freeze (−20 °C). Two samples were quantified in triplicate each month over a period of six months. The stability was expressed as a relative percentage of the initial concentration in QC and in real samples.

2.7. Expression of Analyte Levels

Analyte levels were expressed as mass-normalized response ratios (RR/m), RR for the ratio between peak areas of the ion and the internal standard. This method allows valid results when [14,21–23] it is not possible to have analyte recoveries from bone tissue that provide accurate data. RR/m values were expressed in concentration units (ng/mg).

3. Results

3.1. GC-MS

The chromatogram of the drug-free bone pool samples did not show any background of endogenous substances once the extraction was performed (Figure 1A). This chromatogram was certified as representative. Furthermore, in Figure 1B, a representative chromatogram for an extract of 0.3 g spiked with 50 ng of carbamazepine. The peak for carbamazepine usually is set at minute 12, and its mass fragment is 193 *m/z*. We did not see traces of carryover after the calibration curve's highest point in any controlled sample.

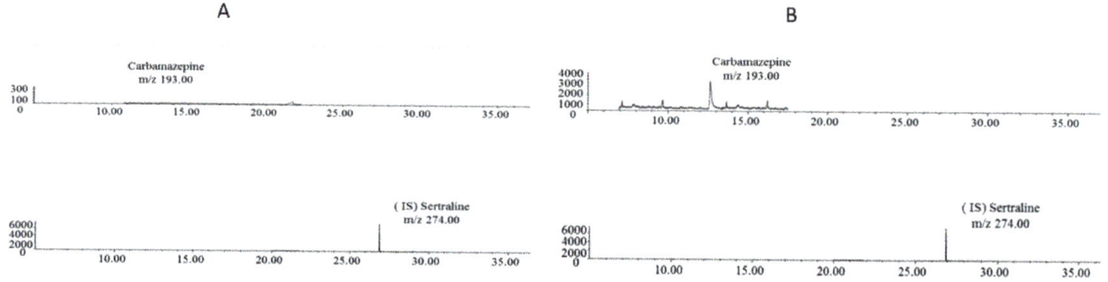

Figure 1. (**A**) Representative chromatograms obtained following the extraction of 0.3 g of drug-free bone pool. (**B**) SIM chromatogram of an extract of 0.3 g of drug-free bone pool spiked with 50 ng of carbamazepine.

3.2. Validation Results

The determination coefficient (r^2) for the linear calibration curve was 0.999 up to 500 ng/mg in the sample studied. We obtained a LOD smaller than 0.1 ng/mg and a LOQ of 0.3 ng/mg. The precision obtained intra- and inter-day was not bigger than 2.5% for all the collected data injected, which assure repeatability. We also repeatedly obtained a result of over 14% for the inter-and intra-assay accuracy values (Table 3). We found an analytical recovery of 92.6%, which confirms a proper extraction activity. The matrix effect was also calculated, resulting in 78.8%. Because of this, the matrix did not significantly change the intensity of the signal. Regarding efficiency, our results showed 73%. We also saw that the QC samples were stable during all the cycles (3 freeze/thaw). We had differences in concentration under 10% if we compare with the value at time 0. Regarding the stability of the samples at mid-term, we also noted a difference below 10%. This allows the samples to be stored until the analysis in the different institutes of legal medicine.

Table 3. Intra- and inter-assay ($n = 3$) precision and accuracy obtained for carbamazepine.

Analyte	Intra-Assay Precision (RSD)			Intra-Assay Accuracy (ABS%Error)			Inter-Assay Precision (RSD)			Inter-Assay Accuracy (ABS%Error)		
	* QCL	** QCM	*** QCH	QCL	QCM	QCH	QCL	QCM	QCH	QCL	QCM	QCH
Carbamazepine	1.4	2.3	0.4	13.6	3.3	1.9	1.3	1.4	0.9	6.9	0.2	1.0

* QCL: 10 ng/mg. ** QCM: 150 ng/mg. *** QCH: 400 ng/mg.

3.3. Application to Real Samples

Once the method was tested and validated, we performed it to see the results in a forensic case with a blood-positive result for carbamazepine. The sample was obtained from a Caucasian male aged 41-years-old who probably died due to chronic ischemic heart disease and had a post-mortem interval of approximately 13 h. The result for the concentration of carbamazepine in blood was 3750 ng/mL, which is within the therapeutic blood range [25]. It was also detected in the bone sample at 46 ng/mg. A representative chromatogram after this extraction is shown in Figure 2.

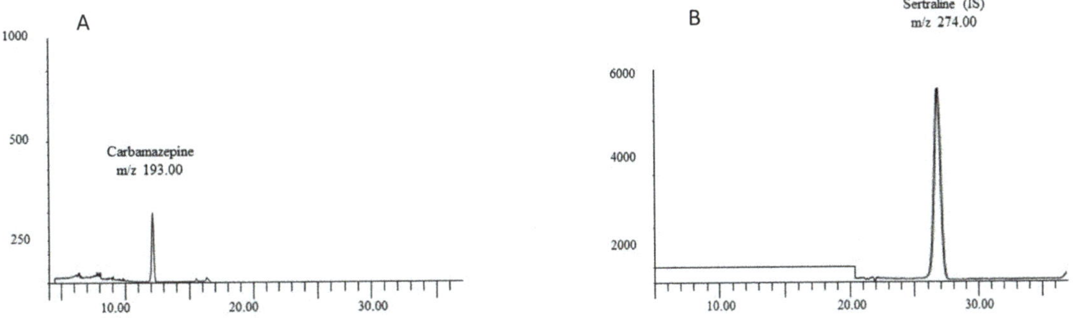

Figure 2. (**A**) SIM chromatogram of bone extracts from the real case containing approximately 46 ng/mg bone of carbamazepine. (**B**) SIM chromatogram for sertraline (IS) of bone extracts from the real case.

4. Discussion

This is the first time in the literature that carbamazepine was detected in bone; therefore, these results demonstrate that carbamazepine may be detected in bone tissue in forensic cases. We have previously validated a method to detect different drugs in bones. The method has been tested in this case study and seems to be valid, reliable, and trustworthy, although more studies should be performed. A procedure that includes the detection of this drug in bone is interesting since it is an increasingly used substance prescribed for multiple therapeutic indications, but especially for psychiatric diseases. Carbamazepine is used in some cases by patients suffering from schizophrenia, bipolar disorder, mania, or major depression, which are disorders characterized by unstable behaviors, abrupt changes in mood, or hallucinations in some cases. These situations may lead to cases of medico-legal interest such as suicides, aggressions, or murders since these mental disorders have been associated with the risk of premature death from suicide and other causes [26], violence, and violent offending, particularly homicide [27], and repeat incarcerations [28].

Postmortem toxicological results in bone are hard to understand since there is no standardized data about toxic, therapeutic, or even lethal concentrations of drugs in bone. It is important to clarify that quantitative data about drugs in bone would not give more information than qualitative data. If a database were developed with all these parameters, this interpretation would be much easier. The problem is that the mentioned database exists only for blood matrix, so the correlation of drug levels between blood and bone would also give interpretative value to quantitative data in bone.

5. Conclusions

This method for the detection of carbamazepine in human bone was tested and validated, providing satisfactory results in a real forensic case. Although there is a huge lack of results in bone matrix, detection of the different drugs could help to establish a correlation between results in blood and bone, allowing forensics to know the cause of death even when the victims have been buried or have been disappeared for a long period of time. We encourage other researchers to expand the number of substances detected in bone in order to make this matrix a valid tool for every case in the future.

Author Contributions: J.-P.H.d.R. extracted the samples. L.F.-L. treated the samples, R.M., M.F. and M.-C.R. were responsible for the study concept and design. L.F.-L. and M.F. developed data analysis. L.F.-L. and J.N.-Z. drafted the manuscript. M.F. and R.M. provided critical revisions for the discussion of the manuscript. All authors have read and agreed to the published version of the manuscript.

Funding: This research and APC costs were funded by FUNDACIÓN SÉNECA, 20847/PI/18 and Ministerio de Ciencia e Innovación, PID2020-113081.

Institutional Review Board Statement: The study was conducted in accordance with the Declaration of Helsinki, and approved by the Ethics Committee of the University of Murcia.

Informed Consent Statement: Not applicable.

Data Availability Statement: Data available on request due to restrictions.

Conflicts of Interest: The authors declare no conflict of interest.

References

1. Bridwell, R.E.; Brown, S.; Clerkin, S.; Birdsong, S.; Long, B. Neurologic toxicity of carbamazepine in treatment of trigeminal neuralgia: A case report. *Am. J. Emerg. Med.* **2022**, *55*, 231.e3–231.e5. [CrossRef] [PubMed]
2. Vieta, E.; Cruz, N.; Garcia-Campayo, J.; De Arce, R.; Crespo, J.M.; Vallès, V.; Pérez-Blanco, J.; Roca, E.; Olivares, J.M.; Moríñigo, A.; et al. A double-blind, randomized, placebo-controlled prophylaxis trial of oxcarbazepine as adjunctive treatment to lithium in the long-term treatment of bipolar I and II disorder. *Int. J. Neuropsychopharmacol.* **2008**, *11*, 445–452. [CrossRef] [PubMed]
3. Tondo, L. El tratamiento a largo plazo del trastorno bipolar. *Psicodebate* **2014**, *14*, 83–100. [CrossRef]
4. Gummin, D.D.; Mowry, J.B.; Beuhler, M.C.; Spyker, D.A.; Bronstein, A.C.; Rivers, L.J.; Pham, N.P.T.; Weber, J. 2020 Annual Report of the American Association of Poison Control Centers' National Poison Data System (NPDS): 38th Annual Report. *Clin. Toxicol.* **2021**, *59*, 1282–1501. [CrossRef]
5. Grunze, A.; Amann, B.L.; Grunze, H. Efficacy of Carbamazepine and Its Derivatives in the Treatment of Bipolar Disorder. *Medicina* **2021**, *57*, 433. [CrossRef]
6. Hirsch, A.; Wanounou, M.; Perlman, A.; Hirsh-Raccah, B.; Muszkat, M. The effect of multidrug exposure on neurological manifestations in carbamazepine intoxication: A nested case-control study. *BMC Pharmacol. Toxicol.* **2020**, *21*, 47. [CrossRef]
7. Ghannoum, M.; Yates, C.; Galvao, T.F.; Sowinski, K.M.; Vo, T.H.V.; Coogan, A.; Gosselin, S.; Lavergne, V.; Nolin, T.D.; Hoffman, R.S.; et al. Extracorporeal treatment for carbamazepine poisoning: Systematic review and recommendations from the EXTRIP workgroup. *Clin. Toxicol.* **2014**, *52*, 993–1004. [CrossRef]
8. Tanaka, E. Toxicological Interactions Between Alcohol and Benzodiazepines. *J. Toxicol. Clin. Toxicol.* **2002**, *40*, 69–75. [CrossRef]
9. Hoegberg, L.C.G.; Shepherd, G.; Wood, D.M.; Johnson, J.; Hoffman, R.S.; Caravati, E.M.; Chan, W.L.; Smith, S.W.; Olson, K.R.; Gosselin, S. Systematic review on the use of activated charcoal for gastrointestinal decontamination following acute oral overdose. *Clin. Toxicol.* **2021**, *59*, 1196–1227. [CrossRef]
10. Anand, L.S.; Anand, J.S. Self-poisoning before and during the initial year of the COVID-19 pandemic in northern Poland. *Int. J. Occup. Med. Environ.* **2022**, *35*, 1–9.
11. Ahmed, H.; Larsen, M.; Hansen, M.; Andersen, C. The role of QT-prolonging medications in a forensic autopsy study from Western Denmark. *Forensic Sci. Int.* **2021**, *325*, 110889. [CrossRef] [PubMed]
12. Caplan, Y.H.; Goldberger, B.A. Alternative Specimens for Workplace Drug Testing. *J. Anal. Toxicol.* **2001**, *25*, 396–399. [CrossRef] [PubMed]
13. McGrath, K.K.; Jenkins, A.J. Detection of Drugs of Forensic Importance in Postmortem Bone. *Am. J. Forensic Med. Pathol.* **2009**, *30*, 40–44. [CrossRef] [PubMed]

14. Watterson, J.H.; Botman, J.E. Detection of Acute Diazepam Exposure in Bone and Marrow: Influence of Tissue Type and the Dose-Death Interval on Sensitivity of Detection by ELISA with Liquid Chromatography Tandem Mass Spectrometry Confirmation. *J. Forensic Sci.* **2009**, *54*, 708–714. [CrossRef]
15. McIntyre, I.M.; King, C.V.; Boratto, M.; Drummer, O.H. Postmortem drug analyses in bone and bone marrow. *Ther. Drug Monit.* **2000**, *22*, 79–83. [CrossRef]
16. Fernández, P.; Aldonza, M.; Bouzas, A.; Lema, M.; Bermejo, A.M.; Tabernero, M.J. GC-FID determination of cocaine and its metabolites in human bile and vitreous humor. *J. Appl. Toxicol.* **2006**, *26*, 253–257. [CrossRef]
17. Lin, D.-L.; Chen, C.-Y.; Shaw, K.-P.; Havier, R.; Lin, R.-L. Distribution of Codeine, Morphine, and 6-Acetylmorphine in Vitreous Humor. *J. Anal. Toxicol.* **1997**, *21*, 258–261. [CrossRef]
18. Politi, L.; Groppi, A.; Polettini, A.; Montagna, M.T. A rapid screening procedure for drugs and poisons in gastric contents by direct injection-HPLC analysis. *Forensic Sci. Int.* **2004**, *141*, 115–120. [CrossRef]
19. Fernandez-Lopez, L.; Pellegrini, M.; Rotolo, M.C.; Maldonado, A.L.; Falcon, M.; Mancini, R. Development and validation of a method for analysing of duloxetine, venlafaxine and amitriptyline in human bone. *Forensic Sci. Int.* **2019**, *299*, 154–160. [CrossRef]
20. Raikos, N.; Tsoukali, H.; Njau, S. Determination of opiates in postmortem bone and bone marrow. *Forensic Sci. Int.* **2001**, *123*, 140–141. [CrossRef]
21. Wiebe, T.R.; Watterson, J.H. Analysis of tramadol and O-desmethyltramadol in decomposed skeletal tissues following acute and repeated tramadol exposure by gas chromatography mass spectrometry. *Forensic Sci. Int.* **2014**, *242*, 261–265. [CrossRef] [PubMed]
22. Wille, S.M.R.; Coucke, W.; De Baere, T.; Peters, F.T. Update of Standard Practices for New Method Validation in Forensic Tox-icology. *Curr. Pharm. Des.* **2017**, *23*, 5442–5454. [PubMed]
23. Peters, F.T.; Wissenbach, D.K.; Busardò, F.P.; Marchei, E.; Pichini, S. Method Development in Forensic Toxicology. *Curr. Pharm. Des.* **2017**, *23*, 5455–5467. [CrossRef] [PubMed]
24. Matuszewski, B.K.; Constanzer, M.L.; Chavez-Eng, C.M. Strategies for the Assessment of Matrix Effect in Quantitative Bioanalytical Methods Based on HPLC−MS/MS. *Anal. Chem.* **2003**, *75*, 3019–3030. [CrossRef]
25. Schulz, M.; Schmoldt, A. Therapeutic and toxic blood concentrations of more than 800 drugs and other xenobiotics. *Pharmazie* **2003**, *58*, 447–474.
26. Ösby, U.; Brandt, L.; Correia, N.; Ekbom, A.; Sparén, P. Excess Mortality in Bipolar and Unipolar Disorder in Sweden. *Arch. Gen. Psychiatry* **2001**, *58*, 844–850. [CrossRef]
27. Fazel, S.; Gulati, G.; Linsell, L.; Geddes, J.R.; Grann, M. Schizophrenia and violence: Systematic review and me-ta-analysis. *PLoS Med.* **2009**, *6*, e1000120. [CrossRef]
28. Baillargeon, J.; Binswanger, I.A.; Penn, J.V.; Williams, B.A.; Murray, O.J. Psychiatric Disorders and Repeat Incarcerations: The Revolving Prison Door. *Am. J. Psychiatry* **2009**, *166*, 103–109. [CrossRef]

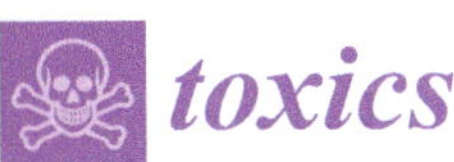

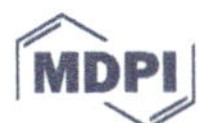

Article

Helium Suicide, a Rapid and Painless Asphyxia: Toxicological Findings

Anna Carfora [1,*], Raffaella Petrella [1], Giusy Ambrosio [1], Pasquale Mascolo [1], Bruno Liguori [1], Christian Juhnke [2], Carlo Pietro Campobasso [1,†] and Thomas Keller [3,†]

[1] Forensic Toxicology Unit, Department of Experimental Medicine, University of Campania "L. Vanvitelli", Via L. Armanni, 5, 80138 Naples, Italy; raffaella.petrella@unicampania.it (R.P.); giusy.ambrosio@studenti.unicampania.it (G.A.); mascolopasquale2@gmail.com (P.M.); bruno.liguori@gmail.com (B.L.); carlopietro.campobasso@unicampania.it (C.P.C.)

[2] Laboratory for Vacuum and Low Temperature Technology, University of Applied Sciences, Nibelungeplatz 1, D-60318 Frankfurt, Germany; juhnke@fb2.fra-uas.de

[3] Institute of Forensic Medicine, University of Salzburg, Ignaz-Harrer-Street, 79, A-5020 Salzburg, Austria; thomas.keller@plus.ac.at

* Correspondence: anna.carfora@unicampania.it; Tel.: +39-0815664107; Fax: +39-0815667720

† These authors contributed equally to this work.

Abstract: Suicide by helium inhalation has become increasingly common in the last few decades in Europe and the US because it produces a quick and painless death. Inhaled-gas suicides can easily be assessed through death scene investigation and autopsy. However, helium is a colorless and odorless inert gas that unfortunately cannot be detected using standard toxicological analysis. A successful gas analysis was performed following the suicide of a 17-year-old female. For the detection of helium, central/peripheral blood samples and gaseous samples from the esophagus, stomach, and upper and lower respiratory airways (from the trachea and the primary left and right bronchia) were collected with a gastight syringe, ensuring minimal dilution. Qualitative analyses were positive in all gaseous samples. Quantitative analyses were performed using a special gas-inlet system with a vacuum by which the sample can be transferred to a mass spectrometer, reducing the risk of contamination. Helium concentrations were 20.16% from the trachea, 12.33% from the right lung, and 1.5% from the stomach. Based on the high levels of helium, the cause and manner of death were assessed as asphyxia suicide by inhalation of helium. Therefore, toxicological analyses should always be applied in order to gain evidence of inhaled gas in gaseous samples.

Keywords: helium; asphyxia; suicide; detection and quantification

Citation: Carfora, A.; Petrella, R.; Ambrosio, G.; Mascolo, P.; Liguori, B.; Juhnke, C.; Campobasso, C.P.; Keller, T. Helium Suicide, a Rapid and Painless Asphyxia: Toxicological Findings. *Toxics* **2022**, *10*, 424. https://doi.org/10.3390/toxics10080424

Academic Editor: Maria Pieri

Received: 30 June 2022
Accepted: 26 July 2022
Published: 28 July 2022

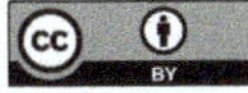

1. Introduction

In the last two decades, an increase in suicides due to gas inhalation has been observed [1–4]. Since 2000, suicide methods using a combination of plastic bag suffocation with inert gas inhalation (e.g., helium, nitrogen, nitrous oxide) have been widely reported around the world [5,6]. Helium is one of the most common inert gases involved in these events, along with propane and nitrogen [7–12]. According to Nowak et al. (2019), suicides due to helium inhalation are very common in Northern and Eastern Europe, but also in South Australia, Hong Kong, and the US. The popularity of asphyxia suicide by gas inhalation has been related to the wide spread of digital and printed publications dealing with this topic [13–16]. In these references, the readers can find all the instructions useful, already applied by the victims who reported the methods on their laptops and smartphones. Similar methods are also described in the so-called right-to-die literature dealing with euthanasia, self-deliverance, and assisted suicide [17,18].

In the inert gas group [19], helium is widely used to commit suicide, due to its characteristics and accessibility. It is an odorless, colorless, and nonflammable gas used to inflate balloons, which makes it extremely easy to get [20–23].

Compared to oxygen, helium has a lower density. When its air concentration increases, it replaces oxygen in the atmospheric air as well as within the lungs, causing hypoxia. With a plastic bag secured over the head by a rope, a rubber band, or adhesive tape fixed around the neck, the flow of helium into the bag can accelerate the removal of oxygen. Therefore, hypoxia is a fast process. It is estimated that loss of consciousness due to oxygen deprivation can occur in 5–10 s and within 60 s cerebral damage can be irreversible due to hypoxia [24].

Helium is very easy to breath but, in case of oxygen replacement by helium, the first symptoms of oxygen deficiency can be observed when oxygen levels go down to 12–16% from the normal oxygen concentrations of atmospheric air (21%). These symptoms are mainly represented by tachypnea, tachycardia, fatigue, and muscular coordination disorders. At lower concentrations of oxygen (6–10% approximately), loss of consciousness can occur and at levels below 6% convulsive movements and gasping breaths can anticipate the death due to brain hypoxic-ischemic injuries [7,25–27].

A peculiar aspect of helium inhalation is the lack of the breathing reflex or the so-called choking feeling, such that the victims do not feel the urge to breathe [15,22,28]. In fact, the breathing reflex is not triggered by oxygen deficiency, but by carbon dioxide excess, which is not present in the case of helium intoxication [28,29]. This is probably the main reason that helium is often used in euthanasia procedures [5]. Helium inhalation can cause painless asphyxia [30–32], which is very attractive to a potential suicide victim, as well as the availability of the gas and equipment.

Unfortunately, helium dissipates rapidly in ambient air and its presence cannot be easily detected postmortem in the blood or in tissue. In cases of helium suicide, the circumstances of disclosure of the corpse and the findings at the death scene are still of utmost importance [19,33], and examination of the cadaver can also provide very useful information [34]. However, according to various analytical processes and methods of detection, few research groups have performed toxicological analysis of helium or other inert gases on biological samples, properly collected, at autopsy. In cases of helium poisonings, the most commonly used detectors are mass spectrometers (MSs) in selected ion monitoring (SIM) mode [9,35–37], and thermal conductivity detectors (TCDs) [38–40], with the modification of mobile phase using the nitrogen or hydrogen as carrier gas.

In this case study, the cause and manner of death was assessed based on the results of the crime scene survey and autopsy findings, including the toxicological analyses. GC-MS and LS-MS/MS analyses on standard biological samples were negative for traditional drugs of abuse, pharmaceuticals, and their metabolites. A special gas-inlet system with a vacuum connected to a mass spectrometer was used for the detection and quantification of helium in gaseous samples, allowing the provision of sufficient evidence of helium inhalation. Helium-induced hypoxia was therefore assessed as the cause of death.

2. Materials and Methods

A 17-year-old female was found dead at home. A plastic bag over her head was fixed by a rope around the neck. Close to the body, there was a container, and a plastic tube was attached to the valve and led into the plastic bag. A forensic autopsy with toxicological analysis was requested.

2.1. Sampling

During the autopsy, biological samples were collected for the standard toxicological analyses. Blood, urine, bile, liver, and brain were sampled in tubes containing sodium fluoride.

Gaseous samples were also collected in order to quantify the helium concentration. For the detection of helium, central/peripheral blood samples and gaseous samples from the esophagus, stomach, and upper and lower respiratory airways (from the trachea and the primary left and right bronchia) were collected with a gastight syringe. Then, the content of the syringe was inserted in closed headspace vials in which the vacuum had already been initiated. All samples were stored in 10 mL headspace vials. These vials are the gold-standard containers for gas samples, as they are closed hermetically with an aluminum cap and a rubber seal with a magnetic crimp cap.

Intratracheal gas was sampled by gas syringe directly in the trachea after clamping. Pulmonary gases were sampled from the right primary bronchia after lung massage and bronchia clamping. Gastric gas was sampled from the stomach after esophageal and duodenal clamping, following the procedure by Varlet et al. [41]. All samples were stored at −20 °C until subsequent analysis.

2.2. Toxicological Analysis

A systematic toxicological analysis (STA) was performed on biological liquids, urine, and blood using gas chromatography coupled with mass spectrometry (GC-MS). In order to fill the gap with respect to thermolabile and nonvolatile analytes, analysis was also performed using liquid chromatography–tandem mass spectrometry (LC-MS/MS) for different classes of drugs of abuse, pharmaceuticals, and their metabolites. Blood was tested for alcohol and other volatile substances by headspace gas chromatography with flame ionization detection (GC-HS/FID). The method used for the analysis of biological matrices is the same reported in Carfora et al. (2018 and 2020) [42,43].

Gas samples were analyzed at the Laboratory for Vacuum and Low Temperature Technology at the Frankfurt University of Applied Sciences, where a special gas-inlet system for the analysis of small amounts of gas is available (Figure 1). It is a receptacle for a gastight syringe that contains the gas sample to be analyzed and a vacuum system by which the sample can be transferred to a mass spectrometer with the least risk of contamination. After a proper calibration curve of helium, oxygen, nitrogen, and carbon dioxide in the spectrometer, the sample's gas composition can be determined quantitatively with an error rate of <1%.

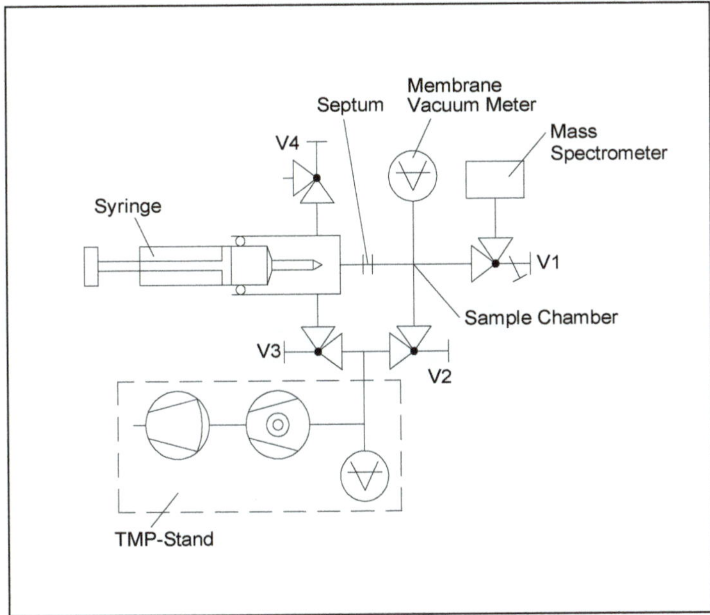

Figure 1. Schematic diagram of gas-inlet system.

2.3. Gas-Inlet System

The syringe is pushed into a Teflon-lined guide tube until the needle protrudes into a vacuum-tight septum made of special rubber. This hermetically seals the gas sample inside the syringe. The space in front of the ultrahigh vacuum (UHV) needle valve V1 is evacuated to a pressure of $<10^{-1}$ mbar via valve V2 with the aid of a turbo molecular pump (TMP) stand. The pressure is controlled by a gas-type independent membrane vacuum meter. Valve V2 is closed again and valve V3 is opened so that the atmospheric air contained in the space in front of the septum gets removed by the TMP stand. Only now is the septum pierced by the tip of the needle so that the gas sample can flow from the syringe into the evacuated sample chamber. The membrane vacuum meter's display indicates if the entire gas sample is contained inside the chamber (volume ~25 cm^3). The tip of the needle is then retracted into the septum so that any air that may enter the syringe does not flow into the chamber. In the event that the septum has a slight leak, sample gas may escape to the outside, but no atmospheric air can flow into the chamber, since the space in front of the septum is continuously being evacuated by the TMP stand. Adulteration of the gas sample's composition is thus made impossible.

3. Results

On external examination of the body, asphyxia signs were observed: conjunctival petechiae and mild facial congestion, slight bruising around the mouth, skin-ligature marking all around the neck reproducing the size of the rope securing the plastic bag, and finally purplish red hypostases in the lowest anatomical areas consistent with the body position. In particular, petechiae of the conjunctiva were not extensive, but represented on both sides by a few areas of scattered pinpoint hemorrhages consistent with an increased venous pressure of the head slightly congested.

At autopsy, no relevant injuries were found, except for a diffuse congestion of internal organs along with cerebral and pulmonary edema, consistent with the suspicion of an asphyxia death. Qualitative and quantitative analyses using GC-MS and LC-MS/MS showed the following results. STA of biological fluids were negative for the most common drugs of abuse and alcohol. Qualitative analyses were positive for helium in all gaseous samples, except for the sample of the left lung, which accidentally was left open during the laboratory procedures. Quantitative analyses were positive for helium from all samples available, collected from the trachea, the right bronchia and the stomach as follows:

- Trachea: 20.16%
- Right lung: 12.33%
- Stomach: 1.5%

In all three positive samples, the helium concentration exceeded the levels normally present in air (0.0005%), but helium was not the only gas detected from the gas samples. The quantitative results of gas analysis showed also additional gases, such as oxygen, nitrogen, and carbon dioxide (Table 1).

Table 1. Results of qualitative and quantitative gases analyses.

	Trachea	Right Bronchus	Stomach
Qualitative Analysis	Positive	Positive	Positive
Helium (He)	20.16%	12.33%	1.5%
Oxygen (O_2)	11.14%	9.37%	—
Nitrogen (N_2)	54.59%	63.06%	—
Carbon Dioxide (CO_2)	13.14%	14.50%	—

Figure 2 shows the chromatograms of qualitative and quantitative analyses from gas samples collected from the trachea and the right lung. Based on these results, the cause of death was related to the lack of oxygen due to helium inhalation. The manner of death was suicide.

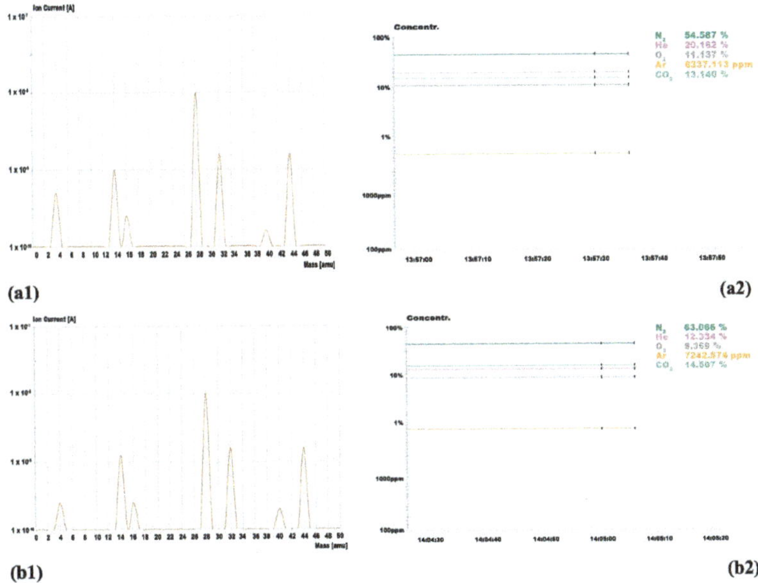

Figure 2. Qualitative and quantitative results of the gas analyses from the trachea sample (**a1**,**a2**) and the right lung (**b1**,**b2**).

4. Discussion

According to Madea et al. [44], asphyxia can be identified as cause of death also in every case of exclusion of oxygen due to the *"depletion and replacement of oxygen by another gas or by chemical interference with oxygen's uptake and utilization by the body"*. In this category, deaths by helium inhalation from a plastic bag, like in the present case, can also be included as lethal events in which oxygen is excluded and carbon dioxide, carbon monoxide, or hydrogen sulfide (toxic gases) enter the body [45,46].

The death of the young teenager has been classified as a suicidal asphyxiation by helium-induced hypoxia, based on the results of the death scene investigation and autopsy findings, including the toxicological analyses. Often, few indicators of hypoxia or suffocation can be found in victims of plastic-bag asphyxiation [47,48]. Although conjunctival petechiae and facial congestion are considered hallmarks of asphyxia deaths, they can be found in a variety of traumatic and natural deaths [49,50] as a result of increased cephalic venous pressure and hypoxic damage to endothelial cells.

The ligature mark can be the only indicator available, but it is not always present, depending on the nature of the rope or tape used to fix the plastic bag [51–53]. If the plastic bag and the other equipment (i.e., the rope fixing the bag over the head or the tube connecting the gas container) are removed at the death scene, the death might appear as being natural [52]. The removal of the equipment can occur when someone tries to hide the real cause of death or for financial reason, when life insurance does not cover a suicide [44,54]. Therefore, the death investigation is at risk due to inaccuracy of cause and manner of death determination. The forensic pathology community is aware that significant discrepancies between external body examination and forensic autopsy are not rare [55]. A violent death can be misclassified as natural if a death scene survey and an autopsy with toxicological analyses are not performed. An autopsy cannot be considered complete without appropriate toxicological analyses [53].

Unfortunately, the toxicological analysis of helium is not easy by standard methods, and a specific sampling procedure must be performed at the autopsy. Furthermore, a special gas-inlet system for the analysis of small amounts of gas is needed similar to the one available in the high-tech laboratory at the Frankfurt University of Applied Sciences.

Quantitative toxicological results for victims of helium inhalation are rare in the literature [39,56]. The reasons are mostly related to the heterogeneous findings due to wrong sampling at autopsy and to the fact that helium can be easily lost during storage and sample preparation. Helium might also not be detected in samples due to its loss while opening the containers to take the subsamples for toxicological analysis, as occurred in one of our samples (the sample collected from the left bronchus).

When the sampling method is carried out properly, helium can still be detected even 3 days after death [39]. In a case reported by Auwaerter et al. [56], helium was detected in samples not only from lung tissue but also from the brain and heart blood in such high concentrations that exceeded those normally present in air (0.0005%) by up to four orders of magnitude. Our results also demonstrate that the helium concentration detected was higher than those reported in literature.

5. Conclusions

Asphyxia by helium inhalation may not leave any physical signs useful to assess the cause and manner of death. Sophisticated forensic toxicological analyses will be able to verify helium exposure prior to death. In suspected unnatural deaths, especially those related to euthanasia or assisted suicide, an accurate sampling procedure using a gastight syringe and closed headspace vials must be considered at autopsy. Helium can be lost if sampling is not performed and processed properly at the laboratory. Furthermore, the toxicological analysis of helium is not easy to perform by standard methods. A special gas-inlet system should be considered crucial to receive reliable results.

Author Contributions: Writing—review and editing, investigation, A.C.; formal analysis, R.P.; writing—original draft preparation, G.A.; autopsy, P.M. and B.L.; methodology and formal analysis, C.J.; writing—review, conceptualization, and supervision, C.P.C.; conceptualization and review, T.K. All authors have read and agreed to the published version of the manuscript.

Funding: This research received no external funding.

Institutional Review Board Statement: The study was conducted in accordance with the Declaration of Helsinki. Approval from the local institutional review board was not necessary, since all analyses were performed in accordance with Prosecutor Office requests.

Conflicts of Interest: The authors declare no conflict of interest.

References

1. Avis, S.P.; Archibald, J.T.; Musshoff, F.; Hagemeier, L.; Kirschbaum, K.; Madea, B. Two cases of suicide by asphyxiation due to helium and argon. *Forensic Sci. Int.* **2012**, *223*, e27–e30.
2. Wick, R.; Gilbert, J.D.; Felgate, P.; Byard, R.W. Inhalant deaths in South Australia: A 20-year retrospective autopsy study. *Am. J. Forensic Med. Pathol.* **2007**, *28*, 319–322. [CrossRef] [PubMed]
3. Gentile, G.; Galante, N.; Tambuzzi, S.; Zoja, R. A forensic analysis on 53 cases of complex suicides and one complicated assessed at the Bureau of Legal Medicine of Milan (Italy). *Forensic Sci. Int.* **2021**, *319*, 110662. [CrossRef] [PubMed]
4. Avis, S.P.; Archibald, J.T. Asphyxial suicide by propane inhalation and plastic bag suffocation. *J. Forensic Sci.* **1994**, *39*, 253–256. [CrossRef]
5. Gallagher, K.; Smith, D.M.; Mellen, P. Suicidal Asphyxiation by Using Pure Helium Gas Case Report, Review, and Discussion of the Influence of the Internet. *Am. J. Forensic Med. Pathol.* **2003**, *24*, 361–363. [CrossRef]
6. Austin, A.; Winskog, C.; van den Heuvel, C.; Byard, R.W. Recent trends in suicides utilizing helium. *J. Forensic Sci.* **2011**, *56*, 649–651. [CrossRef]
7. Frost, J. Death by self-inflicted asphyxia with helium—First case reports from Norway and review of the literature. *Scand. J. Forensic Sci.* **2013**, *19*, 52–54.
8. Nowak, K.; Szpot, P.; Zawadzi, M. Suicidal deaths due to helium inhalation. *Forensic Toxicol.* **2019**, *37*, 273–287. [CrossRef]
9. Wiergowski, M.; Kaliszan, M.; Suminska-Ziemann, B.; Gos, T.; Jankowski, Z. Helium detection in the lungs in case of suicide by helium inhalation-case report and literature review. *Rom. J. Leg. Med.* **2014**, *22*, 153–156.
10. Smedra, A.; Szustowski, S.; Jurczyk, A.P.; Klemm, J.; Szram, S.; Berent, J. Suicidal asphyxiation by using helium-two case reports. *Arch. Med. Sad. Kryminol.* **2015**, *65*, 37–46.

11. Konopka, T.; Strona, M.; Ksiezniak-Baran, D.; Wojton, D. Plastic bag suffocation in material collected by Department of Forensic Medicine in Krakow. *Arch. Med. Sad. Kryminol.* **2013**, *63*, 93–98.
12. Barnung, S.K.; Feddersen, C. Selvmord ved hjaelp af helium og en plastikpose [Suicide by inhaling helium inside a plastic bag]. *Ugeskr. Laeger* **2004**, *166*, 3506–3507. [PubMed]
13. Marzuk, P.M.; Tardiff, K.; Hirsch, C.S.; Leon, A.C.; Stajic, M.; Hartwell, N.; Portera, L. Increase in suicide by asphyxiation in New York City after the publication of Final Exit. *N. Engl. J. Med.* **1993**, *329*, 1508–1510. [CrossRef]
14. Marzuk, P.M.; Tardiff, K.; Leon, A.C. Increase in fatal suicidal poisonings and suffocations in the year Final Exit was published: A national study. *Am. J. Psychiatry* **1994**, *151*, 1813–1814.
15. van den Hondel, K.E.; Punt, P.; Dorn, T.; Ceelen, M.; Aarts, F.; van der Zande, D.; van Kuijk, S.; Duijst, W.; Stumpel, R.; van Mesdag, T.; et al. Suicide by helium inhalation in the Netherlands between 2012 and 2019. *Forensic Sci. Int.* **2021**, *318*, 110566. [CrossRef]
16. Ogden, R.D.; Hassan, S. Suicide by Oxygen Deprivation with Helium: A Preliminary Study of British Columbia Coroner Investigations. *Death Stud.* **2011**, *35*, 338–364. [CrossRef]
17. Humphry, D. *Final Exit the Practicalities of Self-Deliverance and Assisted Suicide for the Dying*, 3rd ed.; Delta Trade Paperback: New York, NY, USA, 2002.
18. Humphry, D. *Supplement to Final Exit: The Latest How-To and Why of Euthanasia/Hastened Death*; Norris Lane Press: Eugene, OR, USA, 2000.
19. Gilson, T.; Parks, B.O.; Porterfield, C.M. Suicide with inert gases: Addendum to Final Exit. *Am. J. Forensic Med. Pathol.* **2003**, *24*, 306–308. [CrossRef]
20. Berganza, C.J.; Zhang, J.H. The role of helium gas in medicine. *Med. Gas Res.* **2013**, *3*, 18. [CrossRef]
21. Byard, R.W. Changing trends in suicides using helium or nitrogen—A 15-year study. *J. Forensic Leg. Med.* **2018**, *58*, 6–8. [CrossRef]
22. Chang, S.S.; Cheng, Q.; Lee, E.S.; Yip, P.S. Suicide by gassing in Hong Kong 2005–2013: Emerging trends and characteristics of suicide by helium inhalation. *J. Affect. Disord.* **2016**, *192*, 162–166. [CrossRef]
23. Fink, J.B. Opportunities and risks of using heliox in your clinical practice. *Respir. Care* **2006**, *51*, 651–660.
24. Ogden, R.D.; Hamilton, W.K.; Witcher, C. Assisted suicide with oxygen deprivation with helium at a Swiss right-to-die organization. *J. Med. Ethics* **2010**, *36*, 174–179. [CrossRef]
25. Ogden, R.D. Observation of Two Suicides by Helium Inhalation in a Prefilled Environment. *Am. J. Forensic Med. Pathol.* **2010**, *31*, 156–161. [CrossRef]
26. Di Maio, D.J.; Di Maio, V.J.M. Asphyxia. In *Forensic Pathology*; Elsevier: New York, NY, USA, 1989; pp. 207–251.
27. Spitz, W.U. Asphyxia. In *Spitz and Fisher's Medicolegal Investigation of Death: Guidelines for the Application of Pathology to Crime Investigation*, 3rd ed.; Charles C Thomas: Springfield, IL, USA, 1993; pp. 444–497.
28. Grassberger, M.; Krauskopf, A. Suicidal asphyxiation with helium: Report of three cases. *Wien. Klin. Wochenschr.* **2007**, *119*, 323–325. [CrossRef]
29. O'Higgins, J.W.; Guillen, J.; Aldrete, J.A. The effect of helium inhalation on asphyxia in dogs. *J. Thorac. Cardiovasc. Surg.* **1971**, *61*, 870–874. [CrossRef]
30. Ogden, R.D. Non-physician assisted suicide: The technological imperative of the deathing counterculture. *Death Stud.* **2001**, *25*, 387–401. [PubMed]
31. Werth, J.L., Jr. Policy and psychosocial considerations associated with non-physician assisted suicide: A commentary on Ogden. *Death Stud.* **2001**, *25*, 403–411. [PubMed]
32. Lubell, K.M.; Swahn, M.H.; Crosby, A.E.; Kegler, S.R. Methods of Suicide Among Persons Aged 10–19 Years—United States, 1992–2001. *JAMA J. Am. Med. Assoc.* **2004**, *292*, 427–428.
33. Byard, R.W. Further observations on plastic bag asphyxia using helium gas. *Aust. J. Forensic Sci.* **2017**, *49*, 483–486. [CrossRef]
34. Borowska-Solonynko, A.; Dabkowska, A. Gas embolism as a potential cause of death by helium poisoning-postmortem computed tomography changes in two cases of suicidal helium inhalation. *Leg. Med.* **2018**, *31*, 59–65. [CrossRef]
35. Malbranque, S.; Mauillon, D.; Turcant, A.; Rouge-maillart, C.; Mangin, P.; Varlet, V. Quantification of fatal helium exposure following self-administration. *Int. J. Leg. Med.* **2016**, *130*, 1535–1539. [CrossRef]
36. Cuypers, E.; Rosier, E.; Loix, S.; Develter, W.; Van Den Bogaert, W.; Wuestenbergs, J.; Van de Voorde, W.; Tytgat, J. Medical Findings and Toxicological Analysis in Infant Death by Balloon Gas Asphyxia: A Case Report. *J. Anal. Toxicol.* **2017**, *41*, 347–349. [CrossRef] [PubMed]
37. Tsujita, A.; Okazaki, H.; Nagasaka, A.; Gohda, A.; Matsumoto, M.; Matsui, T. A new and sensitive method for quantitative determination of helium in human blood by gas chromatography–mass spectrometry using naturally existing neon-21 as internal standard. *Forensic Toxicol.* **2019**, *37*, 75–81. [CrossRef] [PubMed]
38. Schaff, J.E.; Karas, R.P.; Marinetti, L. A Gas Chromatography–Thermal Conductivity Detection Method for Helium Detection in Postmortem Blood and Tissue Specimens. *J. Anal. Toxicol.* **2012**, *36*, 112–115. [CrossRef] [PubMed]
39. Oosting, R.; van der Hulst, R.; Poeschier, L.; Verschraagen, M. Toxicological findings in three cases of suicidal asphyxiation with helium. *Forensic Sci. Int.* **2015**, *256*, 38–41. [CrossRef]
40. Tanaka, N.; Takakura, A.; Jamal, M.; Kumihashi, M.; Ito, A.; Ishimoto, S.; Tsutsui, K.; Kimura, S.; Ameno, K.; Kinoshita, H. Stomach gas as a useful matrix for detecting ante-mortem gas exposure. A case of asphyxia by helium inhalation. *Rom. J. Leg. Med.* **2016**, *24*, 21–22. [CrossRef]

41. Varlet, V.; Iwersen-Bergmann, S.; Alexandre, M.; Cordes, O.; Wunder, C.; Holz, F.; Andersen-Streichert, H.; Bevalot, F.; Dumestre-Toulet, V.; Malbranque, S.; et al. Helium poisoning: New procedure for sampling and analysis. *Int. J. Leg. Med.* **2019**, *133*, 1809–1818. [CrossRef] [PubMed]
42. Carfora, A.; Campobasso, C.P.; Cassandro, P.; Petrella, R.; Borriello, R. Alcohol and drugs use among drivers injured in road accidents in Campania (Italy): A 8-years retrospective analysis. *Forensic Sci. Int.* **2018**, *288*, 291–296. [CrossRef]
43. Carfora, A.; Borriello, R.; Cassandro, P.; Petrella, R.; Campobasso, C.P. Alcohol and drug use in drug-related deaths in campania (Italy): A snapshot study over the years 2008–2018. *J. Integr. OMICS* **2020**, *10*, 10–14. [CrossRef]
44. Madea, B. *Asphyiation, Suffocation, and Neck Pressure Deaths*; Taylor & Francis Inc.: Boca Raton, FL, USA, 2020; p. 191.
45. Carfora, A.; Campobasso, C.P.; Cassandro, P.; La Sala, F.; Maiellaro, A.; Perna, A.; Petrella, R.; Borriello, R. Fatal inhalation of volcanic gases in three tourists of a geothermal area. *Forensic Sci. Int.* **2019**, *297*, e1–e7. [CrossRef]
46. Barbera, N.; Montana, A.; Indorato, F.; Arbouche, N.; Romano, G. Domino effect: An unusual case of six fatal hydrogen sulfide poisonings in quick succession. *Forensic Sci. Int.* **2016**, *260*, e7–e10. [CrossRef]
47. Ogden, R.D.; Wooten, R.H. Asphyxial Suicide with Helium and Plastic Bag. *Am. J. Forensic Med. Pathol.* **2002**, *23*, 234–237. [CrossRef]
48. Saukko, P.; Knight, B. (Eds.) *Knight's Forensic Pathology*, 3rd ed.; Edwards Arnold Publishers: London, UK, 2004.
49. Maxeiner, H.; Bockholdt, B. Homicidal and suicidal ligature strangulation: A comparison of the postmortem findigs. *Forensic Sci. Int.* **2003**, *137*, 60–66. [CrossRef]
50. Ely, S.F.; Hirsch, C.S. Asphyxial deaths and petechiae. *J. Forensic Sci.* **2000**, *45*, 1274–1277. [CrossRef]
51. Grellner, W.; Anders, S.; Tsokos, M.; Wilske, J. Suicide with exit bags: Circumstances and special problem situations in assisted suicide. *Arch. Kriminol.* **2002**, *209*, 65–75.
52. Bullock, M.J.; Diniz, D. Suffocation using plastic bags: A retrospective study of suicides in Ontario, Canada. *J. Forensic Sci.* **2000**, *45*, 608–613. [CrossRef]
53. Jones, L.S.; Wyatt, J.P.; Busuttil, A. Plastic bag asphyxia in southeast Scotland. *Am. J. Forensic Med. Pathol.* **2000**, *21*, 401–405. [CrossRef]
54. Schön, C.A.; Ketterer, T. Asphyxial Suicide by Inhalation of Helium Inside a Plastic Bag. *Am. J. Forensic Med. Pathol.* **2007**, *26*, 364–367. [CrossRef]
55. Campobasso, C.P.; Laviola, D.; Grattagliano, I.; Strada, L.; Dell'Erba, A.S. Undetected patricide: Inaccuracy of cause of death determination without an autopsy. *J. For. Leg. Med.* **2015**, *34*, 67–72. [CrossRef]
56. Auwaerter, V.; Grosse Perdekamp, M.; Kempf, J.; Schmith, U.; Weinmann, W.; Pollak, S. Toxicological analysis after asphyxia suicide with helium and a plastic bag. *Forensic Sci. Int.* **2007**, *170*, 139–141. [CrossRef]

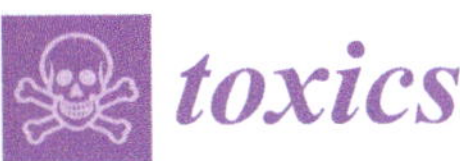 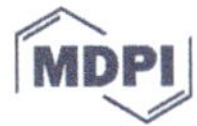

Article

Atypical Fentanyl Transdermal Patch Consumption and Fatalities: Case Report and Literature Review

Federico Manetti [1], Maria Chiara David [2,*], Sara Gariglio [3], Francesca Consalvo [1], Martina Padovano [1], Matteo Scopetti [4], Antonio Grande [5] and Alessandro Santurro [6]

1 Department of Anatomical, Histological, Forensic and Orthopedic Sciences, Sapienza University of Rome, 00185 Rome, Italy
2 Ministry of the Interior, Department of Public Security, Health Central Directorate, State Police, 00185 Rome, Italy
3 DIFAR—Department of Pharmacy, University of Genova, 16148 Genova, Italy
4 Department of Medical Surgical Sciences and Translational Medicine, Sapienza University of Rome, 00189 Rome, Italy
5 Department of Public Security, Anti-Crime Central Directorate, Scientific Police Service, 00174 Rome, Italy
6 Department of Medicine, Surgery and Dentistry, University of Salerno, 84081 Baronissi, Italy
* Correspondence: mariachiara.david@gmail.com

Abstract: Fentanyl is a synthetic L-opioid receptor agonist, approximately 100 times more potent than morphine, that is experiencing an upward trend in the field of abuse. Fentanyl patches' abusive consumption can occur either by transdermal absorption or through other atypical and ingenious routes. In the present case, a 29-year-old man with a history of illicit drug use was found dead in a suburban neighborhood of an Italian city. At autopsy, lungs appeared increased in weight and showed minute subpleural hemorrhages. Airways contained abundant reddish foamy material; in addition, a fentanyl patch protective film was found inside the left main bronchus. Toxicological analysis revealed the presence of morphine, fentanyl, BEG and ethyl alcohol in peripheric blood; 6-MAM was also revealed in urine. Findings collected during post-mortem investigations allowed us to identify fentanyl consumption as the cause of death. Fentanyl consumption presumably took place by chewing of a transdermal patch, with subsequent aspiration of the protective film. The pathophysiology of death can be identified as combined respiratory failure—both central suppression and a fentanyl-induced increase in muscular stiffness; a further minor contribution may be identified in the mechanical airflow obstruction caused by the presence of the protective film at the bronchial level.

Keywords: fentanyl; morphine; transdermal patch; protective film; autopsy; forensic toxicology; forensic pathology

Citation: Manetti, F.; David, M.C.; Gariglio, S.; Consalvo, F.; Padovano, M.; Scopetti, M.; Grande, A.; Santurro, A. Atypical Fentanyl Transdermal Patch Consumption and Fatalities: Case Report and Literature Review. *Toxics* **2023**, *11*, 46. https://doi.org/10.3390/toxics11010046

Academic Editor: Maria Pieri

Received: 21 November 2022
Revised: 27 December 2022
Accepted: 27 December 2022
Published: 31 December 2022

1. Introduction

Fentanyl is a synthetic L-opioid receptor agonist, approximately 100 times more potent than morphine per dose [1,2], widely used as a narcotic supplement in anesthesia and in the management of acute and severe chronic pain [3]. However, by virtue of its effectiveness and diffusion, fentanyl is experiencing an important upward trend also in the field of abuse, to the point of constituting, alongside the well-known classical opioids, a current and concrete problem of public order in many countries [4–12].

The consumption of fentanyl for recreational use includes its addition to other illicit drugs (such as heroin and cocaine) in order to enhance their effect at a low cost, as well as the use of formulations for medical purposes available on the market [3]. As regards the latter aspect, a characteristic and recurrent feature detectable in the international forensic toxicological literature is the widespread use of fentanyl transdermal patches, not only as a prescription in home therapies for the control of chronic pain, but also for recreational consumption.

In the presented case, the orientation towards a diagnosis of death due to the intake of a fentanyl transdermal patch by an atypical route of administration was provided by the typical signs of acute respiratory failure referable to exogenous intoxication, and the finding of a patch protective film inside the left main bronchus; subsequent histological and toxicological investigations, corroborated by available scientific evidence, allowed us to confirm the hypothesis proposed at the autoptic table.

2. Case Report

A 29-year-old man with a history of illicit drug use was found dead in a suburban neighborhood of an Italian major city. At the time of scene investigation, the corpse was laid on a wooden table, along a sidewalk, in lateral decubitus. Early-stage postmortem lividity was expressed consistently with the position assumed by the body. Clear residues of vomit, not observed elsewhere on the scene, were detected on the face and the clothes; whitish foamy material was found in proximity to nasal orifices. At the clothes' examination, a pack of alprazolam and four doses of hashish were found in the right pocket of the sweatshirt.

Preliminary judicial investigations made it possible to suspect that the man was abandoned along the sidewalk after he lost consciousness, while attending a party in which illicit drug consumption had taken place. Judicial autopsy was disposed by the prosecutor and performed approximately 48 h after the discovery of the corpse, in order to clarify the causes of death and exclude criminal conduct.

On external examination, his body was 173 cm in height and 80 kg in weight. Any type of lesion attributable to violent causes was excluded during the inspection.

At autopsy, brain weight was within normal limits (1325 g) and showed on its surface, besides congestion of leptomeningeal vessels, flattening of convolutions and superficialization of sulci, suggestive of cerebral edema. Trachea contained reddish foamy material and minute blood clots.

Lungs appeared increased in weight (848 g and 827 g, respectively, left and right), were regular in size and shape, and showed minute subpleural hemorrhages (Figure 1A). The opening of the airways allowed us to detect abundant reddish foamy material; in addition, a plastic protective film with the inscription "entan" was found inside the left main bronchus (Figure 1B,C). Edema and vascular congestion were revealed at the examination of the parenchyma.

The stomach contained 50 mL of undifferentiated food material; it was not possible to detect the presence of pills or other findings attributable to drugs.

Examination of other organs revealed non-specific signs of asphyxia and marked vascular congestion, in the absence of further noteworthy or pathological findings. Immunochemical drug screening for urine samples was positive for cocaine, morphine, methadone, cannabinoids (THC), and benzodiazepines.

During the investigations, biological samples were taken for histopathological and quantitative toxicological tests. Microscopic investigation of formalin-fixed paraffin-embedded (FFPE) tissue specimens after section and hematoxylin and eosin (H&E) staining allowed us to confirm the generalized vascular congestion macroscopically detected. Brain samples showed both intracellular and extracellular cerebral edema. Heart specimens were characterized by a moderate increase in perivascular and interstitial fibrous connective tissue representation, histologically relevant in consideration of the young age of the man. Lungs were characterized by the presence of abundant amorphous eosinophilic material in alveoli, indicative of alveolar edema, sometimes associated with erythrocyte alveolar infiltrations; in some fields, spots of acute emphysema were also noticed. No further findings of interest were revealed at the examination of the remaining tissue samples. In light of the aforementioned findings, the death was therefore attributed to acute respiratory failure referable to exogenous intoxication.

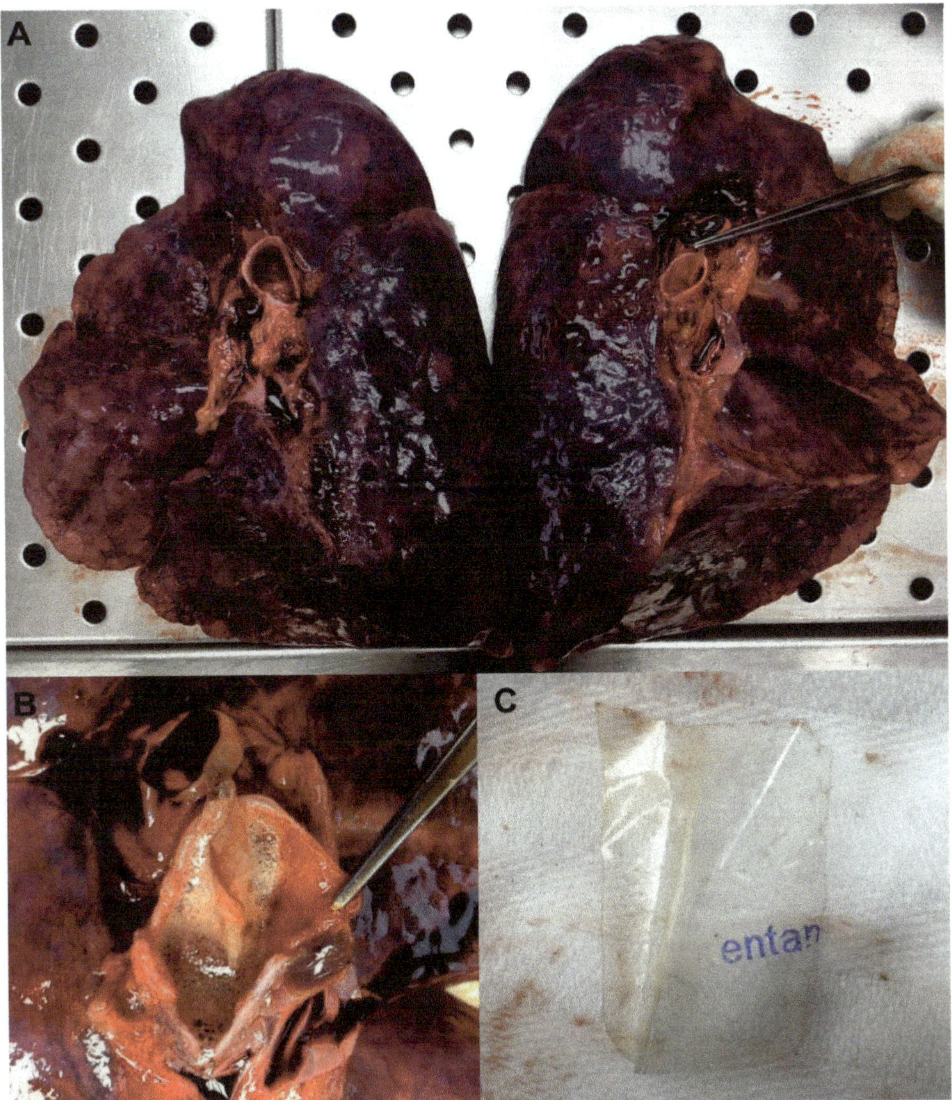

Figure 1. Autopsy Findings: (**A**) Macroscopic aspect of lungs. (**B**) Detail of left bronchus with fentanyl patch protective film. (**C**) Fentanyl patch protective film.

3. Materials and Methods

The toxicological investigations carried out concerned the search for the most common substances of forensic toxicological interest, and were conducted in accordance with the indications of the Group of Italian Forensic Toxicologists (GIFT) and the scientific evidence inferable from the international literature [13–21].

3.1. Chemicals and Reagents

Methanol solutions of fentanyl, methadone, EDDP, morphine, 6-monoacetylmorphine (6-MAM), cocaine, benzoilecgonine, and alprazolam and internal standard solutions of fentanyl-d5, methadone-d9, EDDP-d3, morphine-d3, 6-MAM-d3, cocaine-d3, benzoilecgonine-d3, and alprazolam-d4 (0.1 mg/mL), were purchased from Lipomed AG (Arlesheim, Switzerland). All solutions were stored in the refrigerator at +2–+4 °C when not in use. Mixed working standard solutions were prepared by combining the standards and aliquots of each primary solution and diluting them with methanol. Methanol, dichlormethane, isopropanol, ammonium hydroxide, and others were purchased from Carlo Erba Reagents (Val-de-Reuil, France). Extraction Columns Clean Screen XCEL I and Selectra-SIL BSTFA w/1%TMCS were purchased from UCT (Bristol, PA, USA).

3.2. *Calibration Curves*

All calibration curves were prepared by spiking blank blood with appropriate volumes of standard and internal standard solutions. The amount of internal standard used was the same for the calibration curve and the real samples. Calibration curves were prepared on 0.5 mL of matrix; appropriate dilutions were applied if needed for the analysis of real samples.

3.2.1. Blood Alcohol

Calibration curve points were 0.25, 0.5, 1, 2, 4 g/L.

3.2.2. Fentanyl

Calibration curve points were 2.5, 5, 10, 50, 100 ng/mL.

3.3. *Sample Pretreatment*

3.3.1. Fentanyl, Cocaine, Benzoylecgonine, Morphine, 6-Monoacetylmorphine

Samples were extracted using the extraction column Screen XCEL I (UCT). The extraction procedure was as follows: an appropriate volume of sample was diluted with phosphate buffer (pH 6) and added directly to the column without any preconditioning, allowed to flow by gravity, dried for 1 min, washed with 1 mL of 2% glacial acetic acid/98% methanol, dried for 5 min, and eluted with dichloromethane/isopropanol/ammonium hydroxide (78/20/2). The eluate was then evaporated to dryness under a gentle stream of N_2 gas at 40 °C, and the residue was derivatized with 50 µL of BSTFA 1% TMCS 70 °C per 20 min. Finally, 1 µL of the solution was injected into the GC-MS.

3.3.2. Alprazolam

Samples were extracted using the extraction column Screen XCEL I (UCT). The extraction procedure was as follows: an appropriate volume of sample was diluted with phosphate buffer (pH 6) and added directly to the column without any preconditioning, allowed to flow by gravity, dried for 1 min, washed with 1 mL of dichloromethane, dried for 5 min, and eluted with ethyl acetate:ammonia (98:2). The eluate was then evaporated to dryness under a gentle stream of N_2 gas at 40 °C, and the residue was derivatized with 50 µL of BSTFA 1% TMCS 70 °C per 20 min. Finally, 1 µL of the solution was injected into the GC-MS.

3.3.3. Methadone, EDDP

An appropriate volume of sample was diluted with 0.5 mL deionized water and combined with 50 µL of 10 M ammonium hydroxide aqueous solution and an appropriate amount of internal standard. After vortexing for 30 mins 3 mL of ethyl acetate was added as an extraction solvent. Liquid–liquid extraction (LLE) was carried out by stirring the sample for 15 min on an automatic vortex and then centrifuging it at 3000 RPM for 5 min. The organic phase was recovered, transferred into a disposable vial, and evaporated to dryness with a flow of N_2. The samples were reconstituted using 50 µL of ethyl acetate. Finally, 1 µL of the solution was injected into the GC-MS.

3.3.4. Blood Alcohol

First, 0.5 mL of sample was added to a glass vial for head space analysis and mixed with 0.5 mL of a 1 g/L solution of isopropylic alcohol as an internal standard. The sample was then closed with a tight stopper and mixed.

3.4. GC-MS Conditions

All analyses were performed with a GC system, the Agilent 7820 A, coupled with a single quadrupole mass spectrometer, MSD-5975. Chromatographic separation was conducted with an Agilent GC Column HP-5MS (0.25 μm, 0.2 mm i.d., 20 m) (Agilent Technologies, Santa Clara, CA, USA).

3.4.1. Fentanyl

The injection temperature was 280 °C and the injection volume was 1 μL. The injection mode was split 15:1. The oven was programmed from 160 °C for 1 min, ramped at 20 °C/min to 290 °C, and held for 10 min. Fentanyl retention time was 8.02; Select Ion Monitoring (SIM) values were m/z 189, 194, 146, 151 (qualifiers), and m/z 245 (quantifier); fentanyl-d5 SIM was m/z 250 (quantifier).

3.4.2. Cocaine, Benzoylecgonine, Morphine, 6-Monoacethylmorphine, Methadone, EDDP

The injection temperature was 280 °C and the injection volume was 1 μL. The injection mode was split 15:1. The oven was programmed from 140 °C for 1 min, ramped at 20 °C/min to 290 °C, and held for 6 min. EDDP retention time was 5.90 min; its SIM values were m/z 277, 262 (qualifiers), and m/z 276 (quantifier). Methadone retention time was 6.42 min; its SIM values were m/z 223, 294 (qualifiers), and m/z 72 (quantifier). Methadone-d9 SIM was m/z 78 (quantifier). Cocaine retention time was 6.70 min; its SIM values were m/z 272, 82 (qualifiers) and m/z 303 (quantifier). Cocaine-d3 SIM was m/z 306 (quantifier). Benzoylecgonine retention time was 7.00 min; its SIM values were m/z 240, 82 (qualifiers), and m/z 361 (quantifier). Bezoylecgonine-d3 SIM value was m/z 364 (quantifier). Morphine retention time was 7.99 min; its SIM values were m/z 236, 401 (qualifiers), and m/z 429 (quantifier); morphine-d3 was m/z 433 (quantifier). 6-Monoacetylmorphine retention time was 8.25 min; its SIM values were m/z 340, 287 (qualifiers), and m/z 399 (quantifier); morphine-d3 was m/z 402 (quantifier).

3.4.3. Alprazolam

The injection temperature was 260 °C and the injection volume was 1 μL. The injection mode was split 15:1. The oven was programmed from 120 °C for 1 min, ramped at 15 °C/min to 290 °C, and held for 5 min. Alprazolam retention time was 13.41 min; its SIM values were m/z 279, 204 (qualifiers), and m/z 308 (quantifier). Alprazolam-d5 SIM was m/z 313 (quantifier).

3.5. HS-GC-FID Conditions

Analyses were performed with a GC system, the Agilent 7820A, coupled with a HS Agilent 7694. Chromatographic separation was performed with an Agilent GC Column HP-B ALC (0.32 μm, 0.2 mm i.d., 7.5 mt) (Agilent Technologies, Santa Clara, CA, USA). The manifold temperature was 75 °C, the head-space (HS) temperature was 70 °C, and the oven was programmed at 85 °C and held for 5 min, which was also the total duration of analysis. Ethanol retention time was 0.76 min; IS retention time was 1.26 min.

3.6. Method Validation

The method for fentanyl analysis was validated for this study according to the guidelines of the Group of Italian Forensic Toxicologists (GIFT) [22]. Calibration curves revealed good linearity ($R^2 > 0.997$). The recovery ranged from 80 to 89%. Fentanyl's lower limit of quantification (LLOQ) was 2.5 ng/mL, while the limit of detection (LOD) was 1.5 ng/mL. The LOD was defined as the lowest concentration giving a response at least three times higher than the average of the baseline noise, while the LLOQ was defined as the lowest concentration that could be measured with an intra-assay precision CV% and relative bias less than 20%. The LLOQ also matches the last level of the calibration curve. The results obtained with this method using whole blood were linear and sensitive; the accuracy and precision of validation data were within +/− 15%.

All other methods were already in use in the laboratory of this group prior to this study. All LODs and LOQs can be found in Table 1.

Table 1. LODs and LOQs for all substances analyzed in the study.

Compound	LOD	LOQ
Methadone	5 ng/mL	15 ng/mL
EDDP	5 ng/mL	15 ng/mL
Morphine	5 ng/mL	15 ng/mL
6-MAM	5 ng/mL	15 ng/mL
Fentanyl	1.5 ng/mL	2.5 ng/mL
Alprazolam	3 ng/mL	10 ng/mL
Cocaine	5 ng/mL	15 ng/mL
BEG	10 ng/mL	30 ng/mL
Ethyl alcohol	0.05 g/L	0.1 g/L

4. Results

The results revealed the presence of ethyl alcohol, methadone, 2-ethylidine-1,5-dimethyl-3,3-diphenylpyrrolidine (EDDP), morphine, 6-monoacetylmorphine (6-MAM), cocaine, benzoylecgonine (BEG), fentanyl, and alprazolam, as reported in Table 2.

Table 2. Results of toxicological analysis.

Compound	Femoral Blood	Urine
Methadone	<LOD	195 ng/mL
EDDP	<LOD	285 ng/mL
Total morphine	133 ng/mL	5553 ng/mL
Free morphine	<LOD	995 ng/mL
6-MAM	<LOD	182 ng/mL
Fentanyl	50 ng/mL	73 ng/mL
Alprazolam	<LOD	96 ng/mL
Cocaine	<LOD	994 ng/mL
BEG	91 ng/mL	4967 ng/mL
Ethyl alcohol	0.22 g/l	-

5. Discussion

Fentanyl patches are available in different dosages and formulations. "Membrane-controlled" patches consist of a reservoir (hence the name of "reservoir design") containing the active ingredient in gel form in a formulation containing ethanol USP and hydroxycellulose, with a rate-limiting membrane and an adhesive layer on the skin side. The "matrix design" (or "drug-in-adhesive") formulation, on the other hand, consists of an adhesive layer of solid silicone in which the substance is suspended [23]. The two formulations have a similar substance release pattern and are both widely used for the management of chronic pain in out-of-hospital settings.

These devices are certainly suitable for abusive consumption, which can occur either by transdermal absorption or through other atypical and sometimes notably inventive routes of administration [24,25]. Atypical methods of consumption described in the literature involve the application of the patch on the buccal mucosa, ingestion, or chewing it, combining mechanical and thermal effects in increasing the release of the substance with a notably higher rate of absorption [26–30]. Following the massive release of the substance from the patch, in fact, this is rapidly absorbed through biological barriers constituted by the digestive tract mucosa, which is intrinsically much more permeable and vascularized than the superficial layers of the skin. Moreover, a portion of the substance is absorbed through the oral mucosa and is not affected by the first pass effect through the portal circulation, typical in the case of gastrointestinal absorption, resulting in even higher bioavailability.

Similar mechanisms intervene in the case of transrectal absorption, also described in the case of death from a fentanyl overdose [31]. Another group of atypical routes of administration, on the other hand, is characterized by the extraction of the substance from the patch and its subsequent consumption. In the case of a "reservoir design" patch, it is easily accessible and extractable using a needle [32]. In the case of a "matrix design" patch, as it is not possible to directly aspirate the compound, its extraction is carried out with other methods, such as simmering in hot water [33]; other substances (such as citric acid added to sterile water, methanol, ethanol, dichloromethane, and hot acetone) are also reported to be used as solvents [34]. The substance thus obtained is commonly directly injected intravenously, drunk, or inhaled by volatilization [35–38]. Finally, some cases of "vaporization", performed by cutting a frozen patch into pieces, placing it in an aluminum foil, and heating it, are reported in the scientific literature [34,35] (Table 3).

In all the listed cases, however, the intake of large quantities of fentanyl (between 2.5 and 10 mg per dose), capable of guaranteeing therapeutic dosages for around 72 h with the proper administration route, occurs in a rapid and uncontrolled manner. In particular, the application of fentanyl patches on broken skin is able to provide 5-fold faster absorption, increased to approximately 30-fold through tissues without a stratum corneum (such as oral or respiratory mucosa) [39–41]. These absorption pathways guarantee the achievement of high blood concentrations in short time intervals and allow the achievement of the psychotropic and/or analgesic effects sought by consumers/abusers; on the other hand, associated with the drug's narrow therapeutic window, it exposes them to a high risk of acute toxicity and death from overdose [42,43].

Regarding the post-mortem blood concentration, a retrospective study conducted on fentanyl-related deaths in the province of Ontario showed that, in cases in which fentanyl was recognized as the sole cause of death ($n = 54$), the blood concentration of this substance showed considerable variability, ranging from 3 to 383 ng/mL, with an average value of 25 ng/mL. Furthermore, a partial overlap was found with the blood values relating to cases of death due to natural causes, in which the finding of fentanyl was considered accidental ($n = 12$, range: 2.7–33 ng/mL, mean 12 ng/mL) [44].

Thompson et al. analyzed a 23-case series, divided into three groups based on the role of fentanyl in the determination of death [45]. In the group of fentanyl-only overdose and mixed-drug overdose, the blood concentration of fentanyl ranged from 5 to 120 ng/mL ($n = 8$, mean 36 ng/mL) and from 5 to 152 ng/mL ($n = 11$, mean 31 ng/mL), respectively. Values from the group with the incidental finding of fentanyl (in which death occurred due to natural causes and fentanyl was mainly administered for chronic pain therapy) showed some overlap in concentrations with the other two groups ($n = 4$, range 2–15 ng/mL, mean 5 ng/mL). In this regard, evidence from clinical practice suggests that effective postoperative analgesia is guaranteed for lower serum concentrations in opioid-naive subjects (0.63–1.5 ng/mL); suppressive effects on respiratory function, in the same category, are already observable from concentrations higher than 1.5 ng/mL, while deeper sedation, apnea, and loss of protective airway reflexes occur at concentrations higher than 3 ng/mL [41].

Table 3. Different methods of extraction/consumption of fentanyl contained in an adhesive patch.

Extraction/Consumption Method	Characteristics
Application of a patch on cutaneous surface	- Release of the substance occurs in a controlled manner, guaranteeing approximately constant absorption for a few days; - Heating or applying a patch on broken skin slightly increases the absorption rate.
Chewing or ingestion of a patch—Application of a patch to buccal or rectal mucosa	- Release of the substance from the patch is slightly increased due to the combination of mechanical and thermal effects; - Substance is rapidly absorbed through digestive tract mucosa, which is intrinsically much more permeable and vascularized than the skin; - A variable portion of substance is absorbed through oral or rectal mucosa and is not affected by first pass effect.
Needle extraction of fentanyl from a patch	- Only viable for "reservoir design" patches; - Pharmacokinetics strictly depends on the following consumption method.
Extraction by simmering in hot water	- Also viable for "matrix design" patches; - Release of substance from the patch is mainly determined by thermal effect; - Pharmacokinetics strictly depends on the following consumption method.
Extraction using other solvents	- Also viable for "matrix design" patches; - Citric acid added to sterile water, methanol, ethanol, dichloromethane, and hot acetone are frequently used; - Pharmacokinetics strictly depends on the following consumption method.
Patch smoking or "vaporization"	- Performed by cutting a frozen patch into pieces, heating it, and inhaling the vapors; - Effects of inhaled vapors appear rapidly; on the other hand, only a portion of the substance is absorbed.

The presence of such considerable variability in concentration, as well as the finding of high values of blood fentanyl even in subjects consuming fentanyl who die from other causes, constitute two major issues in the interpretation of fentanyl-related deaths, resulting in the difficulty of identifying a quantitative cut-off above which fentanyl's contribution in the determination of death can be considered relevant.

This aspect can be justified by the presence of tolerance phenomena in habitual consumers, but also by the presence of demonstrated post-mortem redistribution phenomena already consistent in the first few hours following death, difficult to predict and quantify [46,47].

For this reason, in order to confirm the effective role of exogenous intoxication in the determination of death and exclude the existence of further competing elements, the finding of a high concentration of blood fentanyl should not be considered alone, but must necessarily be contextualized with the circumstantial, pharmacological, toxicological, and forensic pathological elements available [46].

The high mortality rate among abusive users, on the other hand, cannot be justified solely by the high dosage used and has led to the deepening of the most intimate pharmacokinetic and pharmacodynamic mechanisms [48]. First of all, it was noticed that respiratory depression induced by fentanyl not only affects the respiratory rate, but also the tidal volume [48]. This effect is thought to be a consequence of an increase in thoracic muscular stiffness, resulting in an important obstacle to the physiological respiratory mechanics [49–51]. Fentanyl-induced lethal respiratory failure generally occurs significantly faster than with classic opioids for abuse, appearing in approximately two minutes after intravenous injection [52]. Moreover, the effects of fentanyl are less easily antagonized by the administration of naloxone [53,54], while maintaining good sensitivity to the effects of diprenorphine. These last two elements clearly pose objective difficulties in rescuing overdosed subjects, as the intervention of health professionals must be very timely and requires rapid recognition of the consumed substances. In view of its highly intrinsic effect, fentanyl also appears to be able to partially bypass the tolerance mechanisms induced by abused opioids [48,55], easily causing respiratory failure even in regular users. Finally, it should be remembered that the consumption of fentanyl is generally associated with the intake of other psychotropic substances, which can enhance or play a synergistic role in its deleterious effects.

According to a recent systematic review conducted on fentanyl-related deaths, in fact, simultaneous drug use was commonly reported; in detail, other opiates (37% of the total deaths), antidepressant/antipsychotic drugs (17%), cocaine (15%), and benzodiazepines (14%) were the most frequently associated substances in the case of fatality [56].

In the present case, findings collected during post-mortem investigations allowed us to identify a decisive role of fentanyl consumption in the cause of death. In fact, the blood concentration of fentanyl was, consistently with the scientific literature, adequate to trigger lethal respiratory suppression. This finding is, moreover, consistent with the set of toxicological and circumstantial data, and with the evidence of forensic pathological nature, which reflects the more classic alterations related to cases of intoxication by opioids or opioid receptor agonists.

In contrast, the concentration of ethyl alcohol was low and not associated with death; at the same time, the positivity for BEG in blood and urine, and cocaine in urine, was suggestive of previous cocaine consumption without any toxicological effects involved in the cause of death. The same can be said about morphine and 6-monoacethylmorphine: the presence of free morphine and 6-monoacethylmorphine only in urine can be attributed to the previous consumption of heroin, while the presence of conjugated morphine (positive total morphine) in the blood may be due to post-mortem redistribution from enterohepatic circulation. The intake of fentanyl presumably took place via the chewing of a transdermal patch with the protective film still attached; following the aspiration of the protective film in the left main bronchus, the transdermal patch was probably eliminated by vomiting. The pathophysiology of death can be identified as combined respiratory failure, in which both central suppression and a fentanyl-induced increase in muscular stiffness played a substantial role; a further contribution, albeit minor, in determining a mechanical obstruction to the flow of air in the airways could have been caused by the presence of the protective film at the bronchial level.

6. Conclusions

According to a comprehensive diagnosis based on the autopsy findings and toxicological analyses, the cause of death has been identified as fentanyl intoxication. This is an unusual autopsy case of intoxication capable of shedding light on some worrying aspects of drug abuse in the present era. In fact, the abusive use of fentanyl is a considerably important issue, burdened by a high rate of complications and lethality for the aforementioned pharmacological reasons [4]; the assumption of this substance through an atypical route of consumption is, on the other hand, a rare but increasing occurrence, which can remain unrecognized in the course of clinical evaluation or post-mortem investigation.

From this point of view, in fact, the role of pathology and forensic toxicology must not end at the collection and documentation of scientific evidence for justice purposes, but should also guarantee the provision of a window on some underestimated social and health problems in order to address the necessary social and health policies [57–65].

Author Contributions: Conceptualization, A.S. and A.G.; methodology, A.G. and M.C.D.; investigation, F.M., M.C.D., S.G., F.C., M.P., M.S., A.G. and A.S.; data curation, F.M., F.C., and M.P.; writing—original draft preparation, F.M. and S.G.; supervision, M.S., A.G. and A.S. All authors have read and agreed to the published version of the manuscript.

Funding: This research received no external funding.

Institutional Review Board Statement: The study was conducted in accordance with the Declaration of Helsinki. Approval from the local institutional review board was not necessary, since all analyses were performed in accordance with Prosecutor Office requests.

Informed Consent Statement: Not applicable.

Data Availability Statement: The data used to support the findings of this study are available from the corresponding author upon request.

Conflicts of Interest: The authors declare no conflict of interest.

References

1. Schug, S.A.; Ting, S. Fentanyl Formulations in the Management of Pain: An Update. *Drugs* **2017**, *77*, 747–763. [CrossRef]
2. Peng, P.W.; Sandler, A.N. A review of the use of fentanyl analgesia in the management of acute pain in adults. *Anesthesiology* **1999**, *90*, 576–599. [CrossRef]
3. Kuczyńska, K.; Grzonkowski, P.; Kacprzak, Ł.; Zawilska, J.B. Abuse of fentanyl: An emerging problem to face. *Forensic Sci. Int.* **2018**, *289*, 207–214. [CrossRef] [PubMed]
4. D'Errico, S. Commentary. Fentanyl-related death and the underreporting risk. *J. Forensic Leg. Med.* **2018**, *60*, 35–37. [CrossRef] [PubMed]
5. Phalen, P.; Ray, B.; Watson, D.P.; Huynh, P.; Greene, M.S. Fentanyl related overdose in Indianapolis: Estimating trends using multilevel Bayesian models. *Addict. Behav.* **2018**, *86*, 4–10. [CrossRef]
6. Lavonas, E.J.; Dezfulian, C. Impact of the Opioid Epidemic. *Crit. Care Clin.* **2020**, *36*, 753–769. [CrossRef] [PubMed]
7. Upp, L.A.; Waljee, J.F. The Opioid Epidemic. *Clin. Plast. Surg.* **2020**, *47*, 181–190. [CrossRef]
8. Sinicina, I.; Sachs, H.; Keil, W. Post-mortem review of fentanyl-related overdose deaths among identified drug users in Southern Bavaria, Germany, 2005–2014. *Drug Alcohol Depend.* **2017**, *180*, 286–291. [CrossRef]
9. Spencer, M.R.; Warner, M.; Bastian, B.A.; Trinidad, J.P.; Hedegaard, H. Drug Overdose Deaths Involving Fentanyl, 2011–2016. *Natl. Vital Stat. Rep.* **2019**, *68*, 1–19.
10. Bardwell, G.; Wood, E.; Brar, R. Fentanyl assisted treatment: A possible role in the opioid overdose epidemic? *Subst. Abuse Treat. Prev. Policy* **2019**, *14*, 50. [CrossRef]
11. Han, Y.; Yan, W.; Zheng, Y.; Khan, M.Z.; Yuan, K.; Lu, L. The rising crisis of illicit fentanyl use, overdose, and potential therapeutic strategies. *Transl. Psychiatry* **2019**, *9*, 282. [CrossRef] [PubMed]
12. Manetti, F.; Scopetti, M.; Santurro, A.; Consoloni, L.; D'Errico, S. Widespread septic embolization in injection drug use mitro-aortic infective endocarditis as a remote cause of death. *Int. J. Legal Med.* **2020**, *134*, 1345–1351. [CrossRef] [PubMed]
13. Juhascik, M.P.; Jenkins, A.J. Comparison of liquid/liquid and solid-phase extraction for alkaline drugs. *J. Chromatogr. Sci.* **2009**, *47*, 553–557. [CrossRef] [PubMed]
14. Black, D.A.; Clark, G.D.; Haver, V.M.; Garbin, J.A.; Saxon, A.J. Analysis of urinary benzodiazepines using solid-phase extraction and gas chromatography-mass spectrometry. *J. Anal. Toxicol.* **1994**, *18*, 185–188. [CrossRef] [PubMed]
15. Stout, P.R.; Horn, C.K.; Klette, K.L. Solid-phase extraction and GC-MS analysis of THC-COOH method optimized for a high-throughput forensic drug-testing laboratory. *J. Anal. Toxicol.* **2001**, *25*, 550–554. [CrossRef] [PubMed]
16. Polettini, A.; Groppi, A.; Vignali, C.; Montagna, M. Fully-automated systematic toxicological analysis of drugs, poisons, and metabolites in whole blood, urine, and plasma by gas chromatography-full scan mass spectrometry. *J. Chromatogr. B Biomed. Sci. Appl.* **1998**, *713*, 265–279. [CrossRef] [PubMed]
17. Alexandridou, A.; Mouskeftara, T.; Raikos, N.; Gika, H.G. GC-MS analysis of underivatised new psychoactive substances in whole blood and urine. *J. Chromatogr. B Analyt. Technol. Biomed. Life Sci.* **2020**, *1156*, 122308. [CrossRef]
18. Abusada, G.M.; Abukhalaf, I.K.; Alford, D.D.; Vinzon-Bautista, I.; Pramanik, A.K.; Ansari, N.A.; Manno, J.E.; Manno, B.R. Solid-phase extraction and GC/MS quantitation of cocaine, ecgonine methyl ester, benzoylecgonine, and cocaethylene from meconium, whole blood, and plasma. *J. Anal. Toxicol.* **1993**, *17*, 353–358. [CrossRef]
19. Weinmann, W.; Renz, M.; Vogt, S.; Pollak, S. Automated solid-phase extraction and two-step derivatisation for simultaneous analysis of basic illicit drugs in serum by GC/MS. *Int. J. Legal Med.* **2000**, *113*, 229–235. [CrossRef]
20. Meatherall, R. GC-MS quantitation of codeine, morphine, 6-acetylmorphine, hydrocodone, hydromorphone, oxycodone, and oxymorphone in blood. *J. Anal. Toxicol.* **2005**, *29*, 301–308. [CrossRef]
21. Armbruster, D.A.; Tillman, M.D.; Hubbs, L.M. Limit of detection (LQD)/limit of quantitation (LOQ): Comparison of the empirical and the statistical methods exemplified with GC-MS assays of abused drugs. *Clin. Chem.* **1994**, *40*, 1233–1238. [CrossRef] [PubMed]
22. GIFT—Group of Italian Forensic Toxicologists. Linee Guida per i Laboratori Di Analisi Di Sostanze D'abuso Con Finalità Tossicologico-Forensi e Medico-Legali—2010. Available online: https://www.gtfi.it/wp-content/uploads/2015/07/LG2010.pdf (accessed on 7 March 2022).
23. Palmer, R.B. Fentanyl in postmortem forensic toxicology. *Clin. Toxicol.* **2010**, *48*, 771–784. [CrossRef] [PubMed]
24. Geile, J.; Maas, A.; Kraemer, M.; Doberentz, E.; Madea, B. Fatal misuse of transdermal fentanyl patches. *Forensic Sci. Int.* **2019**, *302*, 109858. [CrossRef] [PubMed]

25. Kuhlman, J.J., Jr.; McCaulley, R.; Valouch, T.J.; Behonick, G.S. Fentanyl use, misuse, and abuse: A summary of 23 postmortem cases. *J. Anal. Toxicol.* **2003**, *27*, 499–504. [CrossRef] [PubMed]
26. Liappas, I.A.; Dimopoulos, N.P.; Mellos, E.; Gitsa, O.E.; Liappas, A.I.; Rabavilas, A.D. Oral transmucosal abuse of transdermal fentanyl. *J. Psychopharmacol.* **2004**, *18*, 277–280. [CrossRef]
27. Thomas, S.; Winecker, R.; Pestaner, J.P. Unusual fentanyl patch administration. *Am. J. Forensic Med. Pathol.* **2008**, *29*, 162–163. [CrossRef]
28. Woodall, K.L.; Martin, T.L.; McLellan, B.A. Oral abuse of fentanyl patches (Duragesic): Seven case reports. *J. Forensic Sci.* **2008**, *53*, 222–225. [CrossRef]
29. Zhang, Q.; Murawsky, M.; LaCount, T.D.; Hao, J.; Ghosh, P.; Raney, S.G.; Kasting, G.B.; Li, S.K. Evaluation of Heat Effects on Fentanyl Transdermal Delivery Systems Using In Vitro Permeation and In Vitro Release Methods. *J. Pharm. Sci.* **2020**, *109*, 3095–3104. [CrossRef]
30. Prodduturi, S.; Sadrieh, N.; Wokovich, A.M.; Doub, W.H.; Westenberger, B.J.; Buhse, L. Transdermal delivery of fentanyl from matrix and reservoir systems: Effect of heat and compromised skin. *J. Pharm. Sci.* **2010**, *99*, 2357–2366. [CrossRef]
31. Coon, T.P.; Miller, M.; Kaylor, D.; Jones-Spangle, K. Rectal insertion of fentanyl patches: A new route of toxicity. *Ann. Emerg. Med.* **2005**, *46*, 473. [CrossRef]
32. Krinsky, C.S.; Lathrop, S.L.; Crossey, M.; Baker, G.; Zumwalt, R. A toxicology-based review of fentanyl-related deaths in New Mexico (1986-2007). *Am. J. Forensic Med. Pathol.* **2011**, *32*(4), 347–351. [CrossRef] [PubMed]
33. Schauer, C.K.; Shand, J.A.; Reynolds, T.M. The Fentanyl Patch Boil-Up—A Novel Method of Opioid Abuse. *Basic Clin. Pharmacol. Toxicol.* **2015**, *117*, 358–359. [CrossRef] [PubMed]
34. Kacela, M.; Wojcieszak, J.; Zawilska, J.B. Use of fentanyl, butyrfentanyl and furanylfentanyl as discussed on Polish online forums devoted to 'designer drugs'. Używanie fentanylu, butyrylofentanylu i furanylofentanylu w opinii użytkowników polskich forów internetowych poświęconych „dopalaczom". *Psychiatr. Pol.* **2022**, *56*, 355–372. [CrossRef] [PubMed]
35. Marquardt, K.A.; Tharratt, R.S. Inhalation abuse of fentanyl patch. *J. Toxicol. Clin. Toxicol.* **1994**, *32*, 75–78. [CrossRef]
36. Barrueto, F., Jr.; Howland, M.A.; Hoffman, R.S.; Nelson, L.S. The fentanyl tea bag. *Vet. Hum. Toxicol.* **2004**, *46*, 30–31.
37. Carson, H.J.; Knight, L.D.; Dudley, M.H.; Garg, U. A fatality involving an unusual route of fentanyl delivery: Chewing and aspirating the transdermal patch. *Leg. Med.* **2010**, *12*, 157–159. [CrossRef]
38. Rahman, S.; Trussell, A.; Pearson, S.A.; Buckley, N.A.; Karanges, E.A.; Cairns, R.; Litchfield, M.; Todd, A.; Gisev, N. Trends in transdermal fentanyl utilisation and fatal fentanyl overdose across Australia (2003–2015). *Drug Alcohol Rev.* **2022**, *41*, 435–443. [CrossRef]
39. Björkman, S.; Stanski, D.R.; Verotta, D.; Harashima, H. Comparative tissue concentration profiles of fentanyl and alfentanil in humans predicted from tissue/blood partition data obtained in rats. *Anesthesiology* **1990**, *72*, 865–873. [CrossRef]
40. Guitton, J.; Buronfosse, T.; Désage, M.; Lepape, A.; Brazier, J.L.; Beaune, P. Possible involvement of multiple cytochrome P450S in fentanyl and sufentanil metabolism as opposed to alfentanil. *Biochem. Pharmacol.* **1997**, *53*, 1613–1619. [CrossRef]
41. Nelson, L.; Schwaner, R. Transdermal fentanyl: Pharmacology and toxicology. *J. Med. Toxicol.* **2009**, *5*, 230–241. [CrossRef]
42. Tharp, A.M.; Winecker, R.E.; Winston, D.C. Fatal intravenous fentanyl abuse: Four cases involving extraction of fentanyl from transdermal patches. *Am. J. Forensic Med. Pathol.* **2004**, *25*, 178–181. [CrossRef] [PubMed]
43. Jumbelic, M.I. Deaths with transdermal fentanyl patches. *Am. J. Forensic Med. Pathol.* **2010**, *31*, 18–21. [CrossRef] [PubMed]
44. Martin, T.L.; Woodall, K.L.; McLellan, B.A. Fentanyl-related deaths in Ontario, Canada: Toxicological findings and circumstances of death in 112 cases (2002–2004). *J. Anal. Toxicol.* **2006**, *30*, 603–610. [CrossRef] [PubMed]
45. Thompson, J.G.; Baker, A.M.; Bracey, A.H.; Seningen, J.; Kloss, J.S.; Strobl, A.Q.; Apple, F.S. Fentanyl concentrations in 23 postmortem cases from the hennepin county medical examiner's office. *J. Forensic Sci.* **2007**, *52*, 978–981. [CrossRef]
46. Andresen, H.; Gullans, A.; Veselinovic, M.; Anders, S.; Schmoldt, A.; Iwersen-Bergmann, S.; Mueller, A. Fentanyl: Toxic or therapeutic? Postmortem and antemortem blood concentrations after transdermal fentanyl application. *J. Anal. Toxicol.* **2012**, *36*, 182–194. [CrossRef]
47. Moore, P.W.; Palmer, R.B.; Donovan, J.W. Fatal fentanyl patch misuse in a hospitalized patient with a postmortem increase in fentanyl blood concentration. *J. Forensic Sci.* **2015**, *60*, 243–246. [CrossRef]
48. Hill, R.; Santhakumar, R.; Dewey, W.; Kelly, E.; Henderson, G. Fentanyl depression of respiration: Comparison with heroin and morphine. *Br. J. Pharmacol.* **2020**, *177*, 254–266. [CrossRef]
49. Kinshella, M.W.; Gauthier, T.; Lysyshyn, M. Rigidity, dyskinesia and other atypical overdose presentations observed at a supervised injection site, Vancouver, Canada. *Harm Reduct. J.* **2018**, *15*, 64. [CrossRef]
50. Burns, G.; DeRienz, R.T.; Baker, D.D.; Casavant, M.; Spiller, H.A. Could chest wall rigidity be a factor in rapid death from illicit fentanyl abuse? *Clin. Toxicol.* **2016**, *54*, 420–423. [CrossRef]
51. Pergolizzi, J.V., Jr.; Webster, L.R.; Vortsman, E.; Ann LeQuang, J.; Raffa, R.B. Wooden Chest syndrome: The atypical pharmacology of fentanyl overdose. *J. Clin. Pharm. Ther.* **2021**, *46*, 1505–1508. [CrossRef] [PubMed]
52. Green, T.C.; Gilbert, M. Counterfeit Medications and Fentanyl. *JAMA Intern. Med.* **2016**, *176*, 1555–1557. [CrossRef] [PubMed]
53. Fairbairn, N.; Coffin, P.O.; Walley, A.Y. Naloxone for heroin, prescription opioid, and illicitly made fentanyl overdoses: Challenges and innovations responding to a dynamic epidemic. *Int. J. Drug Policy* **2017**, *46*, 172–179. [CrossRef] [PubMed]

54. Peterson, A.B.; Gladden, R.M.; Delcher, C.; Spies, E.; Garcia-Williams, A.; Wang, Y.; Halpin, J.; Zibbell, J.; McCarty, C.L.; DeFiore-Hyrmer, J.; et al. Increases in Fentanyl-Related Overdose Deaths—Florida and Ohio, 2013–2015. *MMWR Morb. Mortal. Wkly Rep.* **2016**, *65*, 844–849. [CrossRef] [PubMed]
55. Bobeck, E.N.; Schoo, S.M.; Ingram, S.L.; Morgan, M.M. Lack of Antinociceptive Cross-Tolerance with Co-Administration of Morphine and Fentanyl into the Periaqueductal Gray of Male Sprague-Dawley Rats. *J. Pain* **2019**, *20*, 1040–1047. [CrossRef]
56. Cheema, E.; McGuinness, K.; Hadi, M.A.; Paudyal, V.; Elnaem, M.H.; Alhifany, A.A.; Elrggal, M.W.; Al Hamid, A. Causes, Nature and Toxicology of Fentanyl-Associated Deaths: A Systematic Review of Deaths Reported in Peer-Reviewed Literature. *J. Pain Res.* **2020**, *13*, 3281–3294. [CrossRef]
57. Manetti, F.; Chericoni, S.; Marrocco, A.; Scopetti, M.; Padovano, M.; Santurro, A.; Frati, P.; Gabbrielli, M.; Fineschi, V. Cannabis and Driving: Developing Guidelines for Safety Policies. *Curr. Pharm. Biotechnol.* **2022**. *ahead of print*. [CrossRef]
58. Scopetti, M.; Morena, D.; Manetti, F.; Santurro, A.; Fazio, N.D.; D'Errico, S.; Padovano, M.; Frati, P.; Fineschi, V. Cannabinoids and brain damage: A systematic review on a frequently overlooked issue. *Curr. Pharm. Biotechnol.* **2022**. *ahead of print*. [CrossRef]
59. Padovano, M.; Aromatario, M.; D'Errico, S.; Concato, M.; Manetti, F.; David, M.C.; Scopetti, M.; Frati, P.; Fineschi, V. Sodium Nitrite Intoxication and Death: Summarizing Evidence to Facilitate Diagnosis. *Int. J. Environ. Res. Public Health* **2022**, *19*, 13996. [CrossRef]
60. Tadrous, M.; Greaves, S.; Martins, D.; Nadeem, K.; Singh, S.; Mamdani, M.M.; Juurlink, D.N.; Gomes, T. Evaluation of the fentanyl patch-for-patch program in Ontario, Canada. *Int. J. Drug Policy* **2019**, *66*, 82–86. [CrossRef]
61. Guliyev, C.; Tuna, Z.O.; Ögel, K. Fentanyl use disorder characterized by unprescribed use of transdermal patches: A case report. *J. Addict. Dis.* **2002**, *40*, 285–290. [CrossRef]
62. La Russa, R.; Catalano, C.; Di Sanzo, M.; Scopetti, M.; Gatto, V.; Santurro, A.; Viola, R.V.; Panebianco, V.; Frati, P.; Fineschi, V. Postmortem computed tomography angiography (PMCTA) and traditional autopsy in cases of sudden cardiac death due to coronary artery disease: A systematic review and meta-analysis. *Radiol. Med.* **2019**, *124*, 109–117. [CrossRef]
63. Gatto, V.; Scopetti, M.; La Russa, R.; Santurro, A.; Cipolloni, L.; Viola, R.V.; Di Sanzo, M.; Frati, P.; Fineschi, V. Advanced Loss Eventuality Assessment and Technical Estimates: An Integrated Approach for Management of Healthcare-Associated Infections. *Curr. Pharm. Biotechnol.* **2019**, *20*, 625–634. [CrossRef] [PubMed]
64. Busardò, F.P.; Frati, P.; Santurro, A.; Zaami, S.; Fineschi, V. Errors and malpractice lawsuits in radiology: What the radiologist needs to know. *Radiol. Med.* **2015**, *120*, 779–784. [CrossRef] [PubMed]
65. Santurro, A.; Vullo, A.M.; Borro, M.; Gentile, G.; La Russa, R.; Simmaco, M.; Frati, P.; Fineschi, V. Personalized Medicine Applied to Forensic Sciences: New Advances and Perspectives for a Tailored Forensic Approach. *Curr. Pharm. Biotechnol.* **2017**, *18*, 263–273. [CrossRef] [PubMed]

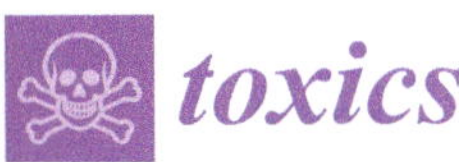

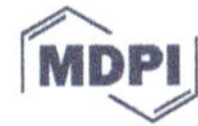

Article

UPLC-MS/MS Based Identification and Quantification of a Novel Dual Orexin Receptor Antagonist in Plasma Samples by Validated SWGTOX Guidelines

Muzaffar Iqbal [1,*], Abdullah Alshememry [2], Faisal Imam [3], Mohd Abul Kalam [2], Ali Akhtar [4] and Essam A. Ali [1]

1 Department of Pharmaceutical Chemistry, College of Pharmacy, King Saud University, Riyadh 11451, Saudi Arabia
2 Department of Pharmaceutics, College of Pharmacy, King Saud University, Riyadh 11451, Saudi Arabia
3 Department of Pharmacology and Toxicology, College of Pharmacy, King Saud University, Riyadh 11451, Saudi Arabia
4 College of Pharmacy, King Saud University, Riyadh 11451, Saudi Arabia
* Correspondence: muziqbal@ksu.edu.sa

Abstract: Lemborexant (LEM) is a novel dual orexin receptor antagonist (DORA), recently approved for the treatment of insomnia. As with other DORAs, LEM has potential of abuse and therefore placed in Schedule IV class by the United States Drug Enforcement Administration (USDEA). In this study, a sensitive and accurate UPLC-MS/MS assay was developed for the quantification of LEM in human plasma sample using losartan as an internal standard (IS). The chromatographic separation was performed by using gradient elution of mobile phase, comprising of 10 mM ammonium acetate and acetonitrile with a flow rate of 0.3 mL/min. An Acquity UPLC BEH C_{18} (1.7 µm, 2.1 × 50 mm) column was used for separation of LEM and IS by maintaining the oven temperature of 40 °C. The electrospray ionization in positive mode was used for sample ionization. The precursor to product ion transition of 411.12 > 175.09 (qualifier) and 411.1 > 287.14 (quantifier) was used for detection and quantification of LEM, respectively, in multiple reaction monitoring mode. Being a drug of abuse, the assay was validated according to "Scientific Working Group for Toxicology" (SWGTOX) guidelines, including limit of detection (LOD), limit of quantification (LOQ), precision and bias, calibration model, interferences, carry-over effects, matrix effects, and stability parameters. The LOD and LOQ of the assay were 0.35 and 1.0 ng/mL, respectively. The linear range was between 1–300 ng/mL with correlation coefficient of ≥0.995. The method was also cross validated in rat plasma samples with acceptable ranges of precision and accuracy before its application for pharmacokinetic study in rats.

Keywords: Lemborexant; insomnia; abuse; UPLC-MS/MS; SWGTOX; DORA

Citation: Iqbal, M.; Alshememry, A.; Imam, F.; Kalam, M.A.; Akhtar, A.; Ali, E.A. UPLC-MS/MS Based Identification and Quantification of a Novel Dual Orexin Receptor Antagonist in Plasma Samples by Validated SWGTOX Guidelines. *Toxics* **2023**, *11*, 109. https://doi.org/10.3390/toxics11020109

Academic Editors: Andrey Toropov and Maria Pieri

Received: 17 November 2022
Revised: 11 January 2023
Accepted: 19 January 2023
Published: 23 January 2023

1. Introduction

Insomnia is a most common sleep–wake disorder, affecting 30–50% of the adult population across the globe [1]. Benzodiazepines and sedative/hypnotics are the most commonly used pharmacological intervention for the management of insomnia. However, their use has been now restricted due to their adverse sleep related behaviors and cognitive/psychomotor impairment [2,3]. Orexin-1 and orexin-2 receptors (OX1R and OX2R), which are apparently expressed in various regions of brain, are recently considered as novel target for the treatment of insomnia [4]. Lemborexant (LEM) is the second approved dual orexin receptor antagonist (DORA) for the treatment of adult patients with insomnia as per the United States Prescribing Information (USPI) [5,6]. It has fast association and dissociation from the OX1R and OX2R in compared to other DORA, and therefore sleep can be achieved quickly and maintained throughout the night while avoiding next morning sleepiness or residual effects [7]. Moreover, it has been reported that LEM has a low propensity to impair next-day functioning among healthy subjects and the subjects suffering with insomnia [8]. The recommended dose of LEM for insomnia disorder is 5 mg to 10 mg daily before going to sleep. In various randomized clinical controlled trails, LEM significantly improved the sleep onset and sleep maintenance by approved dose and without producing residual morning sleepiness [9,10]. Recently, acute cognitive effects of LEM have been also reported in recreational sedative patients [11].

LEM is rapidly absorbed after oral administration of tablet form in humans with peak plasma concentration (C_{max}), which was achieved within 1–3 h. The mean C_{max} and area under-curve ($AUC_{0\text{–}24\,h}$) increased slightly less than in proportion to dose after administration of 2.5 to 75 mg of LEM and the extent of accumulation was 1.5 to three-fold across the dose range at steady-state level. The volume of distribution for LEM is high (1970 L) with clearance rate of 32.8 L/h. The half-life ($T\frac{1}{2}$) is 15–17 h with 94% plasma protein binding [6]. It is mainly excreted through the feces (≈57.4%) and urine (≈29.1%), with around 1% as in unchanged form. It is lipophilic in nature, primarily metabolized by CYP3A4 enzyme. The C_{max} and AUC of LEM were increased by 1.4- to 1.6 time and 3.7- to 4-time by co-administration with itraconazole or fluconazole (strong to moderate CYP3A inhibitor). Similarly, its C_{max} and AUC were reduced by 90% when co-administered with rifampin (strong CYP3A inducer). Therefore, it is recommended to avoid the concomitant administration of LEM with strong or moderate inhibitors or inducers of CYP3A enzyme [12].

LEM is appeared to have similar abuse potential profile to suvorexant and zolpidem and therefore placed in Schedule IV controlled substance [13]. Being a drug of abuse, and also predominantly metabolized by CYP3A4 enzyme, a sensitive bioanalytical assay of LEM is necessary for the testing of drug of abuse in forensic toxicology, therapeutic drug monitoring, and to check or avoid any pharmacokinetic interaction. Until now, only one LC-MS/MS assay has been identified in the literature for the determination of LEM in human plasma, which was applied to an ex vivo protein binding study [14]. The purpose of our study was to develop a UPLC-MS/MS method for determination of LEM in human plasma. Due to abuse potential of LEM, the assay was validated by following the "Scientific Working Group for Toxicology" (SWGTOX) guidelines so that it could also be used for forensic laboratory testing in futuristic study [15]. Assay validation of schedule IV (suvorexant, eluxadoline, lorcaserin) controlled substances has been previously reported by our laboratory by following SWGTOX guidelines [16–19]. For proof of applicability, the validated method was successfully applied by analyzing rat plasma samples to support a pharmacokinetic study.

2. Materials and Methods

2.1. Chemicals and Reagents

LEM (purity; ≥99.0%) was purchased from "Beijing Mesochem Technology Co. Ltd. Beijing, China". Losartan, used as internal standard (IS, purity > 98%) was from "Amriya Pharmaceutical Industries, Cairo, Egypt" (Figure 1). The HPLC grade methanol, acetonitrile (ACN) and ethyl acetate were purchased from "Fisher Scientific Limited, Leicestershire, UK". The AR grade of ammonium acetate and dimethyl sulphoxide (DMSO), were procured from "Loba Chemie Pvt. Ltd. Mumbai, India". The ultrapure deionized water dispensed by "Milli-QR Gradient A10R, Millipore, Moscheim Cedex, France" was used for aqueous solution preparation.

2.2. Instrumentation and Chromatographic Conditions

The UPLC-MS/MS system composed of an Acquity triple quadrupole (TQD) mass spectrometer with Acquity H-Class UPLC system (Waters® Corporation, Milford, MA, USA). An electrospray ionization (ESI) probe operated in positive mode was used as ion source for sample ionization. The detection and quantification were performed under multiple reaction monitoring (MRM) mode using precursor to product ion transition of 411.12 > 175.09 as qualifier ion and 411.12 > 287.14 as quantifier ions for LEM. Quantifier-to-qualifier ion ratio was expected to be within 20% of those in QC samples. The optimized capillary voltage was 0.53 kV, while source and desolvation temperature were 150 °C and 350 °C, respectively. Ultrapure nitrogen (flow rate: 650 L/h) was used as desolvation gas and argon (0.17 mL/min) for collision gas, respectively. The optimized compound specific parameters are presented in Table 1.

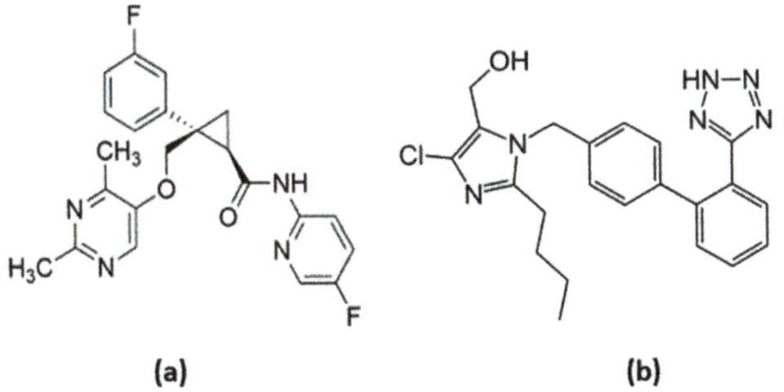

Figure 1. Chemical structure of LEM (**a**) and losartan (**b**).

Table 1. Optimized UPLC-MS/MS parameters for LEM and IS.

Compound	t_R (min)	Q1 [M+H]$^+$	CV (V)	Q3 [M+H]$^+$	CE (eV)	dt (s)
Lemborexant	2.36	411.12	26	287.14	14	0.106
				175.09 *	28	0.106
IS	1.86	423.1	22	207.1	20	0.106

t_R = retention time; Q1 = precursor ion; CV = cone voltage; dt = dwell time; Q3 = product ion [M+H]$^+$, CE = collision energy), * Qualifier ion.

The chromatographic separation of LEM and IS were achieved on Acquity UPLC BEH^{TM} C_{18} column (2.1 × 50 mm; 1.7 μm). The mobile phase comprising of 10 mM ammonium acetate (solvent A) and ACN (solvent B) was pumped in gradient mode at 0.3 mL/min of flow rate. The gradient condition of mobile phase used for sample separation is presented in Table 2. The column temperature was fixed to 40 ± 5 °C, whereas the auto-sampler temperature was 15 ± 5 °C during analysis. The variations of retention times for both LEM and IS were acceptable within ± 2%. The volume of each injection was 5 μL, and the total run time for each analysis was 4 min. The MassLynx software (Version 4.1) with Target Lynx^{TM} program was used to acquired and process all experimental data, respectively.

Table 2. Gradient condition of mobile phase used for sample separation.

Time (min)	Flow (mL/min)	Solvent A	Solvent B	Curve
initial	0.3	80	20	
0.50	0.3	20	80	6
1.00	0.3	50	50	6
1.50	0.3	80	20	6
4.00	0.3	80	20	6

2.3. Stock Solution, Calibration Standards (CSs) and Quality Controls (QCs) Sample Preparation

The stock solution of LEM and IS were prepared by dissolving their requisite amount in DMSO and methanol, respectively, to achieve 1 mg/mL concentration. The stock solution of LEM was further diluted with ACN: water (50:50, *v*/*v*) to prepare working solutions for CSs. The blank plasma matrix was fortified with these working solutions to achieve eight CSs of 1, 2.84, 9.45, 31.5, 63, 126, 210, and 300 ng/mL. Similarly, QCs samples were prepared by fortifying the plasma matrix with working solutions to achieve concentrations of 3, 50, and 250 ng/mL and were treated as low (LQC), middle (MQC), and high (HQC)

QC concentration, respectively. The stock solution of IS was diluted with ACN: water (50:50, *v*/*v*) to prepare a solution of 4 μg/mL concentration. All aqueous solutions were stored at 2–8 °C, while the fortified plasma matrix samples were placed in −80 °C during valid period.

2.4. Sample Extraction Procedure

In 150 μL of fortified plasma sample, 15 μL of IS (4 μg/mL) was added except the blank sample and vortexed each for 30 s. Thereafter, 1 mL of the ethyl acetate was added into each sample and again vortexed followed by cold centrifugation at 10,500× *g* at 4 °C. Then 800 μL of the supernatant organic layer was transferred to a fresh 1.5 mL capacity Eppendorf tubes. All the tubes were placed into sample concentrator and dried for 45 min. The remaining residue in tubes were reconstituted with 150 μL of pure acetonitrile (ACN) and 5 μL of this was injected into the UPLC-MS/MS for analysis.

2.5. Assay Validation

The validation was carried out as per the international parameters set by the SWGTOX in the Standard Practices for Method Validation in Forensic Toxicology [15]. The parameters included for evaluation were: limit of detection (LOD), limit of quantification (LOQ), interferences, calibration model, precision and accuracy, carry-over effects, recovery and matrix effects, dilution integrity, and stability studies.

2.5.1. LOD and LOQ Determination

The LOD was considered as the lowest concentration of the calibrator for which signal-to-noise ratio (S/N) of the qualifier MRM transition was 3. It was determined by analyzing decreasing concentration of LEM to establish the lowest possible concentration that can be distinguished reliably from the limit of blank and the concentration at which detection was feasible. The LOQ was considered as the lowest concentration of calibrator with S/N ratio of 10 for the qualifier MRM transition. Furthermore, the LOQ should be the lowest concentration that can be quantified with acceptable precision and accuracy with a relative standard deviation (RSD) of <20%.

2.5.2. Interference Studies

Interferences of endogenous substances form matrix was evaluated by analyzing the blank matrices which obtained from 10 different sources. The responses in blank matrices were compared with LOD and LOQ responses of the assay.

2.5.3. Calibration Model

An appropriate calibration model is necessary for accurate and reliable quantitative determination. The linear regression using least square method was used to establish the calibration model of this assay. For this, eight different concentrations of CSs samples were analyzed by five replications in different run. The linearity was determined by plotting the calibration curve between the area ratios of analyte and IS versus nominal concentration of CSs. The coefficient of correlation (*r*) for the calibration curves should be ≥0.99. Further weighing factor of $1/X$, $1/X^2$ and none were used to adjust the best fitting of the curve.

2.5.4. Carry-Over Effects

The carry-over effects were evaluated by analyzing the blank plasma matrices, injected in triplicate just after the highest concentration of CSs sample. No significant peaks (≥20% of LOQ) should be observed in blank matrices samples to ensure the assay free from carry-over effects.

2.5.5. Precision and Bias

Precision and bias studies have been evaluated concurrently by using LOQ and all three QC samples. It was measured in pooled fortified matrix using five replicates for each concentration in three batches for over three consecutive days. Precision is expressed as the relative standard deviation (%RSD) and was determined by calculating the mean and standard deviation of the response for each concentration. The bias is expressed as relative error (%RE), which was calculated by measuring the percentage difference in the calculated values for each concentration in compared to the nominal concentration divided by nominal concentration. Both intra- and inter-day variation in the precision and bias were determined and their acceptable criteria were $\leq$20% and $\pm$20%, respectively.

2.5.6. Matrix Effects

The enhancement or suppression of LEM ionization due to presence of co-eluting substances in matrices were evaluated by post extraction addition approach method. This approach is also known as quantitative method as amount of ionization or enhancement is assessed. For this, two different set of samples were prepared. Set one consists of neat solution of all three QC concentration levels, while set two consists of post extracted six different lot of matrix fortified with all three QC concentrations. The average area of each post extracted samples was calculated and compared with neat solution area to evaluate the ion suppression/enhancement effects. Same procedure was followed for IS matrix effects determination. The average suppression/enhancement effects must be $\leq$25%, and the %RSD value should not be >15% to ensure the assay is free from matrix effects.

2.5.7. Assay Recovery

The recovery of LEM and IS were evaluated in plasma matrix at all three QC concentration in six replicates. For this, two sets of samples were prepared. One set consisting of plasma matrix fortified with QC concentration before extraction, while the other set of samples was fortified after post extraction. The percentage difference was calculated to determine the % recovery of LEM and same procedure was followed for IS recovery determination.

2.5.8. Stability

This was designed to address the stability of LEM in plasma matrix at different storage conditions and sample processing procedure during laboratory operation. It was performed by analyzing plasma matrix fortified by two QC (LQC, HQC) concentrations. The short-term stability was evaluated by putting the samples for 8 h at ambient temperature before processing, while the autosampler stability was evaluated by analyzing the processed samples after keeping them in autosampler plate for 24 h at 15 °C temperature. The freeze-thaw stability was evaluated by analyzing the fortified QC samples after completion of three times freezing and thawing cycle. The long-term stability of the samples was performed by analyzing the fortified QC samples stored at −80 °C for 60 days.

2.6. *Pharmacokinetic Study in Rats*

The developed and validated assay was applied to a single dose pharmacokinetic study in rats. Male Wistar albino rats (weighing 250–300 gm) were received from "Animal Care Centre, College of Pharmacy, King Saud University, Riyadh KSA". The animal experiment was performed in accordance with the guidelines of the "Experimental Animal Care and Use Committee of College of Pharmacy, King Saud University Riyadh", and the experimental protocol was approved by "The Research Ethics Committee, King Saud University", (Approval No. KSU-SE-22-17, dated 24/03/2022). After 12 h of fasting, rats were given LEM (10 mg/kg, i.g. dissolved in CMC), and blood samples ($\approx$400 μL) were collected from the retro-orbital plexus into the heparinized tubes at 0, 0.25, 0.5, 1, 2, 4, 12 and 24 h). Plasma samples were harvested by centrifuging the blood at 4500$\times$ *g* for 8 min at 4 °C and kept at -80 ± 2 °C till the analysis was conducted. The pharmacokinetic parameters C_{max}, T_{max}, AUC, $T\frac{1}{2}$, mean residence time (MRT), and elimination rate constant (K_{el}) were calculated by non-compartmental model using WinNonlin Software (version 4.0.1).

3. Results and Discussion

3.1. Mass Spectrometric Condition Optimization

Optimization of mass spectrometric condition was initially performed by standard solution tuning using IntelliStart method. MRM mode was used to carry out the quantitative analyses to achieve high selectivity and sensitivity. An aqueous standard solution of LEM and IS (500 ng/mL) were infused in both positive and negative mode by using combined flow system. It was observed that the ion intensity of LEM and IS were more intense in positive mode as compared to the negative mode. During fragmentation processing, the more abundant product ion of LEM was selected for quantitation (quantifier ion) and the less abundant product ion as qualifier for confirmation. Further mass spectrometric (general and molecule specific) parameters were optimized to achieve maximum possible ion intensity as presented in Table 1. The precursor and precursor to product ion transition spectra of LEM in ESI positive mode are well represented in Figure 2.

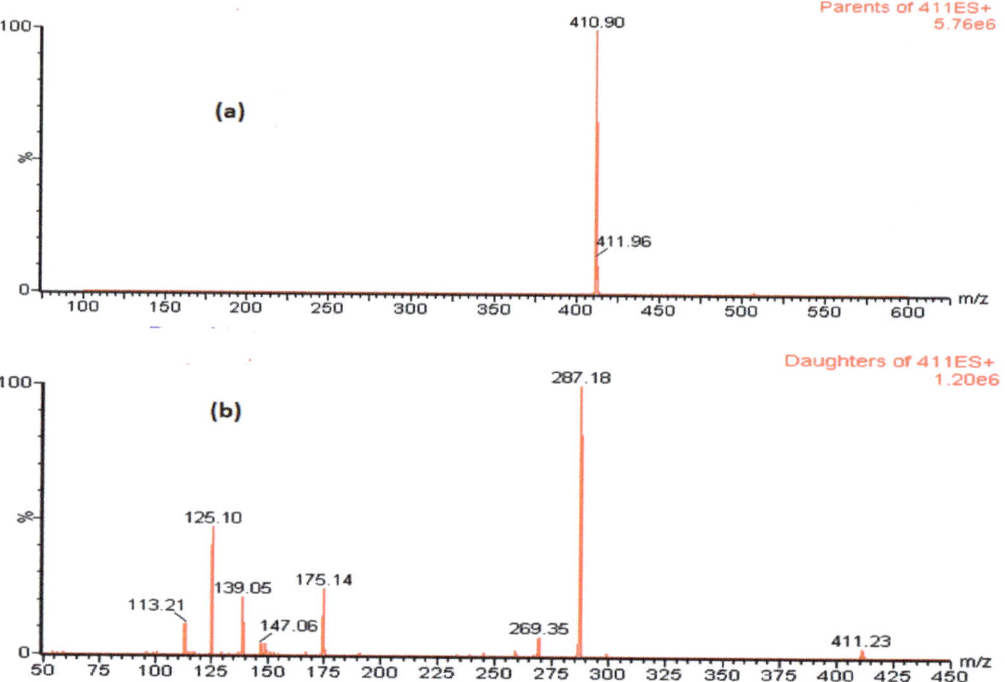

Figure 2. Representative LEM mass spectra of precursor ion (**a**) and precursor to product ion (**b**) in ESI positive mode.

3.2. Chromatographic Condition Optimization

Due to hydrophobic nature of analyte, Acquity CSH and BEH column of different size (2.1 × 50 and 2.1 × 100 mm) with common particle size (1.7 µm) were tried for separation of analyte and IS. The result with Acquity BEH column of 2.1 µm × 50 mm size was better among them and was selected for chromatographic elution optimization. Initially, mobile phase comprising of ammonium acetate, formic acid with organic modifiers of methanol and ACN were tried for chromatographic elution in isocratic mode. Although ammonium acetate together with ACN produced better separation, both analyte and IS were eluted within 0.65 min of time, which reflects non-proper retention of molecules in stationary phase. Therefore, we switched to gradient elution mode, and it produced better separation of both with best resolution as described in Table 2. Usually, analyte labeled stable isotope is best choice for IS in order to minimize the difference in extraction recovery and matrix effects. Unfortunately, deuterated form of LEM is not commercially available in market and therefore we have tried here some common and easily available molecules with same ionization pattern and elution properties. In this regard, losartan produced better separation with optimized chromatographic condition and column and therefore selected as IS of this method.

3.3. *Optimization of Sample Extraction Procedure*

Optimization of sample extraction procedure is an important step for development of a reliable and reproducible bioanalytical assay. An ideal procedure should be simple with easy step, inexpensive, high recovery, and low matrix effects. Initially, protein precipitation method by using ACN, methanol, and its combination were tried. Although the recovery was satisfactory with ACN, the peak intensity was not stable, and the sensitivity was low, which requires further drying and reconstitution step. Then, liquid–liquid extraction was tested by using different organic solvents of dichloromethane, ethyl acetate, n-hexane and diethyl ether. Among these extracting solvents, the recovery with ethyl acetate was higher than others and, hence, it was selected as extracting solvent. Although the mean recovery of this assay (≈74%) was lower than previous reported method [12] by solid phase extraction (SPE), it is an expensive procedure and is of limited availability regarding that setup in maximum laboratory.

3.4. *Method Validation*

3.4.1. LOD and LOQ

In this assay, LEM was detected and quantified down to 0.35 and 1 ng/mL, respectively, with the acceptable S/N ratio and was considered as LOD and LOQ of this assay. Moreover, the determined precision and bias for LOQ were within the acceptable limits (≤20%) as mentioned in SWGTOX guideline [13].

3.4.2. Interference and Selectivity Studies

No significant interfering peaks were observed in the blank plasma chromatograms of all tested transition channels of analyte and IS. The extracted ion chromatograms of blank plasma and plasma spiked at LOD and LOQ concentration are depicted in Figure 3. These results confirm that the method is selective and specific for the analysis of LEM in plasma matrices.

3.4.3. Calibration Model

The calibration curves plotted between area ratio (analyte/IS) versus nominal concentration of LEM were linear over the CSs range of 1.0–300 ng/mL using the propose least square method. The mean value of coefficient of correlation for calibration curves (n = 5) was 0.995 ± 0.002. The weighing factor ($1/X^2$) has shown the best linear fit with lowest bias and was used for back calculation of concentration of the CSs. The deviation in the back calculated concentration of all CSs were found within the acceptable limit of ±15% of the nominal concentration.

3.4.4. Carry-Over Effects

No significant peaks were found in the processed blank plasma matrices, which were analyzed just after the highest CS concentration (300 ng/mL). These results confirmed that the proposed method is free from carry-over effects and expected concentration of analyzed samples were accurate and reliable.

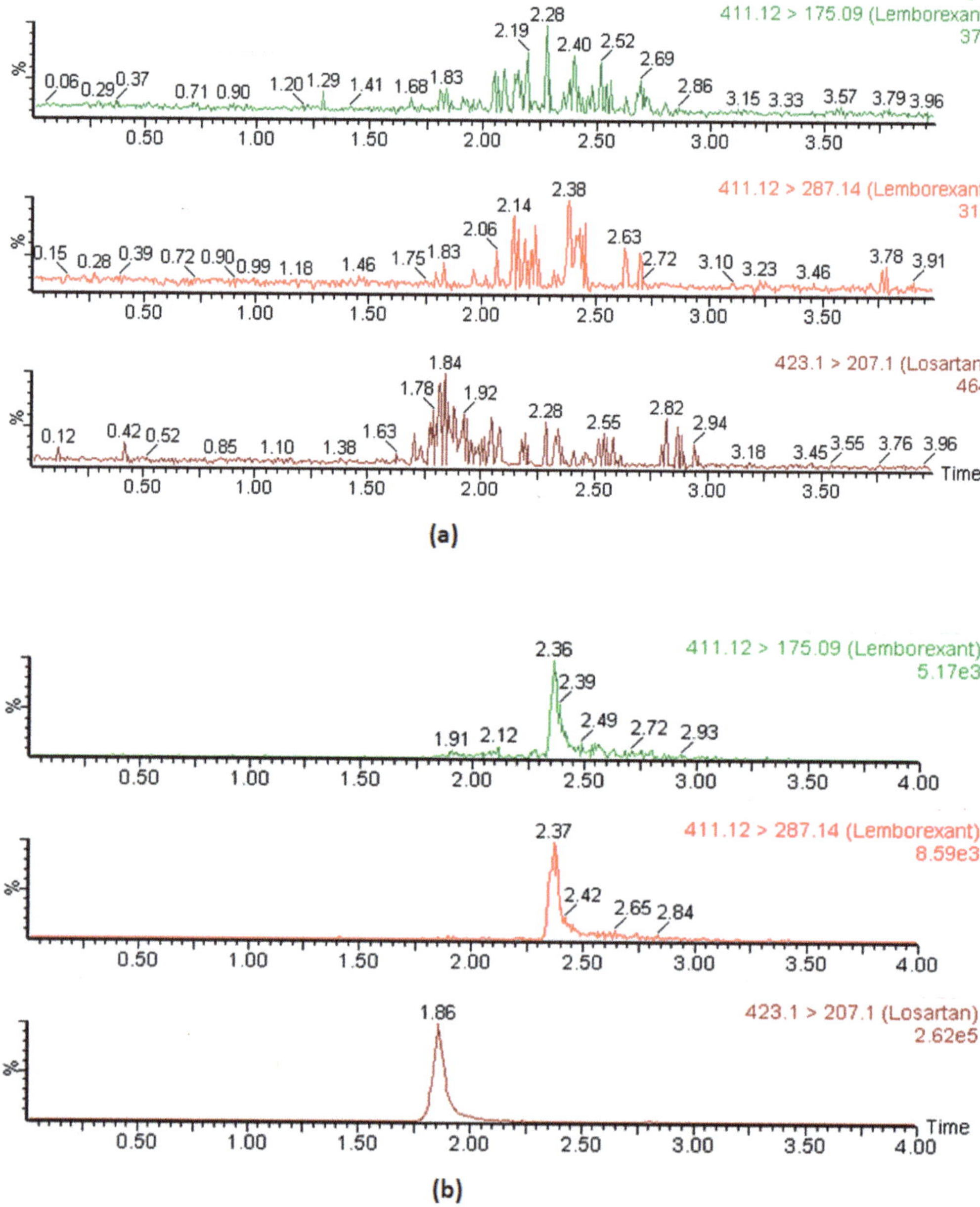

411.12 > 175.09 (Lemborexant) 374

0.06 0.29 0.37 0.71 0.90 1.20 1.29 1.41 1.68 1.83 2.19 2.28 2.40 2.52 2.69 2.86 3.15 3.33 3.57 3.79 3.96

411.12 > 287.14 (Lemborexant) 316

0.15 0.28 0.39 0.72 0.90 0.99 1.18 1.46 1.75 1.83 2.06 2.14 2.38 2.63 2.72 3.10 3.23 3.46 3.78 3.91

423.1 > 207.1 (Losartan) 464

0.12 0.42 0.52 0.85 1.10 1.38 1.63 1.78 1.84 1.92 2.28 2.55 2.82 2.94 3.18 3.45 3.55 3.76 3.96

Time

0.50 1.00 1.50 2.00 2.50 3.00 3.50

(a)

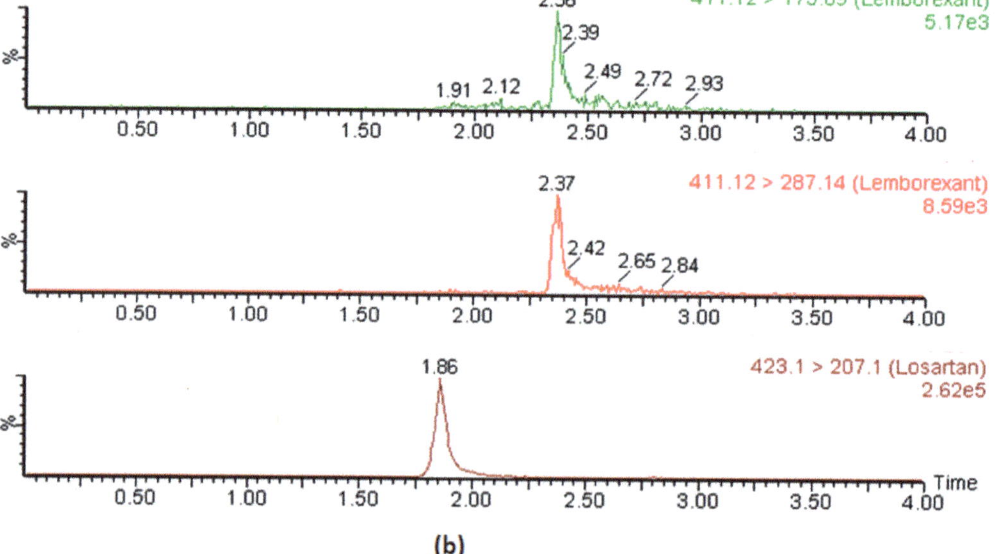

Figure 3. Representative MRM chromatogram of LEM and IS in blank plasma (**a**) and plasma fortified at LOQ level concentration (**b**). [411.12 > 175.09 → Qualifier ion; 411.12 > 287.14 → Quantifier ion; 423.1 > 207.1 → IS].

3.4.5. Precision and Bias

The precision and bias results for LOQ and all three QC$_s$ (LQC, MQC and HQC) concentrations processed in human plasma matrix are displayed in Table 3. The mean value of intra- and inter-day precision (% RSD) were ≤11.49 and ≤9.35%, respectively.

The measured mean value of intra- and inter-day bias were ranged in −10.03% to 6.99% and −9.12% to 10.74%, respectively. All of these data ranges were within 15% of the limit, indicating acceptable bias and precision according to the SWGTOX guideline.

Table 3. Intra- and inter-day precision and bias data of LEM in human plasma samples.

Nominal QC (ng/mL)	Precision (RSD, %)		Bias (RE, %)	
	Intra-Day	Inter-Day	Intra-Day	Inter-Day
1.0	11.49	9.35	6.99	10.74
3.0	5.91	5.79	−10.03	−9.12
50	3.60	3.35	2.25	1.66
250	1.68	4.85	−8.77	−6.12

3.4.6. Recovery and Matrix Effects

The extraction recovery and matrix effects results for LEM and IS are displayed in Table 4. As evident form the results, the overall mean recovery of LEM form plasma matrix was 73.9% with 5.68% of RSD, using ethyl acetate as extraction solvents. Although the % recovery is lower than the previous reported SPE method, the results were consistent and concentration independent between all three QC concentration [12].

Table 4. Matrix effects and recovery percentage of LEM and IS in plasma (n = 6).

Compound	Nominal QC (ng/mL)	Matrix Effects		Extraction Recovery	
		% Mean	RSD, %	% Mean	RSD, %
LEM	3.0	106.8	2.95	79.1	6.54
	50	93.3	5.18	67.8	3.97
	500	87.4	9.65	74.7	9.49
Overall mean		95.8	10.4	73.9	5.68
IS	400	86.9	6.95	80.7	7.39

During matrix effects evaluation, ion suppression effects were observed with MQC (93.3%) and HQC (87.4%) concentration, while ion enhancement effects (106.8%) were observed with LQC concentration, indicating minimal ion suppression/enhancement effects. The overall mean value was 95.8% and were under the limits of SWGTOX guideline [13].

3.4.7. Stability

The stability of LEM fortified in plasma matrix using LQC and MQC concentration at different anticipated conditions are presented in Table 5. The results demonstrated that LEM is stable, up to 8 h after keeping the sample at bench top position before processing, in processed plasma samples after three freeze/thaw cycles, in processed plasma samples stored in autosampler up to 24 h, and after processing the fortified plasma samples stored for two months in deep freezer (−80 °C). It is concluded that the plasma samples can be stored in deep freezer (−80 °C) up to two months from their collection time to analysis. The aqueous standard solutions of LEM and IS were also stable for 15 days at refrigerator temperature.

Table 5. Stability data of LEM in human plasma.

Stability	Nominal Concentration (ng/mL) (n = 6)	Precision (RSD, %)	BIAS (RE, %)
Bench top (8 h)			
	3.0	4.80	9.22
	250	6.75	−6.40
Freeze thaw (3 cycle)			
	3.0	8.15	12.11
	250	−5.56	−3.93
Auto-sampler (24 h)			
	3.0	6.41	2.06
	250	9.07	4.87
60 days at −80 °C			
	3.0	5.13	−6.78
	250	9.53	−9.73

3.5. *Application in Pharmacokinetic Study in Rats*

To ensure the reliability of the assay, the validated method was applied in pharmacokinetic study of LEM in rats. Usually, human plasma is a unique matrix, which can be considered to analyze samples from other species, e.g., rats also. Although a slight difference is sometimes noted in the matrices among different species in the case of analysis by using TQD, a cross-validation in term of precision and bias was also performed in rat plasma matrix to ensure the robustness of the method. The results of basic pharmacokinetic parameters are presented in Table 6. The mean value of C_{max} and $AUC_{0\text{–}24\,h}$ of 39.69 ng/mL and 109.16 ng.h/mL, respectively, were achieved after intragastrical administration of 10 mg/kg of LEM. The elimination $T\frac{1}{2}$ and MRT value were 3.78 h and 4.41 h, respectively. These results are comparable to previously reported data of innovator submitted in USFDA [5], which further ensure the reliability of the assay. The plasma concentration versus time profile and representative MRM chromatograms of LEM in rats are presented in Figure 4.

Table 6. Pharmacokinetic parameters of LEM in male rats (n = 6) after single dose administration (10 mg/kg p. o.).

Pharmacokinetic Parameters	Unit	Values (mean ± SD)
C_{max}	ng/mL	39.69 ± 11.69
T_{max}	h	0.25
AUC_{0-t}	ng.h/mL	109.16 ± 21.06
$T^{1/2}$	h	3.78 ± 1.07
Kel	h	0.19 ± 0.04
MRT	h^{-1}	4.41 ± 1.0

3.6. *Limitation of the Study*

The limitation of this study is that it not directly applied in real human plasma samples due to unavailability of approved formulation in kingdom. Upcoming studies are considered necessary to conduct application in human samples to ensure more reliability of the proposed assay.

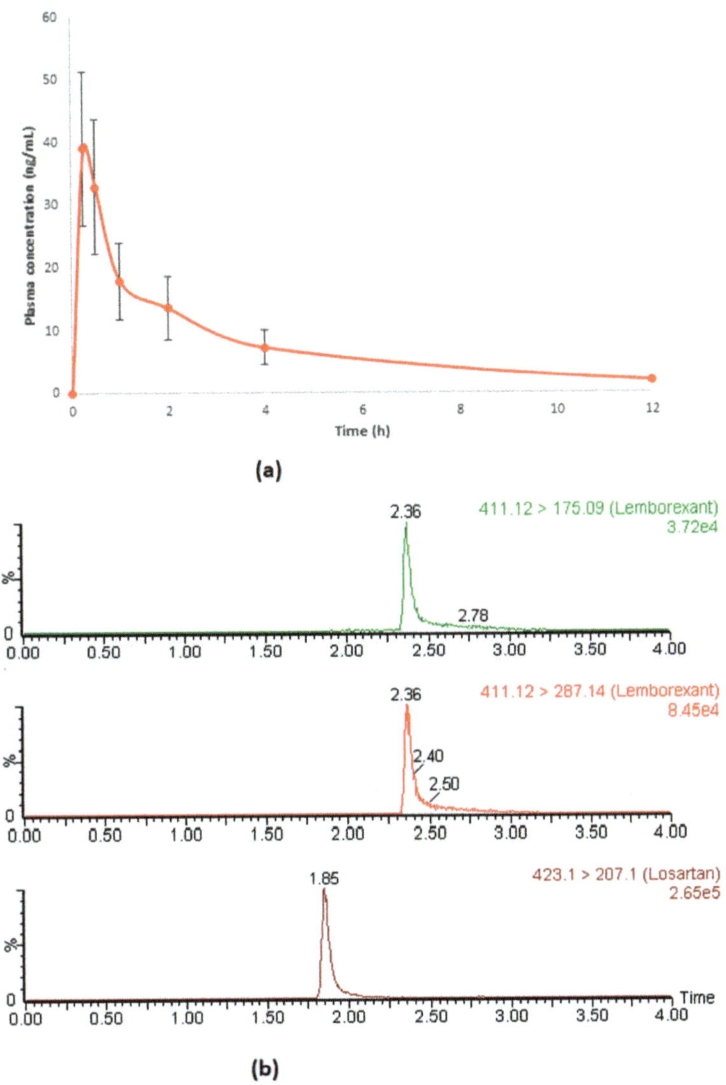

Figure 4. Plasma concentration versus time profile of LEM (**a**) and representative MRM chromatogram of LEM and IS (**b**) in rat after oral administration of 10 mg/kg LEM. [411.12 > 175.09 → Qualifier ion; 411.12 > 287.14 → Quantifier ion; 423.1 > 207.1 → IS].

4. Conclusions

A sensitive and reliable assay was developed and validated for the detection and quantification of LEM in plasma matrix. Being a drug of abuse, the assay was validated following the SWGTOX guidelines, which are able be to used for both detection and quantification of LEM in blood samples. All validation parameters were within the acceptable ranges and linear between the concentration range of 1–300 ng/mL, which is sufficient to detect intoxicating or fatal concentrations of LEM. The assay was successfully applied in pharmacokinetic study of LEM in rats. Moreover, the assay could be used for futuristic forensic toxicology testing, therapeutic drug monitoring, and pharmacokinetics drug interaction studies after conducting its application in real human samples.

Author Contributions: Conceptualization, M.I; methodology, E.A.A.; A.A. (Ali Akhtar); validation, M.A.K. and E.A.A.; formal analysis, A.A. (Abdullah Alshememry); investigation, F.I.; data curation, A.A. (Abdullah Alshememry); writing—original draft preparation, M.I.; writing—review and editing, M.I. and E.A.A.; supervision, M.I.; funding acquisition, M.I. All authors have read and agreed to the published version of the manuscript.

Funding: This work was supported by the Deputyship for Research & Innovation, Ministry of Education in Saudi Arabia (Project No. IFKSURG-2-299).

Institutional Review Board Statement: The research was approved by the Research Ethics Committee of King Saud University College of Pharmacy Riyadh, Saudi Arabia (KSU-SE-22-17).

Informed Consent Statement: Not applicable.

Data Availability Statement: All the data generated from the study are clearly presented in the manuscript.

Acknowledgments: The authors extend their appreciation to the Deputyship for Research & Innovation, Ministry of Education in Saudi Arabia for funding this research work through the project no. IFKSURG-2-299.

Conflicts of Interest: The authors declare no conflict of interest.

References

1. Chung, K.F.; Yeung, W.F.; Ho, F.Y.; Yung, K.P.; Yu, Y.M.; Kwok, C.W. Cross-cultural and comparative epidemiology of insomnia: The Diagnostic and statistical manual (DSM), International classification of diseases (ICD) and International classification of sleep disorders (ICSD). *Sleep Med.* **2015**, *16*, 477–482. [CrossRef] [PubMed]
2. Asnis, G.M.; Thomas, M.; Henderson, M.A. Pharmacotherapy Treatment Options for Insomnia: A Primer for Clinicians. *Int. J. Mol. Sci.* **2015**, *17*, 50. [CrossRef] [PubMed]
3. Sateia, M.J.; Buysse, D.J.; Krystal, A.D.; Neubauer, D.N.; Heald, J.L. Clinical Practice Guideline for the Pharmacologic Treatment of Chronic Insomnia in Adults: An American Academy of Sleep Medicine Clinical Practice Guideline. *J. Clin. Sleep Med.* **2017**, *13*, 307–349. [CrossRef] [PubMed]
4. Kumar, A.; Chanana, P.; Choudhary, S. Emerging role of orexin antagonists in insomnia therapeutics: An update on SORAs and DORAs. *Pharmacol. Rep.* **2016**, *68*, 231–242. [CrossRef] [PubMed]
5. Centre for Drug Evaluation and Research. US FDA Approves Eisai's DAYVIGOtm (Lemborexant) for the Treatment of Insomnia in Adult Patients. NDA 212028 Multi-Disciplinary Review and Evaluation DAYVIGO (Lemborexant). 2018. Available online: https://www.accessdata.fda.gov/drugsatfda_docs/nda/2019/212028Orig1s000MultidisciplineR.pdf (accessed on 10 December 2022).
6. Prescribing Information for DAYVIGO®(Lemborexant) Tablets, for Oral Use, CIV Initial U.S. Approval: 2019. 2019. Available online: https://www.accessdata.fda.gov/drugsatfda_docs/label/2019/212028s000lbl.pdf (accessed on 10 December 2022).
7. Beuckmann, C.T.; Suzuki, M.; Ueno, T.; Nagaoka, K.; Arai, T.; Higashiyama, H. In Vitro and In Silico characterization of lemborexant (E2006), a novel dual orexin receptor antagonist. *J. Pharmacol. Exp. Ther.* **2017**, *362*, 287–295. [CrossRef] [PubMed]
8. Moline, M.; Zammit, G.; Yardley, J.; Pinner, K.; Kumar, D.; Perdomo, C.; Cheng, J.Y. Lack of residual morning effects of lemborexant treatment for insomnia: Summary of findings across 9 clinical trials. *Postgrad. Med.* **2021**, *133*, 71–81. [CrossRef] [PubMed]
9. Mayleben, D.; Rosenberg, R.; Pinner, K.; Hussein, Z.; Moline, M. Assessment of morning sleep propensity with lemborexant in adults with insomnia disorder in a randomized, placebo-controlled crossover study. *Sleep Adv.* **2021**, *2*, zpab011. [CrossRef]
10. Murphy, P.; Moline, M.; Mayleben, D.; Rosenberg, R.; Zammit, G.; Pinner, K.; Dhadda, S.; Hong, Q.; Giorgi, L.; Satlin, A. Lemborexant, A Dual Orexin Receptor Antagonist (DORA) for the Treatment of Insomnia Disorder: Results From a Bayesian, Adaptive, Randomized, Double-Blind, Placebo-Controlled Study. *J. Clin. Sleep Med.* **2017**, *13*, 1289–1299. [CrossRef] [PubMed]
11. Landry, I.; Hall, N.; Alur, J.; Filippov, G.; Reyderman, L.; Setnik, B.; Henningfield, J.; Moline, M. Acute Cognitive Effects of the Dual Orexin Receptor Antagonist Lemborexant Compared With Suvorexant and Zolpidem in Recreational Sedative Users. *J. Clin. Psychopharmacol.* **2022**, *42*, 374–382. [CrossRef] [PubMed]
12. Landry, I.; Aluri, J.; Nakai, K.; Hall, N.; Miyajima, Y.; Ueno, T.; Dayal, S.; Filippov, G.; Lalovic, B.; Moline, M.; et al. Evaluation of the CYP3A and CYP2B6 Drug-Drug Interaction Potential of Lemborexant. *Clin. Pharmacol. Drug Dev.* **2021**, *10*, 681–690. [CrossRef] [PubMed]
13. Landry, I.; Hall, N.; Aluri, J.; Filippov, G.; Reyderman, L.; Setnik, B.; Henningfield, J.; Moline, M. Abuse Potential of Lemborexant, a Dual Orexin Receptor Antagonist, Compared With Zolpidem and Suvorexant in Recreational Sedative Users. *J. Clin. Psychopharmacol.* **2022**, *42*, 365–373. [CrossRef] [PubMed]
14. Mano, Y.; Ueno, T.; Hotta, K. Establishment of a simultaneous assay for lemborexant, a novel dual orexin receptor antagonist, and its three metabolites, and its application to a clinical protein binding study. *J. Pharm. Biomed. Anal.* **2020**, *187*, 113359. [CrossRef] [PubMed]
15. Scientific Working Group for Forensic Toxicology. Scientific Working Group for Forensic Toxicology (SWGTOX) standard practices for method validation in forensic toxicology. *J. Anal. Toxicol.* **2013**, *37*, 452–474. [CrossRef]
16. Iqbal, M.; Ezzeldin, E.; Al-Rashood, K.A. UPLC-MS/MS assay for identification and quantification of brivaracetam in plasma sample: Application to pharmacokinetic study in rats. *J. Chromatogr. B Anal. Technol. Biomed. Life Sci.* **2017**, *1060*, 63–70. [CrossRef] [PubMed]

17. Iqbal, M.; Ezzeldin, E.; Al-Rashood, K.A.; Al-Shdefat, R.; Anwer, M.K. High throughput mu-SPE based elution coupled with UPLC-MS/MS for determination of eluxadoline in plasma sample: Application in pharmacokinetic characterization of PLGA nanoparticle formulations in rats. *J. Pharm. Biomed. Anal.* **2018**, *149*, 172–178. [CrossRef] [PubMed]
18. Iqbal, M.; Ezzeldin, E.; Khalil, N.Y.; Alam, P.; Al-Rashood, K.A. UPLC-MS/MS determination of suvorexant in urine by a simplified dispersive liquid-liquid micro-extraction followed by ultrasound assisted back extraction from solidified floating organic droplets. *J. Pharm. Biomed. Anal.* **2019**, *164*, 1–8. [CrossRef] [PubMed]
19. Iqbal, M.; Khalil, N.Y.; Ezzeldin, E.; Al-Rashood, K.A. Simultaneous Detection and Quantification of Three Novel Prescription Drugs of Abuse (Suvorexant, Lorcaserin and Brivaracetam) in Human Plasma by UPLC-MS-MS. *J. Anal. Toxicol.* **2019**, *43*, 203–211. [CrossRef] [PubMed]

MDPI
St. Alban-Anlage 66
4052 Basel
Switzerland
Tel. +41 61 683 77 34
Fax +41 61 302 89 18
www.mdpi.com

Toxics Editorial Office
E-mail: toxics@mdpi.com
www.mdpi.com/journal/toxics

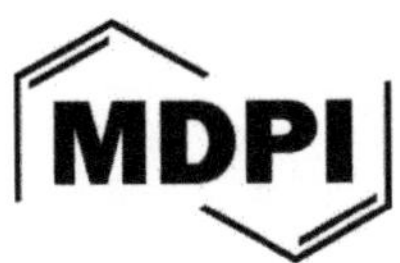

www.ingramcontent.com/pod-product-compliance
Lightning Source LLC
LaVergne TN
LVHW070854170726
843515LV00005B/646
* 9 7 8 3 0 3 6 5 7 9 6 6 5 *